# Graves' Orbitopathy
## A Multidisciplinary Approach

# Graves' Orbitopathy

## A Multidisciplinary Approach

Editors

*Wilmar M. Wiersinga*, Amsterdam
*George J. Kahaly*, Mainz

83 figures, 47 in color, and 38 tables, 2007

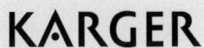

Basel · Freiburg · Paris · London · New York ·
Bangalore · Bangkok · Singapore · Tokyo · Sydney

**Wilmar M. Wiersinga, MD, PhD**
Department of Endocrinology and Metabolism
Academic Medical Center, University of Amsterdam
Meibergdreef 9
NL–1105 AZ Amsterdam
The Netherlands

**George J. Kahaly, MD, PhD**
Department of Medicine I, Gutenberg University Hospital
Langenbeckstrasse 1
DE–55131 Mainz
Germany

Library of Congress Cataloging-in-Publication Data

Graves' orbitopathy : a multidisciplinary approach / editors, Wilmar M. Wiersinga, George J. Kahaly.
   p. ; cm.
  Includes bibliographical references and indexes.
  ISBN 978-3-8055-8342-8 (hard cover : alk. paper)
 1. Thyroid eye disease. I. Wiersinga, Wilmar M. II. Kahaly, George J.
  [DNLM: 1. Graves Ophthalmopathy–diagnosis. 2. Graves Ophthalmopathy–therapy. 3. Diagnosis, Differential. 4. Ophthalmologic Surgical Procedures. WK 265 G7765 2007]
   RE715.T48G75 2007
   617.7–dc22
                                  2007026922

Disclaimer. The statements, options and data contained in this publication are solely those of the individual authors and contributors and not of the publisher and the editor(s). The appearance of advertisements in the book is not a warranty, endorsement, or approval of the products or services advertised or of their effectiveness, quality or safety. The publisher and the editor(s) disclaim responsibility for any injury to persons or property resulting from any ideas, methods, instructions or products referred to in the content or advertisements.

Drug Dosage. The authors and the publisher have exerted every effort to ensure that drug selection and dosage set forth in this text are in accord with current recommendations and practice at the time of publication. However, in view of ongoing research, changes in government regulations, and the constant flow of information relating to drug therapy and drug reactions, the reader is urged to check the package insert for each drug for any change in indications and dosage and for added warnings and precautions. This is particularly important when the recommended agent is a new and/or infrequently employed drug.

All rights reserved. No part of this publication may be translated into other languages, reproduced or utilized in any form or by any means electronic or mechanical, including photocopying, recording, microcopying, or by any information storage and retrieval system, without permission in writing from the publisher.

© Copyright 2007 by S. Karger AG, P.O. Box, CH–4009 Basel (Switzerland)
www.karger.com
Printed in Switzerland on acid-free and non-aging paper (ISO 9706) by Reinhardt Druck, Basel
ISBN 978–3–8055–8342–8

# Contents

**XIII Preface**
Wiersinga, W.M. (Amsterdam); Kahaly, G.J. (Mainz)

Diagnosis and Pathogenesis

**1 Clinical Manifestations**
Dickinson, A.J. (Newcastle upon Tyne)
1 What Are the Common Symptoms of Graves'Orbitopathy?
1 What Are the Common Signs of Graves'Orbitopathy?
2 What Signs Are Unusual in Graves'Orbitopathy?
4 Are There Racial Differences in How Graves'Orbitopathy Manifests?
4 Is the Presentation of Graves'Orbitopathy Different in Older Compared to Younger Patients?
5 Why Can the Clinical Presentation of Graves'Orbitopathy Be So Variable?
5 Can You Give Me a Short Mechanistic Explanation for All These Clinical Manifestations?
6 What Do the Terms 'Activity' and 'Severity' Denote?
7 Why Is It Important to Distinguish Activity and Severity when Evaluating Patients?
8 What Symptoms and Signs Are Valuable for Assessing Activity?
8 How Are These Signs Assessed?
11 How Reproducible Are These Assessments?
11 What Value Does the 'Clinical Activity Score' Have?
12 Do Patients without Signs of Activity Ever Have Active Disease?
13 What Should I Do if I Am Not Sure whether the Disease Is Active?
13 Are There Any Other Ways to Evaluate Activity Other than Clinical Examination?
13 When Should These Other Methods for Assessing Activity Be Used in Routine Clinical Practice?

V

14 What Signs Are Helpful for Assessing Severity?
14 What Value Does the Mnemonic 'NOSPECS' Have?
14 What Are the Relative Frequencies of Classes I–VI?
16 How Are Signs of Severity Assessed?
20 How Reproducible Are These Assessments?
20 How Do You Decide Whether a Patient Has Dysthyroid Optic Neuropathy?
22 Can Dysthyroid Optic Neuropathy Ever Be Present with Normal Vision?
22 Are Some Patients at Particular Risk?
22 What Other Assessments Are Useful in Evaluating Possible Dysthyroid Optic Neuropathy?
23 Should These Tests Be Performed in All Patients at Every Assessment?
23 References

## 27 Orbit-Thyroid Relationship
Lazarus, J.H. (Cardiff); Marino, M. (Pisa)

27 Should This Condition Always Be Called Graves' Orbitopathy?
27 Does Graves' Orbitopathy Occur in the Absence of Hyperthyroidism?
29 Do All Patients with Graves' Disease Have Graves' Orbitopathy?
29 What Comes First in Graves' Disease? The Eye Changes or the Hyperthyroid Symptoms?
30 Do TSH Receptor Antibodies Also Cause GO?
31 Are There Any Other Extrathyroidal Manifestations of Graves' Disease Apart from Graves' Orbitopathy?
32 References

## 34 Epidemiology
Daumerie, C. (Brussels); Kalmann, R. (Utrecht)

34 What Is the Present Estimated Prevalence of Graves' Orbitopathy? Has It Changed over the Last Decade?
35 Is the Age and Sex Distribution of Graves' Orbitopathy Similar to that of Graves' Disease?
35 Are There Ethnic Differences?
35 What Are the Risk Factors for the Occurrence of Graves' Orbitopathy?
36 Is Tobacco Bad for Graves' Orbitopathy?
37 Is Ocular Co-Morbidity Relevant for Graves' Orbitopathy?
37 Is Elevated Intraocular Pressure Relevant in Graves' Orbitopathy?
38 Is There Significant Non-Ocular Co-Morbidity (Like Diabetes) which Is Relevant for Graves' Orbitopathy?
39 References

## 41 Pathogenesis
Orgiazzi, J. (Lyon)

41 What Are the Pathological Changes in Orbital Tissue of Graves' Orbitopathy?
44 How Do the Pathological Changes Give Rise to the Clinical Manifestations?
45 What Triggers Graves' Orbitopathy?
46 Is Graves' Orbitopathy Triggered by an Autoimmune Phenomenon? If so, what Is the Nature of the Auto-Antigen?

47 Why Is the Orbit a Special Target for Thyroid Autoimmunity?
48 What Kind of Immune Reaction Takes Place within the Orbit?
50 Do Anti-TSH Receptor Antibodies (TRAb) Play a Role in the Onset or Development of Graves'Orbitopathy?
50 Is There a Familial Predisposition to Graves' Orbitopathy? Is There a Specific Genetic Background for Graves' Orbitopathy?
51 Smoking Increases the Risk of Graves'Orbitopathy and Its Severity: What Is the Mechanism for It?
52 How May the Observations Described Above and the Current Understanding of the Disease Lead to More Effective Treatment of Graves'Orbitopathy?
54 References

## 57 Orbital Imaging
Pitz, S. (Mainz)

57 Is Orbital Imaging Always Necessary?
57 What Are the Relative Benefits of Orbital CT and MRI?
59 What Is Apical Crowding?
61 What Is the Place of Orbital Ultrasound?
62 What Lessons Can We Learn from Orbital Octreoscan?
62 What Other Imaging Techniques May Be Useful?
64 Acknowledgments
64 References

## 66 Diagnosis and Differential Diagnosis of Graves' Orbitopathy
Mourits, M.P. (Amsterdam)

66 Can You Give an Overall Scheme for the Diagnosis of Graves' Orbitopathy?
66 Which Clinical Findings Are Helpful in Making a Diagnosis of Graves'Orbitopathy?
70 Can One Make a Diagnosis of Graves'Orbitopathy Based on Medical History and Clinical Picture Alone?
70 Do We Always Need to Order Thyroid Autoantibodies and Thyroid Function Tests?
71 Which Imaging Technique Is Best to Make a Diagnosis of Graves'Orbitopathy and Is Imaging Always Requested?
72 Which Are the Most Frequent Conditions Mimicking Graves'Orbitopathy?
76 Conclusion
76 References

## 78 Natural History
Kendall-Taylor, P. (Newcastle upon Tyne)

78 Does Graves' Orbitopathy Occur at the Same Time as Hyperthyroidism?
78 Does Restoring Euthyroidism Lead to Improvement in Graves'Orbitopathy?
79 What Effect May Hypothyroidism Have?
80 What Is the Typical Course of the Disease?
81 What Is the Difference between Activity and Severity?
83 How Do You Determine which Phase of the Disease the Patient Is Displaying? [see also chapter by Dickinson, pp. 1–26]

83 How Does the Phase of the Disease Influence Choice of Treatment?
84 Will the Graves'Orbitopathy Eventually Burn Itself Out?
84 Will the Orbital Changes Return to Normal when the Condition Eventually Resolves?
85 How Long Is it Likely to Take before the Disease Becomes Inactive?
85 Once the Condition Has Become Inactive (Whether Treated or Untreated) Is it Likely to Flare Up Again?
85 Are There Any Other Factors, Additional to Thyroid Status, which May Influence the Course of the Disease?
86 References

## Management

### 88 General Management Plan
Boboridis, K. (Thessaloniki); Perros, P. (Newcastle upon Tyne)

88 What Are the Priorities when Faced with a New Presentation of Graves'Orbitopathy?
89 How Good Is the Evidence that Quitting Smoking Helps?
89 Does Thyroid Status Affect the Eyes?
90 What Simple Measures Can Help the Eyes?
91 Is There a Place for Botulinum Toxin?
92 How Do You Define Mild, Moderately Severe, and Very Severe Graves'Orbitopathy?
92 Can You Give a Simplified Overall Management Scheme?
93 References

### 96 Combined Thyroid-Eye Clinics
Wiersinga, W.M. (Amsterdam)

96 What Are Combined Thyroid-Eye Clinics?
97 Why Is a Multidisciplinary Approach Recommended?
98 Can Patients-Support Groups Be Helpful?
98 I Have Heard of a Fast-Track Clinic for Graves' Orbitopathy Patients: What Is That?
99 References

### 100 Thyroid Treatment
Marcocci, C.; Pinchera, A. (Pisa)

100 Does It Matter for the Eyes How the Patient Is Rendered Euthyroid?
103 Are There Any Specific Criteria to Prefer One of the Treatment Modalities for Hyperthyroidism in Graves'Orbitopathy?
104 Is There Any Risk Factor which May Predict Worsening of Graves' Orbitopathy after Radioiodine?
105 Should the Presence of Graves' Orbitopathy Limit the Use of Radioiodine Therapy?
105 Does Transient Hypothyroidism following Therapy Influence the Course of Graves' Orbitopathy?
107 Has Total Thyroid Ablation a Role in the Management of Hyperthyroidism in Graves'Orbitopathy?
108 References

## 111 Management of Mild Graves' Orbitopathy
### Salvi, M.; Currò, N. (Milan)

111 What Is the Degree of Intra-Orbital Involvement in Mild Graves'Orbitopathy?
111 Are Mild Forms of Graves'Orbitopathy Likely to Progress to More Severe Graves'Orbitopathy?
112 Is a 'Wait and See'Policy Justified in Mild Graves'Orbitopathy?
114 Are Low-Dosage Oral Steroids Advisable or Is Orbital Irradiation Preferable?
115 Can We Reassure Patients About the Long-Term Safety of Orbital Irradiation?
116 What Is the Rationale for Antioxidant Therapy in GO?
117 References

## 120 Management of Moderately Severe Graves' Orbitopathy
### Kahaly, G.J. (Mainz)

120 Is Immunosuppression Indicated in Moderately Severe Graves' Orbitopathy?
121 What Are the Results of Randomized Trials with Steroids?
131 What Are the Results of Randomized Trials Using Orbital Radiotherapy?
135 Do You Favor Combination Therapy?
138 What Are the Results of Randomized Trials Using Nonsteroid Immunosuppressants?
144 What Are the Results of Randomized Trials Using Somatostatin Analogs?
147 What Should You Do if Steroids Fail?
148 What Are the Actual Evidence-Based Therapeutic Recommendations for Patients with Moderately Severe Graves' Orbitopathy?
149 Acknowledgments
149 References

## 153 Management of Very Severe Graves' Orbitopathy (Dysthyroid Optic Neuropathy)
### Lane, C.M. (Cardiff); Boschi, A. (Brussels)

153 How Do You Define Dysthyroid Optic Neuropathy?
153 Are There Specific Risk Factors for Dysthyroid Optic Neuropathy?
154 Which Symptoms Should Alert Me?
155 What Are the Ophthalmological Signs of Dysthyroid Optic Neuropathy?
156 Are Additional Investigations Helpful?
156 How Fast Can Dysthyroid Optic Neuropathy Develop? Is Urgent Treatment Necessary?
157 What Is the Evidence Base for the Treatment of Dysthyroid Optic Neuropathy?
157 What Is the Role of Surgery in Dysthyroid Optic Neuropathy?
158 How Many Patients Become Blind due to Dysthyroid Optic Neuropathy?
158 References

## 160 Rehabilitative Surgery
### Baldeschi, L. (Amsterdam)

160 Why Is This Chapter Called Rehabilitative Surgery and Not Cosmetic Surgery?
161 What Are the Steps and Timing of Rehabilitative Surgery?
161 How Should Patients Be Selected for Rehabilitative Surgery
162 References

## 163 Orbital Decompression
Baldeschi, L. (Amsterdam)

163  What Is Orbital Decompression?
163  What Are the Aims of Orbital Decompression?
167  Which Surgical Technique Should Be Preferred?
172  What Are the Possible Complications of Orbital Decompression?
172  Can Complications Be Forecasted or Prevented?
173  References

## 176 Eye Muscle Surgery
Nardi, M. (Pisa)

176  What Is the Cause of Ocular Motility Impairment?
176  How Do You Identify the Affected Muscles?
178  How Can You Avoid Diagnostic Errors in Complex Cases?
179  How Can You Evaluate the Need for Surgery?
182  When Is the Right Time for Surgery?
182  What Can You Realistically Expect from Surgery?
182  How Should You Advise the Patient?
183  The Surgical Plan: What Procedures Are Recommended?
185  What Are the Possible Complications of Surgery and How Can I Avoid or Manage Them?
187  References

## 188 Eyelid Surgery
Neoh, C. (Newcastle upon Tyne); Eckstein, A. (Essen)

188  What Are the Indications for Eyelid Surgery in Patients with Graves' Orbitopathy?
189  Is Botulinum Toxin Useful?
190  Is Surgical Intervention Indicated in Corneal Ulceration Secondary to Exposure Keratopathy?
190  Does Orbital Decompression Have Any Effect on Lid Retraction?
191  Does Squint Surgery Influence the Lid Configuration?
193  What Surgical Procedures Are Available for Correction of Upper Lid Retraction?
195  Are There Complications?
196  What Surgical Procedures Are Available for Correction of Lower Lid Retraction?
196  Should This Be Combined with Horizontal Lid Tightening?
196  Which Materials Are Suitable for Use as Spacers? Should the Use of Allogeneic Grafts Be Avoided?
197  Are There Complications?
198  What About Upper Lid Debulking and Upper and Lower Lid Blepharoplasty?
198  References

*Miscellaneous Issues*

## 201 Quality of Life
Wiersinga, W.M. (Amsterdam)

201  What Is Quality of Life?
201  What Is the Usefulness of Quality of Life Measurements?

203 What Is Known about General Health-Related Quality of Life in Graves' Orbitopathy?
204 Is There a GO-Specific Quality of Life Questionnaire?
206 What Are the Results of the GO-QoL?
206 Can You Explain Response Shift in Quality of Life?
207 Can GO-QoL Be Used as a Separate Outcome Measurement in GO?
208 Is Quality of Life Fully Restored after Treatment of GO?
209 Can I Apply the GO-QoL in My Own Practice?
210 References

## 212 Atypical Manifestations
von Arx, G. (Olten)

212 What Are the Atypical Manifestations of Graves' Orbitopathy?
212 How Do You Explain Unilateral Graves' Orbitopathy (We Don't have Graves' Hyperthyroidism in Just One Thyroid Lobe, Have We?)
216 Will Unilateral Graves' Orbitopathy Proceed to Bilateral Graves' Orbitopathy?
217 Is the Clinical Presentation of Unilateral Graves' Orbitopathy Different from Bilateral Graves' Orbitopathy?
217 How Does Unilaterality Affect Treatment?
218 Is Euthyroid Graves' Orbitopathy a Reason to Refrain from Specific Eye Treatment?
219 What Is Globe Subluxation?
219 References

## 221 Childhood Graves' Orbitopathy
Krassas, G.E. (Thessaloniki)

221 Is Childhood Graves' Orbitopathy Really that Rare?
222 Is the Clinical Presentation of Graves' Orbitopathy in Childhood Different from that in Adulthood?
222 Why Is Graves' Orbitopathy in Children Less Severe than in Adults?
224 What Is the Best Therapeutic Approach for Graves' Orbitopathy in Children and Adolescents?
226 What About Surgical Decompression of the Orbit in Childhood?
226 References

## 229 Prevention
Bartalena, L. (Varese)

229 What Is Primary, Secondary and Tertiary Prevention?
229 Can a General Strategy Be Applied to Prevent Graves' Orbitopathy?
230 What Can Be Done in the Primary Prevention of Graves' Orbitopathy?
231 What Can Be Done in Terms of Secondary Prevention of Graves' Orbitopathy?
233 What About Tertiary Prevention of Graves' Orbitopathy?
234 What Should One Do when Talking to a Graves' Orbitopathy Patient Who Smokes?
234 Acknowledgements
234 References

**237 Future Developments**
   Salvi, M. (Milan); Baldeschi, L. (Amsterdam)
237  Is There Evidence that Steroids in Graves' Orbitopathy Act as True Immunosuppressants and Modify Disease Outcome?
238  What Are the Reasons for Exploring the Potential Efficacy of New Immunosuppressive Medications?
238  Is There Evidence for the Efficacy of New Immunotherapy Agents in Graves' Orbitopathy?
239  Which Anticytokine Treatment Would Be the Most Effective in Your Opinion?
239  What About Rituximab?
241  What About Interfering with the TSH Receptor Pathways?
241  Are Technical Developments in Surgical Approaches to Be Expected?
243  Are Conceptual Developments in Surgical Approaches to Be Expected?
243  References

**246 Historical Notes on Graves' Disease**
   Mourits, M.P. (Amsterdam)
246  Is It Fair to Call Graves' Disease Graves' Disease?
247  Various Eye Signs Carry Specific Names: Are They Still Relevant?
248  How Did Old Theories Explain the Relationship between Hyperthyroidism and Proptosis?
249  Which Are Rundle's Contributions to Our Understanding of Graves' Orbitopathy?
252  Which Are Kriss' Contributions to the Management of Graves' Orbitopathy?
252  When Was Evidence-Based Medicine Incorporated in Graves' Orbitopathy?
253  References

**254 Author Index**

**255 Subject Index**

# Preface

We are very pleased to present *Graves' Orbitopathy: A Multidisciplinary Approach*.

The title of the book is a reflection of our opinion that real progress can be made in understanding thyroid eye disease and in improving outcome of the disfiguring and often invalidating eye changes associated with Graves' orbitopathy only if specialists of various disciplines work closely together. In other words, we favour a multidisciplinary approach in which internists/endocrinologists, ophthalmologists/orbital surgeons and basic scientists combine their forces. This has been the philosophy since the foundation of EUGOGO, the European Group on Graves' Orbitopathy in 1999. The group is currently composed of 13 centres in 8 European countries (Belgium, France, Germany, Greece, Italy, the Netherlands, Switzerland and the United Kingdom), and, in accordance with our philosophy, each centre is represented by specialists in internal medicine and ophthalmology. A further requirement of EUGOGO membership is that each participating centre must have combined thyroid-eye clinics in which the patient can be seen simultaneously by physicians from both disciplines. It is gratifying to note that the number of combined thyroid-eye clinics has been increasing slowly but steadily throughout Europe over the last decade, thereby enhancing the quality of patient care.

EUGOGO meets twice a year, and we have had many lengthy and at times heated discussions on how to assess the eye changes in a most objective manner and what the best treatment should be. It has taken us several years to reach an acceptable degree of agreement among ourselves, again illustrating the many pitfalls in the management of Graves' orbitopathy as well as the importance of using a multidisciplinary approach. Only then could we embark on prospective clinical trials (the size of the group allows completion of clinical studies in a much shorter time than possible for each individual centre), on teaching courses how to investigate and treat the patient with Graves' orbitopathy (so far three courses have been held – Thessalonica 2005, Pisa 2006, and Mainz 2007), and on papers in scientific journals describing the outcome of our studies and recommendations on disease management.

The present book reflects our current thinking on Graves' orbitopathy: all authors are EUGOGO members. The internal consistency between chapters is the result of our ongoing discussions during the annual EUGOGO meetings. The outline of the book is unusual by its choosing the question-and-answer format. The purpose is to enable the book to also be used as a quick reference source for the practicing physician confronted with an ordinary or extraordinary management question: most likely the answer can be found in one of the 194 questions asked in this book. We do not apologise for some overlap between chapters (especially on smoking and thyroid treatment), because these issues are relevant to many aspects of Graves' orbitopathy and it facilitates fast retrieval of the information you are looking for. Topics such as unilateral eye disease, childhood Graves' orbitopathy, and disease-specific quality-of-life assessment which are not easily found elsewhere receive the attention they deserve. The editors welcome feedback from the readership: please send your comments to us; also on how future editions could be improved. You may also consult the EUGOGO website (www.eugogo.org).

We would like to thank the patients with Graves' orbitopathy who cooperated in our endeavours to better understand their disease. We also thank S. Karger AG, Medical and Scientific Publishers, for their efforts to edit, produce, and publish the book within a very short time. Last but not least, we are grateful to the authors for their excellent contributions. It again proves how much can be accomplished by a group of dedicated people.

*Wilmar M. Wiersinga*, President EUGOGO, Editor
*George J. Kahaly*, Treasurer EUGOGO, Co-Editor

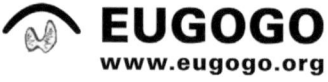

**Diagnosis and Pathogenesis**

Wiersinga WM, Kahaly GJ (eds): Graves' Orbitopathy: A Multidisciplinary Approach.
Basel, Karger, 2007, pp 1–26

# Clinical Manifestations

*A.J. Dickinson*

Eye Department, Claremont Wing, Royal Victoria Infirmary,
Newcastle upon Tyne, UK

### What Are the Common Symptoms of Graves' Orbitopathy?

The most common initial symptom of Graves' orbitopathy (GO) is a change in appearance. In over 70% of the patients, this is due to lid retraction, with or without proptosis or periorbital swelling [1, 2]. During early GO, 40% of patients also develop symptoms that relate to ocular surface irritation comprising a gritty sensation, light sensitivity (photophobia) and excess tearing [1–3]. Double vision is a less common initial symptom, but when it does develop, it is usually first noticed either on waking, when tired, or on extremes of gaze, sometimes accompanied by aching [1, 3, 4]. Orbital ache unrelated to gaze is less common, but can occur with severe orbital congestion [5]. Only about 5% of patients report visual symptoms such as blurring of vision, which may be either patchy or generalised, or alteration in colour perception [1–3]. These latter are potentially significant markers of dysthyroid optic neuropathy (DON), and as they may not be volunteered, they should be specifically elicited from all patients with progressive or otherwise symptomatic disease.

Episodes of globe subluxation (where the eyeball protrudes in front of the eyelids) are extremely alarming for both patient and any witnesses, but fortunately affect only 0.1% of patients [6].

### What Are the Common Signs of Graves' Orbitopathy?

Although GO can present with a number of clinical signs it is very unusual for a patient to present with all of them.

The most frequent sign is of upper eyelid retraction, which affects 90–98% of patients at some stage [2, 7], and frequently varies with attentive gaze (Kocher's

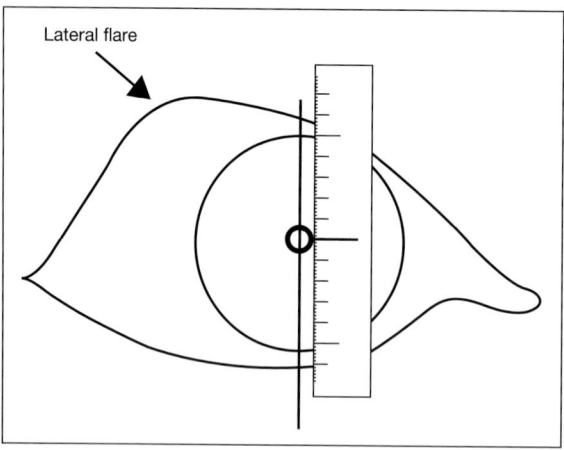

*Fig. 1.* Assessment of the palpebral aperture. The midpoint of the pupil is chosen regardless of lateral flare. In this example, upper eyelid retraction and lower eyelid retraction both measure +1 mm with the limbus as a reference point. Note that the normal adult upper eyelid position would measure – 2 mm.

sign) [8]. Indeed, if upper eyelid retraction is absent then it is appropriate to question the diagnosis [9], and imaging may be required. The contour of the retracted upper eyelid often shows lateral flare (fig. 1) [10], an appearance that is almost pathognomonic for GO. The excursion of the upper eyelid often lags behind eyeball movement on vertical downward pursuit (lid lag) and remains high. Other extremely common signs include the soft tissue signs of peri-orbital swelling and redness, conjunctival swelling and redness, and prominent glabellar rhytids [7]. Proptosis (also known as exophthalmos) is also very frequent and correlates significantly with lower lid retraction [11]; these patients are more likely to show incomplete eyelid closure (lagophthalmos). Many such patients, especially those with a wide palpebral fissure will show punctate inferior corneal staining with fluorescein [11, 12]. Most patients presenting to tertiary centres show restriction of ocular excursions in one or more directions of gaze.

### What Signs Are Unusual in Graves' Orbitopathy?

Less common soft tissue signs include superior limbic keratoconjunctivitis, and inflammation of the caruncle and/or plica [see below 'How are these signs assessed?']. It is also unusual to detect signs of optic neuropathy (DON) as this secondary phenomenon of severe disease only affects around 5% of

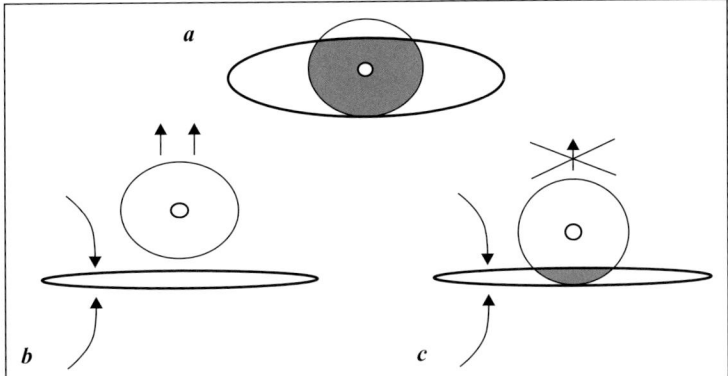

*Fig. 2.* Eyelid closure: lagophthalmos and Bell's phenomenon (*a*) open eye, (*b*) attempted eyelid closure with lagophthalmos, but no corneal exposure due to good Bell's phenomenon rotating the eyeball upwards, and (*c*) attempted eyelid closure with lagophthalmos and no Bell's phenomenon, hence risk of corneal ulceration.

clinical GO. However, detecting subtle evidence of DON is very important and any reduction in corrected vision or colour vision should be elicited. If DON is significantly asymmetrical (30%) then an afferent pupil defect will also be apparent. Sight-threatening corneal ulceration is far less common than DON but presents as an area of corneal staining, sometimes with thinning or abscess and very occasionally perforation. Corneal ulceration can only develop when normal corneal protection is lost. This occurs in those patients who not only cannot close their eyes, but whose cornea remains visible when the eyelids are closed due to absent Bell's phenomenon, the normal protecting upward movement of the eyeball (fig. 2). Although this reflex is absent in 10% of individuals, it is more likely to be lost in GO due to a very tight inferior rectus limiting the upward excursion of the eyeball. It is not known whether patients with extreme eyelid retraction are at greater risk of ulceration, but it is clear that sight-threatening ulceration can develop in patients without severe eyelid retraction.

Although ptosis can develop following longstanding GO, it is very rare for patients to present with ptosis early in the course of their disease: such patient may have concomitant myasthenia gravis and should be appropriately investigated.

Similarly, divergent strabismus does occasionally occur with GO but so rarely that the diagnosis should be questioned and further investigations are required.

## Are There Racial Differences in How Graves' Orbitopathy Manifests?

GO can affect people of all races. Genetic susceptibility to Graves' disease varies between races [13], and there is some evidence that amongst patients with Graves' disease, susceptibility to GO also varies between races. For example, Europeans appear more likely to develop GO than Japanese Asians [14]. There is very little data on racial differences in both prevalence and presentation of GO and the influence of important confounding factors such as smoking needs to be considered.

There is known to be significant variation in normal exophthalmometry values between races [15], with Chinese Asians showing significantly lower values than Caucasians [16], while Negroes have relatively shallow orbits and show higher values. Hence proptosis should be assessed in relation to the normal range for the patient's race and gender.

## Is the Presentation of Graves' Orbitopathy Different in Older Compared to Younger Patients?

There are some important differences in the presentation of GO at different ages and a tendency for overall severity to increase with age, regardless of gender [17].

Children and teenagers with Graves' disease appear as likely as adults to develop GO, particularly in countries where teenagers are more likely to smoke [see chapter by Krassas, pp. 221–228; 18, 19]. However, unlike adults, they rarely develop severe disease and the majority will require no specific treatment [20, 21]. They commonly show a degree of eyelid retraction and mild proptosis but rarely show muscle restriction, corneal ulceration or optic neuropathy.

By contrast, some data suggest that patients over 50 years of age are more likely to have impaired motility than those under 50 (32% vs. 12%, respectively) with greater limitation in upgaze [1] while others show no such difference [17]. However, studies consistently show a significantly higher risk of optic neuropathy with age [1, 22–24]. This may relate at least partly to a higher prevalence of concomitant vascular disease in older patients.

Older patients are also more likely to have unilateral or very asymmetrical disease and are more likely to be euthyroid or hypothyroid at time of presentation [1].

## Why Can the Clinical Presentation of Graves' Orbitopathy Be So Variable?

It is not fully understood why some patients develop one pattern of tissue involvement while others show a different pattern. However, some differences are likely to be due to anatomical variation: the secondary sequelae of GO relate to the interaction between the degree and speed of onset of the inflammation and the anatomical constraints of the orbit, which are at least in part racially determined. It is clear that there is premorbid variation in the relative position of the globe within the orbit and in the laxity of the anterior orbital septum [see next section].

We also know that muscles are asymmetrically involved. While the majority of patients show some muscle involvement on imaging, less than 10% of patients appear to have normal muscle dimensions with expansion of only orbital fat. This can still lead to proptosis; however, restriction of eye movements is uncommon and when it does occur is diffuse rather than localised to one or several muscles. Smoking is associated with more severe GO [see chapters by Daumerie and Kalmann, pp. 34–40 and Orgiazzi, pp. 41–56], but also with chronic skin ageing which may arguably influence the presentation of soft tissue signs.

## Can You Give Me a Short Mechanistic Explanation for All These Clinical Manifestations?

When inflammation develops in orbital soft tissues, particularly muscle and fat, hydrophilic glycosaminoglycans are produced which promote further tissue swelling. Similar inflammation in the eyelids causes visible edema, erythema and festoons. These are the primary effects of GO and when they affect the muscles, they commonly lead to dysfunction due to a failure of relaxation. This limits movement into the field of the ipsilateral antagonist, which, if asymmetrical, causes double vision. Unfortunately, the orbit is a tight space which is completely surrounded by bone except anteriorly. Here, instead of bone, there is a fascial sheet extending across the top and bottom of the orbital opening which is known as the anterior orbital septum (AOS). The AOS limits anterior movement of the orbital contents to a greater or lesser extent. Patients with orbital tissue swelling and a very tight AOS cannot develop significant proptosis, but instead will experience a marked rise in intraorbital pressure. Secondary effects of GO may then ensue, with pressure on the optic nerve leading to loss of vision, colour impairment and altered pupil responses. In contrast, patients with equivalent intraorbital soft tissue swelling but with a lax AOS will 'self-decompress' to develop proptosis (another secondary manifestation) but less rise in intraorbital

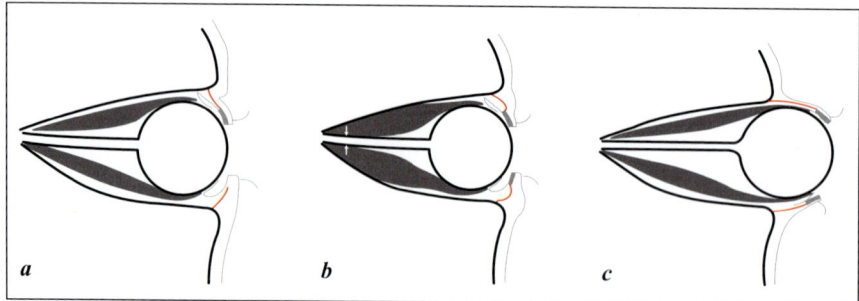

***Fig. 3.*** Diagrammatic representation of secondary effects of GO. Secondary effects depend partly on the laxity of the anterior orbital septum shown in red. *a* Normal relationships of structure within the orbit. *b* Gross compression of the nerve (white arrows) caused by increased orbital muscle volume unaccompanied by significant proptosis: therefore high intraorbital pressure. *c* Gross self-decompression. The optic nerve may be compromised by stretching.

pressure. This is the reason that clinicians should be particularly alert to the risk of DON in patients with muscle restriction but without proptosis and is illustrated diagrammatically in figure 3.

Upper eyelid retraction is multifactorial [3, 11, 25] and due to a combination of increased sympathetic stimulation of Müllers muscle, contraction of the levator muscle due to its direct involvement, and scarring between the lacrimal gland fascia and levator, which specifically gives rise to lateral flare [10]. In addition, tight restriction of the inferior rectus leads to upper eyelid retraction, regardless of upper eyelid pathology [11].

In contrast, lower eyelid retraction correlates with proptosis and may be better described as lower eyelid displacement, as no evidence of direct involvement of the lower lid retractors currently exists.

All corneal signs of GO are secondary phenomena of GO. A wide palpebral aperture leads to increased tear evaporation, which, combined with poor blinking, causes superficial punctate erosions and the symptoms of surface irritation [12]. The mechanism for corneal ulceration is described above in 'What signs are unusual in Graves' orbitopathy?' and arises from lagophthalmos and corneal exposure, due to proptosis, lower lid retraction and/or poor levator function, usually accompanied by a tight inferior rectus [3].

## What Do the Terms 'Activity' and 'Severity' Denote?

During the course of GO, the disease passes through several phases. From the onset, the first phase involves worsening symptoms and signs, often with

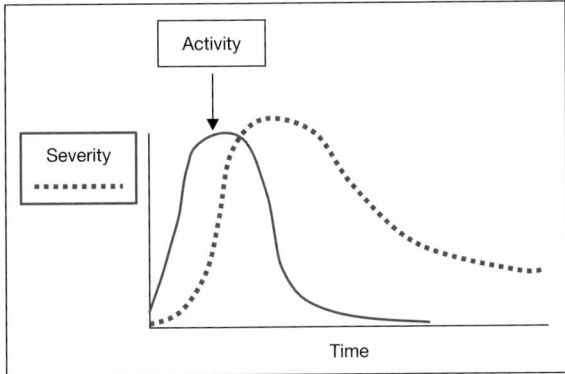

*Fig. 4.* The relationship between activity and severity.

visible evidence of inflammation, followed by a plateau phase during which no further deterioration occurs. A phase of gradual improvement follows until eventually no further change occurs, although permanent abnormalities in both function and appearance may remain. The 'severity' of GO describes the degree of functional or cosmetic deficit at any stage [3, 26]. What is now apparent is that the first three phases represent a time during which there is thought to be inflammation, and these are known as the 'active' phases of GO [3, 4, 27]. Hence 'activity' refers to the presence of inflammation. In contrast, the final stage is not accompanied by further spontaneous change as any inflammation has probably resolved, and this is therefore referred to as the inactive phase of GO. Figure 4 illustrates the relationship between severity and activity.

## Why Is It Important to Distinguish Activity and Severity when Evaluating Patients?

Determining the phase of GO at each clinical assessment is fundamental to formulating an appropriate management plan. This is because immunomodulatory therapies can only be effective while there is active inflammation. On the other hand, certain surgical treatments, e.g. strabismus surgery, should only be undertaken when GO is inactive and there is no further chance of spontaneous change. Furthermore, sight-threatening disease occurs insidiously during active GO; therefore, symptoms and signs of corneal ulceration and DON should be specifically sought during this phase [3].

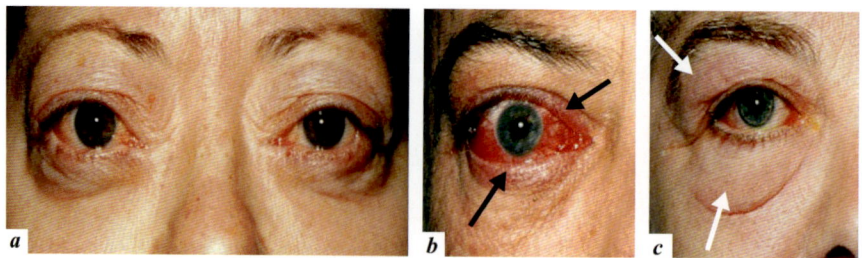

*Fig. 5.* Assessment of eyelid erythema. *a* Normal appearance. *b* Pre-tarsal erythema (black arrows). *c* Pre-septal erythema (white arrows).

## What Symptoms and Signs Are Valuable for Assessing Activity?

The active phase of GO is the period when the patient is most likely to be symptomatic, commonly presenting with grittiness, photophobia, watering, and/or orbital aching – either gaze evoked or spontaneous. Patients will often have noticed a change in the severity of other features over the previous 3 months, e.g. worsening double vision. As we cannot directly identify the degree of orbital inflammation, i.e. activity, the classical signs of inflammation are used as its surrogate markers. In addition, if there has been a change in severity of any feature, worsening or improvement, then this also suggests that the disease is active.

## How Are These Signs Assessed?

In view of their subjective nature, all the features of soft tissue inflammation discussed below are most easily assessed by comparison with an atlas of standard photographs available at www.eugogo.org. Standardisation with careful methodology allows both change and stability of signs to be noted over time, which is essential when determining management options.

*Eyelid Erythema.* The localised eyelid erythema of active GO can affect either the eyelid close to the margin where it may be confused with the much more common condition of blepharitis, or more commonly the area known as the pre-septal eyelid, where maximal swelling occurs (fig. 5). Comparison with the rest of the face helps determine what is abnormal for that individual, and therefore likely to represent active GO. Note that localised eyelid erythema can occasionally persist for years.

*Conjunctival Redness.* This doesn't appear to relate to eyelid retraction and ocular exposure, except where there is actual corneal exposure. Inflammation

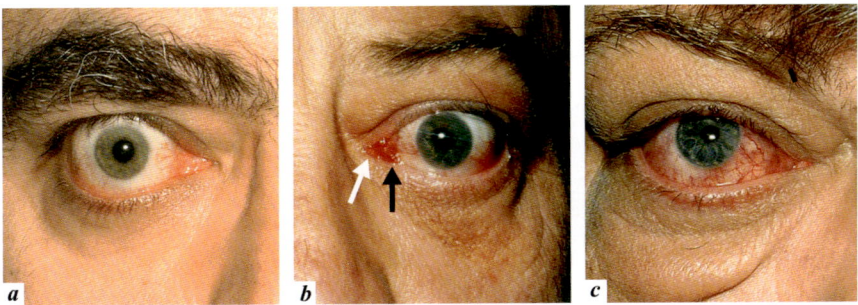

*Fig. 6.* Assessment of conjunctival redness. *a* Normal appearance. *b* Moderate redness, excluding the redness of the caruncle (white arrow) and plica (black arrow). *c* Severe redness.

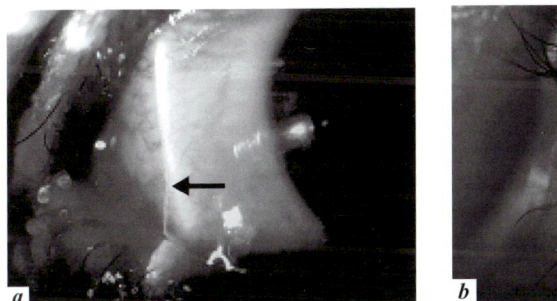 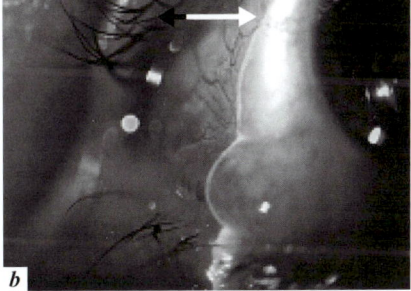

*Fig. 7.* Assessment of chemosis. *a* Normal appearance (conjunctivochalasis). Separation of reflections from conjunctiva and sclera (black arrow) are ≤1/3 total height of palpebral aperture. *b* Chemosis. White arrow shows separation of conjunctival and scleral reflections >1/3 total height of palpebral aperture.

may extend forwards from the insertion of the lateral rectus and can be assessed by comparison with figure 6.

*Chemosis (Conjunctival Edema).* Lesser degrees of chemosis need to be differentiated from the common condition of conjunctivochalasis (redundant folds of conjunctiva) often apparent in older subjects. This requires a slit lamp, and comparative photographs and method are shown in figure 7. However, more severe chemosis can be seen without a slit lamp: simply use a finger to push the lateral lower eyelid upwards over the surface of the eyeball and observe if edematous tissue is displaced.

*Eyelid Swelling.* Assessing eyelid swelling that represents active inflammation is sometimes difficult for several reasons. Periorbital fullness varies

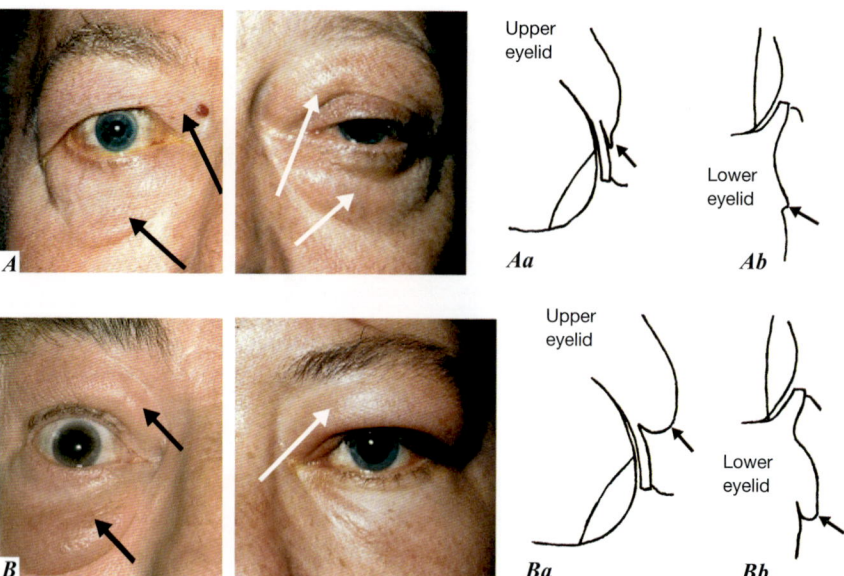

***Fig. 8.*** Assessment of eyelid swelling. ***A*** Moderate active swelling. There is definite subcutaneous fluid (black arrows) or skin thickening (white arrows), but swelling is not tense. This is more than just fat prolapse as the fat pads are not seen distinctly. ***B*** Severe active swelling. There is tense subcutaneous fluid (black arrows) or thickened skin (white arrows). Note that in the upper eyelid, moderate swelling is distinguished from severe swelling by asking the patient to look down slightly: the central part of the skin fold remains a fold and not rounded in moderate swelling (***Aa***), whereas it remains rounded in severe swelling (***Ba***). In the lower eyelid with moderate swelling, the fluid does not fold the skin (***Ab***), whereas it does in severe swelling (***Bb***).

enormously between normal subjects due to age, general body mass and the integrity of the anterior orbital septum (AOS). As the anterior orbital septum weakens with age, a degree of orbital fat prolapse is common. Unfortunately, recent pre-morbid photographs are rarely available to confirm change. Additionally, this anterior displacement of fat and also lacrimal gland may have been exacerbated by GO regardless of whether it is currently active. Hence, assessing what represents active swelling will rely on ascertaining probable recent change and noting signs of either subcutaneous fluid or rather tense skin, usually in the context of other signs of activity as discussed above (fig. 8). Note that subcutaneous fluid bags, known as festoons, occasionally persist for years, implying that their resolution does not mirror the resolution in activity.

*Inflammation of the Caruncle or Plica.* Inflammation of one or both structures is relatively uncommon but easily diagnosed by comparison with figure 9.

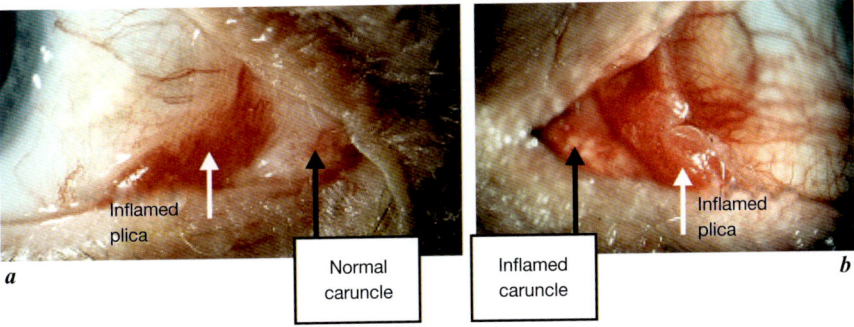

*Fig. 9.* Inflammation of the caruncle and/or plica. Note the difference in colour between the normal caruncle (*a*) and the inflamed caruncle (*b*). Proptosis causes the caruncle to prolapse forwards but does not denote caruncle inflammation.

Either is used in the Clinical Activity Score (CAS): only recently was their differentiation appreciated.

### How Reproducible Are These Assessments?

The assessment of soft tissue signs will always be somewhat subjective, and the validity of attempting to measure them has therefore been called into question [28]. Nevertheless, they remain of great importance, both for patients who endure the disfigurement, as well as for clinicians who need to clarify disease phase. It therefore behoves us to attempt to make their assessment as reproducible as possible. Studies show that reproducibility can be improved by the use of a comparative atlas and careful methodology [29, 30], indeed observers reached agreement in 86%, and kappa values for soft tissue signs were moderate or good for most features. Although far from perfect, photographic comparison remains the most reliable method for assessing soft tissue signs.

### What Value Does the 'Clinical Activity Score' Have?

Mourits et al. [4] devised the Clinical Activity Score (CAS) in 1989. It remains in widespread use, as it is an easy scoring system that allows the majority of patients to be classified as either active or inactive (table 1). Patients seen for the first time are scored for 7 points, 2 symptoms and 5 soft tissue signs. Clarifying the presence or absence of both symptoms and signs is best achieved in conjunction with the protocol and notes of the EUGOGO atlas

*Table 1.* Clinical activity score

- Painful, oppressive feeling on or behind the globe
- Pain on attempted up-, side-, or downgaze
- Redness of the eyelids
- Redness of the conjunctiva
- Chemosis
- Inflammatory eyelid swelling
- Inflammation of caruncle or plica
- Increase of 2 mm or more in proptosis in the last 1–3 months
- Decrease in visual acuity in the last 1–3 months
- Decrease in eye movements of 8° or more in the last 1–3 months

Amended after Mourits et al. [4].
One point is given for each feature.

(www.eugogo.org). On subsequent assessments any significant change in severity is added to the score. Since its inception, it has become apparent that a significant deterioration in any ocular excursion amounts to 8° rather than 5° and the atlas reflects this [see also 'How reproducible are these assessments?', below]. The evidence for the value of the CAS lies in studies correlating pre-treatment CAS and response to immunomodulation. Using a cut-off of at least 4 points, the positive predictive value of the CAS alone was 80% while the negative predictive value was 64% [27]. A further study showed a significant correlation between TSH receptor antibodies and the CAS [31].

The disadvantages of the CAS relate to 2 aspects. Firstly, all features are given equal weighting, and it is not clear whether this is appropriate. Secondly, it is a poor tool for monitoring change as it employs binary scoring, whereby improvement of any feature does not alter the score unless it completely resolves [3].

## Do Patients without Signs of Activity Ever Have Active Disease?

A small minority of patients appear to show no signs of active disease, but subsequently either change spontaneously or respond to immunomodulation. Identifying such patients is of course difficult, however they may have orbital pain or gaze related pain suggesting active disease, and/or describe worsening of severity features usually implying active disease.

### What Should I Do if I Am Not Sure whether the Disease Is Active?

In this situation management will depend on the presenting features and their severity. Unless there is clear evidence to the contrary, all sight-threatening features should be assumed to be of recent onset, implying active disease and a need for urgent intervention. At the other end of the spectrum, patients who present with only eyelid retraction and mild proptosis do not require any urgent intervention, and can safely be sequentially assessed until their disease phase is apparent and any necessary therapy then offered.

### Are There Any Other Ways to Evaluate Activity Other than Clinical Examination?

Over the past 15 years, many other methods have been tried in the hope of evaluating activity more accurately than CAS alone. These include assay of thyrotropin receptor antibodies [31] or measurement of glycosaminoglycans (GAG) in either serum or urine [32]; A-mode ultrasonography [33]; MRI using either STIR sequences [34] or T2 weighted images [35–38]; and scintigraphy using octreotide [39] or gallium [40].

Some studies have also examined the value of noting disease duration when determining whether GO is active [38, 41]. A more recent study examined a wide variety of pre-treatment indices in 66 patients with moderately severe GO undergoing radiotherapy [42]. These comprised disease duration, CAS, GAG excretion, cytokines and other cell factors related to the immune response (IL-6, IL-6R, TNFα RI, TNFα RII, IL-1RA, sIL-2R, sCD30, thyrotropin receptor antibodies (TSI and TBII) plus quantified measurements on A-mode ultrasound, MRI T2 and octreoscan. From this, two models were devised to predict either response or no response to radiation. The 'optimal' model evaluating all indices was compared to the 'practical' model, which evaluated only duration of GO, soft tissue involvement, restriction of elevation and A-mode ultrasound. The discriminative ability of 'practical' approach was 0.82 vs. 0.93 for the 'optimal' approach. Hence, the practical model was significantly more robust than CAS alone in predicting response for an individual.

### When Should These Other Methods for Assessing Activity Be Used in Routine Clinical Practice?

At present we do not know the value of assessing all patients using these additional methods as no data relate to patients with all grades of severity.

Of course all patients in routine clinical practice can have disease duration and soft tissue evaluation without any additional cost or facilities. At present, the place for the other methods described will depend partly on their availability and cost, and partly on the presenting features of an individual patient. There is no proven necessity for additional tests in patients with a very high CAS and severe disease or conversely a very low CAS and very mild disease, as in neither circumstance would the management be influenced. For those patients who have significant but not sight-threatening disease and a low CAS then current evidence favours the use of additional tests if disease-modifying agents are to be considered. An alternative approach is simply to give a short trial of treatment provided the anticipated morbidity for that patient is acceptable.

### What Signs Are Helpful for Assessing Severity?

The following features are quantified to assess severity: eyelid swelling, eyelid aperture, proptosis (exophthalmos), eye motility, visual acuity and colour vision. Pupil responses and the appearance of the cornea and optic discs are also noted.

### What Value Does the Mnemonic 'NOSPECS' Have?

The modified NOSPECS classification (table 2) was devised in 1977 as a way of summarising the severity of GO [43], with an assumed rank order attached to the various clinical features. It is now generally accepted that summary scores are of little value in assessing outcomes [3], and there are 2 further disadvantages to NOSPECS. Firstly, the order of features relates poorly to the order in which an efficient examination is performed: class I eyelid retraction, class II soft tissue involvement, class III proptosis, class IV extraocular muscle involvement, class V corneal involvement, class VI visual loss. Secondly, the features are poorly defined. Without accurate definitions scoring patients remains impossible. Despite this, the mnemonic NOSPECS remains a useful reminder of the features that should be assessed.

### What Are the Relative Frequencies of Classes I–VI?

The prevalence of features comprising NOSPECS classes I–VI is difficult to ascertain with any precision, as most studies relate to tertiary referral populations and some describe only signs at presentation. Nevertheless, there are

*Table 2.* Modified **NOSPECS** classification

| Class | Grade |
|---|---|
| 0 | **N**o physical signs or symptoms |
| I | **O**nly signs |
| II | **S**oft tissue involvement<br>o. Absent<br>a. Minimal<br>b. Moderate*<br>c. Marked* |
| III | **P**roptosis*<br>o. Absent<br>a. Minimal<br>b. Moderate<br>c. Marked |
| IV | **E**xtraocular muscle involvement*<br>o. Absent<br>a. Limitation of motion in extremes of gaze<br>b. Evident restriction of motion<br>c. Fixation of a globe or globes |
| V | **C**orneal involvement<br>o. Absent<br>a. Stippling of the cornea<br>b. Ulceration<br>c. Clouding, necrosis, perforation |
| VI | **S**ight loss (due to optic nerve compression)*<br>o. Absent<br>a. Visual acuity 0.63–0.5<br>b. Visual acuity 0.4–0.1<br>c. Visual acuity <0.1 – no light perception |

After Werner [43].

Note that grades a, b and c within class II, class III and class IV are largely undefined. Severity should be scored by the method given in 'How are signs of severity assessed?'. The severity signs marked with asterisk * are also used to assess activity: namely class IIb and c, or a defined deterioration in class III, IV or VI.

sufficient data to give a picture of the relative frequencies of the different classes and these are as follows: Class I is easily the most common and presents at some stage in 90–98% patients [2]. Class II signs are also extremely common, affecting 32% of an incidence cohort of Graves' patients, but up to 75% of tertiary referrals [1, 2, 44]. The prevalence of class III signs in the EUGOGO series of tertiary referrals was similar to an incidence cohort at 63% [1, 2, 44]. The prevalence of class IV signs depends on assessment method, but is between 40–60% [2, 44]. Class V signs are much less common and although 10–17% of patients will show punctuate staining, the incidence of sight-threatening ulceration was <2% a century ago, and is probably lower now [45]. Class VI affects around 5% of patients, and although it is generally thought to affect 10% of tertiary referrals, in the EUGOGO series 21% of patients had DON [2, 3, 44, 46].

## How Are Signs of Severity Assessed?

A precise and consistent method is required when assessing the various signs of severity. One such method is described in principle below but can be found in more detail at www.eugogo.org. The order of NOSPECS has been used.

(I) Palpebral aperture (fig. 1): The vertical height of the eyelid in the mid-pupil position is noted after first stabilising the patient's head position and fixation to reduce artefacts, and occluding the opposite eye if vertical strabismus is present. Both upper and lower eyelid positions are recorded relative to the respective limbus. Lateral flare is disregarded.

(II) Soft tissue involvement: Although soft tissue involvement indicates activity, the degree of soft tissue swelling also describes severity. The signs are assessed as described above and in figure 8.

(III) Proptosis: This is usually measured clinically using a Hertel exophthalmometer. Unfortunately, the numerous models available give significantly different readings and accuracy will depend on using the same instrument, and ideally the same observer [46]. An intercanthal distance is chosen to fit the instrument snugly against the lateral orbital margins at the level of the lateral canthi and prevent horizontal rotation, and the patient looks at the examiners eye being used to record the position of the corneal apex, i.e. the examiner's right eye for patient's left eye etc. The measurement is taken after aligning the reference points on the instrument (fig. 10). Proptosis is defined as a reading 2 mm greater than the upper limit of normal for that patient's gender, age and race; however, despite many publications reporting normal ranges, the instruments on which they are based are not always described, and meaningful calibration has yet to be achieved [47–49]. It appears true that women have lower measurements than men, and children have lower measurements than adults, although these decline again with age. Asians have lower measurements than Caucasians who have lower measurements than Negros. Until normal ranges are reported for specified and calibrated instruments then the measured change in exophthalmometry is of greatest relevance to monitoring [50].

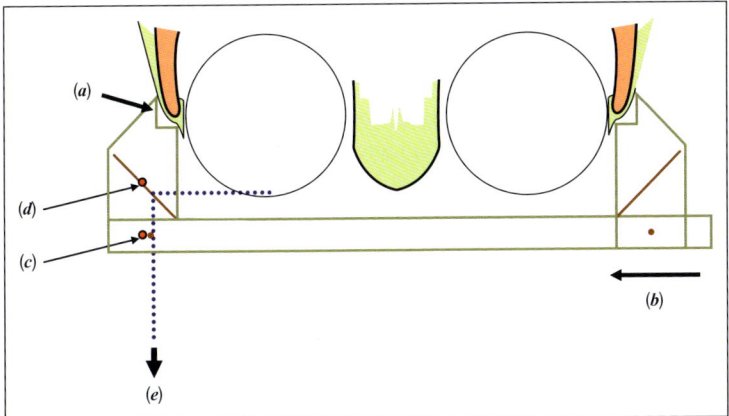

*Fig. 10.* Measurement of proptosis. A Hertel, ideally with a single mirror and straight foot plates is chosen, and the fixed (left) side is positioned fairly firmly against the orbital rim (*a*) before sliding the other (right) side into a similar position (*b*). The reference points in red (*c*) and (*d*) are kept aligned while the position of the corneal surface is read off from the ruler (*e*).

*Table 3.* Scheme for subjectively scoring diplopia: after Bahn and Gorman [51]

| | |
|---|---|
| Grade I | intermittent diplopia, present only when patient fatigued |
| Grade II | inconstant diplopia, present only on lateral or upward gaze |
| Grade III | constant diplopia, present in primary gaze but correctable with prisms |
| Grade IV | constant diplopia, not correctable by prisms |

(IV) Extraocular muscle dysfunction: There are numerous ways of assessing the extraocular muscles, some of which are more relevant to quantifying the severity of GO than others. Subjective diplopia scores [51] are simple and reasonably helpful (table 3); however, significant changes in limitation of motility may go unrecorded. Additionally, it could be argued that grade II may be less severe than grade I. For example, a patient may have severe but asymmetrical bilateral inferior rectus restriction to which they have adapted well owing to a good prism fusion range, but their fusion may break down daily when tired leading to intermittent diplopia. By contrast, a car driver may be very aware of a much smaller restriction in one medial rectus which is evident daily on lateral gaze. Hence, objective assessments are required to assess therapeutic interventions.

*Table 4.* Mean ocular excursions at all ages in degrees

| | |
|---|---|
| Lateral rectus (0°) (abduction) | 46.2*–52[†] |
| Superior rectus (67°)[†] | 43[†] |
| Elevation centrally (90°)* | 33.8* |
| Inferior oblique (141°)[†] | 46[†] |
| Medial rectus (180°) (adduction) | 47.5*–51[†] |
| Superior oblique (216°)[†] | 49[†] |
| Depression centrally (270°)* | 58.4* |
| Inferior rectus (293°)[†] | 62[†] |

Directions of gaze right eye (NB left eye is a mirror image around the vertical axis).
After Mourits et al. [53]* and Haggerty et al. [54][†].

The extraocular muscles may behave quite differently over the course of GO. Hence, uniocular fields of fixation (UFOF) are of value as they independently assess the limitation of excursions of each eye [26, 52–54]. The prism cover test and the field of binocular single vision (BSV) reflect changes in both eyes; however, each retains a valuable place in assessment, the first in planning for strabismus surgery, and the second as a useful way to monitor change. They remain useful when both eyes are abnormal, unlike the Hess-Lees screen [3]. BSV has been shown to be quantifiable and reproducible [55], and to correlate well with the functional deficit from the patient's perspective [56]. UFOF are quantified in either 4 or 6 directions of gaze [53, 54] by using a bowl or arc perimeter, with mean excursions as shown in table 4. An age-related decline in excursions, especially elevation has been noted by some but not all studies [53, 54, 57].

(V) Corneal pathology: While minor corneal pathology requires slit lamp examination to detect punctate fluorescein staining, sight-threatening pathology is evident with simple torch examination. In this situation, the eyelids do not close gently to cover the cornea, which remains visible. The lower conjunctiva is generally red and if ulceration has developed, then a grey opacity or even an abscess will be seen in the inferior cornea. This constitutes an emergency.

(VI) Visual disturbance: Clinical assessments for DON comprise the following:

(a) Best corrected visual acuity of each eye, which is most accurately measured with a Logmar chart, although Snellen charts are more widely available.

(b) Colour vision. Testing in the blue/yellow axis is most likely to pick up early defects of DON; however red-green pseudo-isochromatic charts (e.g. Ishihara) are more readily available and remain very useful in this context

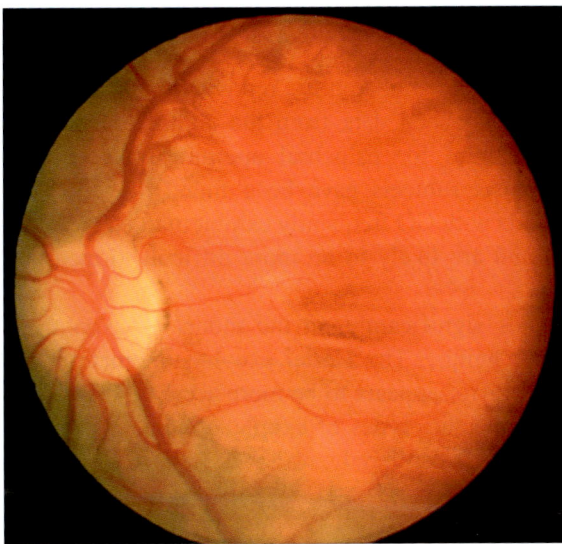

*Fig. 11.* Fundus showing choroidal folds.

[see below, 'How do you decide whether a patient has dysthyroid optic neuropathy']. Each eye is tested separately using a reading correction as required.

(c) Pupil responses are assessed by the swinging flashlight test for a relative afferent pupil defect. Artefacts can easily be produced if a consistent method is not followed, particularly in patients with manifest strabismus. The patient fixates on a distant target and care is taken to give both eyes equal stimulation with the same alignment to the visual axis while the light is moved between alternate eyes.

(d) Fundoscopy will detect abnormal swelling or pallor of the optic disc and the presence of choroidal folds (fig. 11) as well as giving valuable information on confounding pathology such as cataract and glaucoma. Choroidal folds are thought to develop when the eyeball is mechanically deformed by the secondary effects of enlarged rectus muscles in a restricted space. The folds are horizontal, and generally pass straight through the macula unlike retinal folds.

(e) Perimetry. This is reserved for eyes with suspicion of DON. Automated perimetry is most commonly used.

In addition to the above, the intra-ocular pressure is measured. High readings are commonly found in patients with orbital congestion [58], and although these may increase on upgaze in relation to a tight inferior rectus muscle, the reliability of this sign is poor [3].

### How Reproducible Are These Assessments?

There are no peer-reviewed publications on the reproducibility of eyelid dimensions in GO although unpublished data from the author's institution show that the intraclass correlation for palpebral aperture was good at 0.65. Eyelid dimensions in ptosis subjects have been found to be highly repeatable [59]; however, patients with GO frequently exhibit marked variability in upper eyelid positions and are likely to be more difficult to measure accurately.

Proptosis accuracy depends significantly on the model of exophthalmometer used together with technique. The Hertel exophthalmometer with straight footplates and a single mirror appears to be more accurate than other Hertel models [50], and although other types of exophthalmometer may be more reliable [60] they are much less commonly available. Reproducibility to within 2 mm is generally quoted [3, 47, 48] and unpublished data from the author's institution showed the intraclass correlation to be 0.71 for exophthalmometry.

Both UFOF and BSV measurements show high levels of accuracy with UFOF repeatable to within 8° for single muscle measurement [54], and BSV fields accurate to within 4%.

The reproducibility of assessments for DON is unknown.

### How Do You Decide Whether a Patient Has Dysthyroid Optic Neuropathy?

There is no single test that will conclusively establish or refute the diagnosis of DON. Therefore the clinician has to be alert to the possibility of DON in all patients with active disease and look for it in particular when there are certain constellations of other GO features.

Although in theory any patient could develop DON during active GO, unless there is significant motility disturbance or extreme proptosis then they are essentially not at risk. To put it another way, for the optic nerve to be compromised, which is a secondary phenomenon, there has to be evidence of primary tissue involvement that could lead to this as described above 'Can you give me a short mechanistic explanation for all these clinical manifestations?'. There are 2 scenarios: in the majority of patients DON is caused by very large muscles at the orbital apex (especially the medial rectus and inferior rectus) combined with sufficient tension in the anterior orbital septum that the orbit cannot self decompress. In such patients there may be little or no proptosis, although it can still be moderately severe [23, 24, 61]. However, there should always be evidence of restricted motility, very often with a vertical tropia or esotropia [23, 62]. Ballottement of the globe is a crude test, but these patients will have tense rather than soft orbits. In the alternative scenario, there is such extreme proptosis from self-decompression of the orbit that there is no compression of the optic nerve, but rather it is stretched, as are the muscles. In some of these patients there is global restriction of motility. Although in one series this scenario accounted for 24% of DON [61], others have found it to be much less common [23, 24].

The typical presentation of DON is of a symptomatic patient with ocular surface discomfort or aching and evidence of muscle restriction. Soft tissue involvement is often not severe [23, 61, 63] although the CAS is often ≥4 [24]. The onset of DON is usually insidious, but symptoms of blurring, patchy visual loss or colour desaturation can be elicited from up to 80% of affected patients [23, 61]. Nevertheless, visual acuity is often well preserved, and a normal acuity does not exclude DON. DON is usually bilateral (70%) and therefore a relative afferent pupil defect is usually absent. Colour defects are present in most patients [23, 24] and although red-green pseudo-isochromatic colour plates (e.g. Ishihara) are thought to be less sensitive for detecting early DON, a recent study found them to be almost universally abnormal [24]. While 30–40% of eyes with DON may show disc swelling, all studies agree that 40–50% will appear normal. Visual field assessment will detect defects in most patients with other evidence of DON. These are commonly central paracentral and/or inferior [3]. It should be appreciated that these tests can show normal fluctuation and may be very misleading in patients with marked visual loss [64] or confounding pathology such as cataract, age-related maculopathy or glaucoma. Unfortunately, the age of patients at greatest risk of DON makes them more likely to show these confounding pathologies, and indeed a recent study showed confounding pathology in 28% [24]. This may make the signs of DON difficult to interpret.

So, how then can the diagnosis of DON be made with confidence? Recent evidence suggests that the signs with the greatest specificity for DON are impairment of colour perception and optic disc swelling [24]. These signs are least likely to be influenced by confounding pathology, provided the patient is not colour blind. A practical approach would be to diagnose DON on disc swelling alone, provided other causes for this have been excluded. In patients without disc swelling, DON should only be diagnosed when there are at least 2 other features of optic neuropathy: impaired acuity or colour vision, an afferent pupil defect or abnormal perimetry [3]. Patients without significant visual loss who have inconclusive evidence of DON, may not require treatment; however, they should be monitored very carefully.

### Can Dysthyroid Optic Neuropathy Ever Be Present with Normal Vision?

There is clear evidence that DON can be present with normal vision [3, 24]. In some patients, visual acuity of 1.0 may represent a reduction on their normal acuity, while others will truly have no objective reduction by the time DON is diagnosed. Indeed, 50–70% of eyes with DON have acuities of 0.5 or better [61, 65, 66].

### Are Some Patients at Particular Risk?

There is a higher risk of DON in men, and in older patients of either gender. The mean age at presentation of DON is 56–57 years [23, 24] whereas for GO without DON it is 49 years [17, 23]. Other risk factors included diabetes mellitus which constitutes an additional 10-fold risk for DON [67]. Smoking is associated with a greater risk of more severe orbitopathy and may confer a higher risk for DON.

### What Other Assessments Are Useful in Evaluating Possible Dysthyroid Optic Neuropathy?

In addition to the clinical assessments described above, several ancillary tests can also help to identify DON. These include visual-evoked potentials, contrast sensitivity and imaging.

Abnormalities in both latency and amplitude of visual-evoked potentials can be supportive in the diagnosis of DON; however, several issues affect their value in practice. Firstly, they can be affected by thyroid dysfunction, which is frequently present at the time that DON develops [24]. In addition, many laboratories have no normal data for patients over 60 years old, making it hard to interpret findings in those who are already the most difficult to diagnose due to confounding pathology [3]. Hence, they should be interpreted with caution in patients with no other evidence of DON.

Contrast sensitivity, which measures spatial resolution at all levels of contrast, appears to be a sensitive indicator of DON [66]; however, it is less readily available and still subject to confounding pathologies.

Imaging has a very valuable place in supporting the diagnosis of DON. Coronal images on CT or MRI demonstrate apical crowding in the majority of patients. This is defined as the effacement of perineural orbital fat in the posterior orbit. The combination of apical crowding with evidence of fat herniation through the superior orbital fissure seen on axial images is thought to have a specificity of 91% and sensitivity of 94% for DON [68]. Nugent et al. [69] noted mild or no apical crowding in 17% of DON, while 13% had severe apical crowding but no clinical evidence of DON. This emphasises the point that, as with evoked potentials and contrast sensitivity, DON should not be diagnosed from imaging alone. Stretching of the optic nerve is less easy to diagnose without both axial and sagittal images: the latter are not generally available with CT.

### Should These Tests Be Performed in All Patients at Every Assessment?

It is not necessary to perform any of these additional tests in all patients at every assessment. They can be very valuable when there are features suspicious for DON as described above, and, if abnormal, they may be useful for monitoring response to treatment.

### References

1. Kendler DL, Lippa J, Rootman J: The initial clinical characteristics of Graves' orbitopathy vary with age and sex. Arch Ophthalmol 1993;111:197–201.
2. Bartley GB, Fatourechi V, Kadrmas EF, Jacobsen SJ, Ilstrup DM, Garrity JA, Gorman CA: Clinical features of Graves' ophthalmopathy in an incidence cohort. Am J Ophthalmol 1996;121: 284–290.
3. Dickinson AJ, Perros P: Controversies in the clinical evaluation of active thyroid-associated orbitopathy: use of a detailed protocol with comparative photographs for objective assessment. Clin Endocrinol 2001;55:283–303.
4. Mourits MP, Koornneef L, Wiersinga WM, Prummel MF, Berghout A, van der Gaag R: Clinical criteria for the assessment of disease activity in Graves' ophthalmopathy: a novel approach. Br J Ophthalmol 1989;73:639–644.
5. Khan JA, Doane JF, Whitacre MM: Does decompression diminish the discomfort of severe dysthyroid orbitopathy? Ophthal Plast Reconstr Surg 1995;11:109–112.
6. Rubin PA, Watkins LM, Rumelt S, Sutula FC, Dallow RL: Orbital computed tomographic characteristics of globe subluxation in thyroid orbitopathy. Ophthalmology 1998;105:2061–2064.
7. Saks ND, Burnstine MA, Putterman AM: Glabellar rhytids in thyroid-associated orbitopathy. Ophthal Plast Reconstr Surg 2001;17:91–95.
8. Velasco e Cruz AA, Vagner de Oliveira M: The effect of Mullerectomy on Kocher sign. Ophthal Plast Reconstr Surg 2001;17:309–311.
9. Bartley GB, Gorman CA: Diagnostic criteria for Graves' ophthalmopathy. Am J Ophthalmol 1995;119:792–795.
10. Koornneef L: Eyelid and orbital fascial attachments and their clinical significance. Eye 1988;2: 130–134.
11. Frueh BR, Musch DC, Garber FW: Lid retraction and levator aponeurosis defects in Graves' eye disease. Ophthalmic Surg 1986;17:216–220.
12. Gilbard JP, Farris RL: Ocular surface drying and tear film osmolarity in thyroid eye disease. Acta Ophthalmol (Copenh) 1983;61:108–116.
13. Vaidya B, Oakes EJC, Imrie H, Dickinson AJ, Perros P, Kendall-Taylor P, Pearce SHS: CTLA4 gene and Graves' disease: association of Graves' disease with the CTLA4 exon 1 and intron 1 polymorphisms, but not with the promoter polymorphism. Clin Endocrinol 2003;58:732–735.

14 Tellez M, Cooper J, Edmonds C: Graves' ophthalmopathy in relation to cigarette smoking and ethnic origin. Clin Endocrinol 1992;36:291–294.
15 de Juan E, Hurley DP, Sapira JD: Racial differences in normal values of proptosis. Arch Intern Med 1980;140:1230–1231.
16 Tsai CC, Kau HC, Kao SC, Hsu WM: Exophthalmos of patients with Graves' disease in Chinese of Taiwan. Eye 2006;20:569–573.
17 Perros P, Crombie AL, Matthews JNS, Kendall-Taylor P: Age and gender influence the severity of thyroid-associated ophthalmopathy: a study of 101 patients attending a combined thyroid-eye clinic. Clin Endocrinol 1993;38:367–372.
18 Krassas GE, Segni M, Wiersinga WM: Childhood Graves' ophthalmopathy: results of a European questionnaire study. Eur J Endocrinol 2005;153:515–521.
19 Krassas GE, Gogakos A: Thyroid-associated ophthalmopathy in juvenile Graves' disease: clinical, endocrine and therapeutic aspects. J Pediatr Endocrinol Metab 2006;19:1193–1206.
20 Young LA: Dysthyroid ophthalmopathy in children. J Pediatr Ophthalmol Strabismus 1979;16:105–107.
21 Durairaj VD, Bartley GB, Garrity JA: Clinical features and treatment of Graves ophthalmopathy in pediatric patients. Ophthal Plast Reconstr Surg 2006;22:7–12.
22 Trobe JD, Glaser JS, Laflamme P: Dysthyroid optic neuropathy: clinical profile and rationale for management. Arch Ophthalmol 1978;96:1199–1209.
23 Neigel JM, Rootman J, Belkin RI, Nugent RA, Drance SM, Beattie CW, Spinelli JA: Dysthyroid optic neuropathy: the crowded orbital apex syndrome. Ophthalmology 1988;95:1515–1521.
24 McKeag D, Lane C, Lazarus JH, Baldeschi L, Boboridis K, Dickinson AJ, Hullo A, Kahaly G, Krassas G, Marcocci C, Marino M, Mourits M, Nardi M, Neoh C, Orgiazzi J, Perros P, Pinchera A, Pitz S, Prummel MF, Sartini MS, Wiersinga WM: Clinical features of dysthyroid optic neuropathy: a European Group on Graves' Orbitopathy (EUGOGO) survey. Br J Ophthalmol 2007;91:455–458.
25 Mourits MP, Rose GE, Garrity JA, Nardi M, Matton G, Koorneef L: Surgical management of Graves' ophthalmopathy; in Prummel MF (ed): Recent Developments in Graves' Ophthalmopathy. London, Kluwer Academic Publishers, 2000, pp 133–169.
26 Garrity JA, Terwee CB, Feldon SE, Wiersinga WM: Assessment of disease severity; in Prummel MF (ed): Recent Developments in Graves' Ophthalmopathy. London, Kluwer Academic Publishers, 2000, pp 39–57.
27 Mourits MP, Prummel MF, Wiersinga WM, Koornneef L: Clinical activity score as a guide in the management of patients with Graves' ophthalmopathy. Clin Endocrinol 1997;47:9–14.
28 Gorman CA: The measurement of change in Graves' ophthalmopathy. Thyroid 1998;8:539–543.
29 Gerding MN, Prummel MF, Kalmann R, Koornneef L, Wiersinga WM: The use of colour slides in the assessment of changes in soft-tissue involvement in Graves' ophthalmopathy. J Endocrinol Invest 1998;21:459–462.
30 Anderton LC, Neoh C, Walshaw D, Dickinson AJ: Reproducibility of clinical assessment in thyroid eye disease; in Abstract of the European Society of Ophthalmic, Plastic and Reconstructive Surgery, Paris, 2000, p 107.
31 Gerding MN, van der Meer JW, Broenink M, Bakker O, Wiersinga WM, Prummel MF. Association of thyrotrophin receptor antibodies with the clinical features of Graves' ophthalmopathy. Clin Endocrinol (Oxf) 2000;52:267–271.
32 Martins JRM, Furlanetto RP, Oliveira LM, Mendes A, Passerotti CC, Chiamolera MI, Rocha AJ, Manso PG, Nader HB, Dietrich CP, Maciel RMB: Comparison of practical methods for urinary glycosaminoglycans and serum hyaluronan with clinical activity scores in patients with Graves' ophthalmopathy. Clin Endocrinol 2004;60:726–733.
33 Gerding MN, Prummel MF, Wiersinga WM: Assessment of disease activity in Graves' ophthalmopathy by orbital ultrasonography and clinical parameters. Clin Endocrinol 2000;52:641–646.
34 Hiromatsu Y, Kojima K, Ishisaka N, Tanaka K, Sato M, Nonaka K, Nishimura H, Nishida H: Role of magnetic resonance imaging in thyroid-associated ophthalmopathy: its predictive value for therapeutic outcome of immunosuppressive therapy. Thyroid 1992;2:299–305.
35 Just M, Kahaly G, Higer HP, Rösler HP, Kutzner J, Beyer J, Thelen M. Graves ophthalmopathy: role of MRI imaging in radiation therapy. Radiology 1991;179:187–190.

36  Polito E, Leccisotti A: MRI in Graves orbitopathy: recognition of enlarged muscles and prediction of steroid response. Ophthalmologica 1995;209:182–186.
37  Ohnishi T, Noguchi S, Murakami N, Tajiri J, Harao M, Kawamoto H, Hoshi H, Jinnouchi S, Futami S, Nagamachi S, Watanabe K: Extraocular muscles in Graves' ophthalmopathy: usefulness of T2 relaxation time measurements. Radiology 1994;190:857–862.
38  Prummel MF, Gerding MN, Zonneveld FW, Wiersinga WM: The usefulness of quantitative orbital magnetic resonance imaging in Graves' ophthalmopathy. Clin Endocrinol 2001;54:205–209.
39  Gerding MN, van der Zant FM, van Royen EA, Koorneef L, Krenning EP, Wiersinga WM, Prummel MF: Octreotide-scintigraphy is a disease-activity parameter in Graves' ophthalmopathy. Clin Endocrinol 1999;50:373–379.
40  Konuk O, Atasever T, Mehmet U, Ayvaz G, Yetkin I, Cakir N, Arslan M, Hasanreisoglu B: Orbital gallium-67 scintigraphy in Graves' ophthalmopathy: a disease activity parameter that predicts the therapeutic response to immunosuppressive treatment. Thyroid 2005;15:358–363.
41  Gerding MN, Prummel MF, Wiersinga WM: Assessment of disease activity in Graves' ophthalmopathy by orbital ultrasonography and clinical parameters. Clin Endocrinol 2000;52:641–646.
42  Terwee CB, Prummel MF, Gerding MN, Kahaly GJ, Dekker FW, Wiersinga WM: Measuring disease activity to predict therapeutic outcome in Graves' ophthalmopathy. Clin Endocrinol 2005;62: 145–155.
43  Werner SC: Modification of the classification of the eye changes of Graves' disease. Am J Ophthalmol 1977;83:725–727.
44  Prummel MF, Bakker A, Wiersinga WM, Baldeschi L, Mourits MP, Kendall-Taylor P, Perros P, Neoh C, Dickinson AJ, Lazarus JH, Lane CM, Kahaly GJ, Pitz S, Orgiazzi J, Pinchera A, Marcocci C, Sartini MS, Rocchi R, Nardi M, Krassas GE, Halkias A: Multi-center study on the characteristics and treatment strategies of patients with Graves' orbitopathy: the first European Group on Graves' Orbitopathy experience. Eur J Endocrinol 2003;148:491–495.
45  Burch HB, Wartofsky L: Graves' ophthalmopathy: current concepts regarding pathogenesis and management. Endocr Rev 1993;14:747–793.
46  Bartalena L, Wiersinga WM, Pinchera A: Graves' ophthalmopathy: state of the art and perspectives. J Endocrinol Invest 2004;27:295–301.
47  Mourits MP, Lombardo SHC, van der Sluijs FA, Fenton S: Reliability of exophthalmos measurement and the exophthalmometry value distribution in a healthy Dutch population and in Graves' patients: an exploratory study. Orbit 2004;23:161–168.
48  Sleep TJ, Manners RM: Interinstrument variability in Hertel-type exophthalmometers. Ophthal Plast Reconstr Surg 2002;18:254–257.
49  Van den Bosch WA: Normal exophthalmometry values: the need for calibrated exophthalmometers. Orbit 2004;23:147–151.
50  Vardizer Y, Berendschot TTJM, Mourits MP: Effect of exophthalmometer design on its accuracy. Ophthal Plast Reconstr Surg 2005;21:427–430.
51  Bahn RS, Gorman CA: Choice of therapy and criteria for assessing treatment outcome in thyroid-associated ophthalmopathy. Endocrinol Metab Clin N Am 1987;16:391–407.
52  Steel DHW, Hoh HB, Potts MJ, Harrad RA: Uniocular fields of fixation in thyroid eye disease. Eye 1995;9:348–351.
53  Mourits MP, Prummel MF, Wiersinga WM, Koornneef L: Measuring eye movements in Graves' ophthalmopathy. Ophthalmology 1994;101:1341–1346.
54  Haggerty H, Richardson S, Mitchell KW, Dickinson AJ: A modified method for measuring uniocular fields of fixation: reliability in normal subjects and in patients with Graves' orbitopathy. Arch Ophthalmol 2005;123:1–7.
55  Sullivan TJ, Kraft SP, Burack C, O'Reilly C: A functional scoring method for the field of binocular single vision. Ophthalmology 1992;99:575–581.
56  Fitzsimons R, White J; Functional scoring of the field of binocular single vision. Ophthalmology 1990;97:33–35.
57  Clark RA, Isenberg SJ: The range of ocular movements decreases with ageing; in Transactions 25th Meeting European Strabismologicol Association. Jerusalem, 1986, pp 152–157.
58  Kalmann R, Mourits MP: Prevalence and management of elevated intraocular pressure in patients with Graves' orbitopathy. Br J Ophthalmol 1998;82:754–757.

59  Boboridis K, Assi A, Indar A, Bunce C, Tyers AG: Repeatability and reproducibility of upper eyelid measurements. Br J Ophthalmol 2001;85:99–101.
60  Cole HP, Couvillion JT, Fink AJ, Haik BG, Kastl PR: Exophthalmometry: a comparative study of the Naugle and Hertel instruments. Ophthal Plast Reconstr Surg 1997;13:189–194.
61  Trobe JD: Optic nerve involvement in dysthyroidism. Ophthalmology 1981;88:488–492.
62  Feldon SE, Muramatsu S, Weiner JM: Clinical classification of Graves' ophthalmopathy. Identification of risk factors for optic neuropathy. Arch Ophthalmol 1984;102:1469–1472.
63  Ohtsuka K, Nakamura Y: Results of transmedial-canthal ethmoidal decompression for severe dysthyroid optic neuropathy. Jpn J Ophthalmol 1999;43:426–432.
64  Henson DB, Chaudry S, Artes PH, Faragher EB, Ansons A: Response variability in the visual field: comparison of optic neuritis, glaucoma, ocular hypertension, and normal eyes. Invest Ophthalmol Vis Sci 2000;41:417–421.
65  Kennerdell JS, Rosenbaum AE, El-Hoshy MH: Apical optic nerve compression of dysthyroid optic neuropathy on computed tomography. Arch Ophthalmol 1981;99:807–809.
66  Suttorp-Schulten MS, Tijssen R, Mourits MP, Apkarian P: Contrast sensitivity function in Graves' ophthalmopathy and dysthyroid optic neuropathy. Br J Ophthalmol 1993;77:709–712.
67  Kalmann R, Mourits MP: Diabetes mellitus: a risk factor in patients with Graves' orbitopathy. Br J Ophthalmol 1999;83:463–465.
68  Birchall D, Goodall KL, Noble JL, Jackson A: Graves' ophthalmopathy: intracranial fat prolapse on CT images as an indicator of optic nerve compression. Radiology 1996;200:123–127.
69  Nugent RA, Belkin RI, Neigel JM, Rootman J, Robertson WD, Spinelli J, Graeb DA: Graves' orbitopathy: correlation of CT and clinical findings. Radiology 1990;177:675–682.

Dr. A. Jane Dickinson
Eye Department, Claremont Wing, Royal Victoria Infirmary
Queen Victoria Road
Newcastle upon Tyne, NE1 4LP (UK)
Tel. +44 191 282 4410, Fax +44 191 2825446
E-Mail Jane.Dickinson@nuth.nhs.uk

… … … … … … … …
# Orbit-Thyroid Relationship

*J.H. Lazarus*[a], *M. Marino*[b]

[a]Centre for Endocrine and Diabetes Sciences, Cardiff University, Cardiff, UK;
[b]Department of Endocrinology, University of Pisa, Pisa, Italy

## Should This Condition Always Be Called Graves' Orbitopathy?

The eye disease generally associated with Graves' disease has been known by many names [1]. This is not surprising as the disease has been referred to by its clinical features, by a relation to Graves' disease (or von Basedow's disease) and also just in relation to thyroid in general (table 1). These terms indicate firstly that the aetiopathogenesis of the condition is not fully elucidated and secondly that the disease has many and varied clinical presentations and some features are more sight-threatening than others. We believe that the term Graves' orbitopathy (GO) is an accurate reflection of the condition in the majority of patients. It does usually occur in the context of Graves' disease although there are exceptions. It does involve contents of the orbit so that it is reasonable to use the term orbitopathy. However, it could be argued that in the mild form of the condition, where the symptoms and signs are predominantly related to periorbital soft tissues, the term orbitopathy may be an alarming misnomer. From a practical point of view, in the Graves' eye clinic the term GO is appropriate.

## Does Graves' Orbitopathy Occur in the Absence of Hyperthyroidism?

Around 80% of cases of GO occur in association with hyperthyroidism although not all coincide with the onset of hyperthyroid symptoms. In relation to hyperthyroidism, GO may present well before the onset of thyroid dysfunction, during thyroid dysfunction or when the patient is euthyroid following

*Table 1.* Synonyms for Graves' orbitopathy

Graves' eye disease
Graves' ophthalmopathy
Ophthalmic Graves' disease
Thyroid-associated ophthalmopathy (TAO)
Thyroid exophthalmos
Thyroid eye disease (TED)
Thyroid-related eye disease
Von Basedow's ophthalmopathy

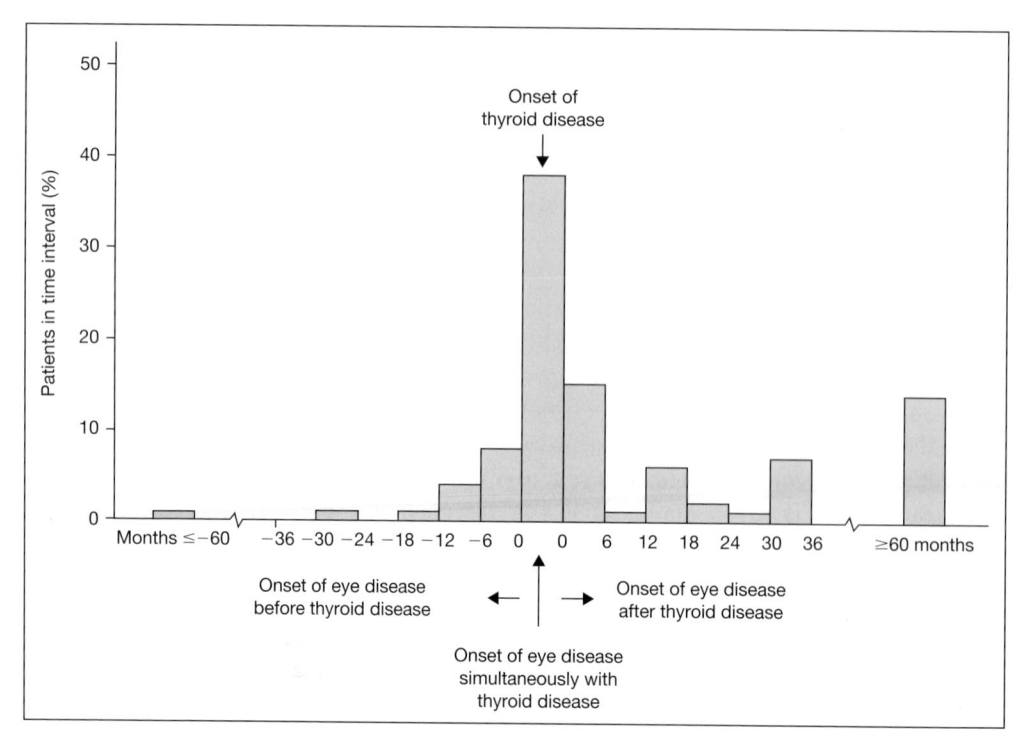

*Fig. 1.* Temporal relationship between the onset of Graves' hyperthyroidism and the onset of Graves' ophthalmopathy in 99 patients [2].

therapy (fig. 1). Similar data have also been found by the Pisa group [3]. In a pooled analysis over 40% of Graves patients developed orbitopathy after the onset of hyperthyroidism [4].

Patients may also develop GO in the absence of hyperthyroidism and never develop the high circulating thyroid hormone levels at all. This euthyroid GO (also called ophthalmic Graves' disease) occurs in 5–10% of patients. However, when these patients are extensively evaluated they are often found to have some features of thyroid disease, ranging from a positive family history through to the presence of TSH-receptor-stimulating antibodies. In addition, they may have isolated positive TPO antibodies or an abnormal response to TRH. Up to 50% of these initially euthyroid patients will develop hyperthyroidism within 18 months of presentation [4]. In addition to the euthyroid group around 10% of GO patients have primary autoimmune hypothyroidism characterised by the presence of moderate or high titres of TPO antibodies. These patients are receiving levothyroxine substitution therapy and are usually found to have TSH receptor antibodies. The severity of the orbitopathy in patients with primary hypothyroidism is as great or sometimes greater than that seen in those with overt Graves' hyperthyroidism [5].

### Do All Patients with Graves' Disease Have Graves' Orbitopathy?

The prevalence or orbitopathy in Graves' disease depends on the sensitivity of the testing methodology, the inclusion of patients with lid changes only and selection bias of patients.

About 30% of unselected patients with Graves' disease will have clinical evidence of GO. This may consist of mild symptomatology such as irritation, watering and discomfort or more significant complaints of ocular protrusion, diplopia and pain on eye movement or even at rest. The remainder of the patients are asymptomatic from the eye point of view and careful clinical examination does not reveal any obvious sign of GO. However, an abnormal elevation of intraocular pressure on upgaze has been found in 68% of patients without gross evidence of ophthalmopathy [6]. Imaging studies have shown extraocular muscle involvement in 90.5% of Graves' patients when assessed by CT [7] but the generally accepted figure is that CT abnormalities occur in about 2/3 of the patients.

### What Comes First in Graves' Disease? The Eye Changes or the Hyperthyroid Symptoms?

As indicated above, a small proportion of patients do develop eye changes prior to the onset of hyperthyroidism but in the majority of patients with GO the eye symptoms occur concurrently with the hyperthyroidism or after treatment has been started (fig. 1). Note that in euthyroid GO, an analysis has shown that 89% may have any thyroid abnormality [4].

## Do TSH Receptor Antibodies Also Cause GO?

It has been long debated whether GO and Graves' disease share a common cause, namely autoimmunity against the same antigens. Thus, most investigators believe that the reason why GO and Graves' disease are associated relies on the fact that either the same proteins or proteins that are similar in their structure are expressed both in the thyroid gland and in orbital tissues, thereby representing a common target for the immune system [8]. Among the various proteins that have been involved, the most reasonable candidate is the TSH receptor, which is well known to be the major target of the immune system in Graves' disease [9]. Several studies have shown that the TSH receptor is actually expressed in orbital tissues, especially fibroadipose cells. Thus, mRNA encoding the TSH receptor can be found there by RT-PCR [9]. However, TSH receptor mRNA was also found in unrelated tissues [10], raising the question whether its presence in orbital tissue actually reflects a true expression of the receptor or if it may be due to technical artifacts, such as the so-called illegitimate transcription. In this regard, a key point is to understand whether the protein (i.e. the TSH receptor itself) rather than the mRNA encoding it is expressed in orbital tissues. In fact, studies performed with several antibodies against the TSH receptor, either polyclonal or monoclonal, have generated conflicting results [9]. A piece of evidence in support of the expression of TSH receptor in orbital tissues is provided by functional studies in cultured fibroblasts. When primary cultures of fibroblasts derived from fibroadipose orbital tissues of GO patients are cultured under certain conditions, they undergo profound changes, resulting in a pre-adipocyte or adipocyte-like phenotype, following which a higher expression of TSH receptor can be observed together with a functional TSH-receptor-like response [11]. Thus, when challenged with TSH or TSH-receptor stimulating antibodies, differentiated fibroblasts show an increased release of cyclic AMP, suggesting an activation of the cyclic AMP cascade, as it occurs in thyroid cells once the TSH receptor is stimulated. When dealing with autoimmune diseases, the best way to show that a given protein is the responsible autoantigen is to reproduce the disease in animals immunized with the same protein. However, evidence is not available concerning the TSH receptor in GO. Although in some studies genetic immunization of mice with the TSH receptor resulted to some extent in a Graves' like phenotype (hyperthyroidism), certain eye changes that had been originally interpreted as resembling GO [12] were confirmed only in part in subsequent studies [13]. It is unquestionable that GO is almost always associated with the presence of autoantibodies against the TSH receptor in the serum, and that these also correlate with the stage of GO [14]. Based on all the above considerations, it remains uncertain whether the TSH receptor is the antigen responsible for GO. Although the functional receptor is

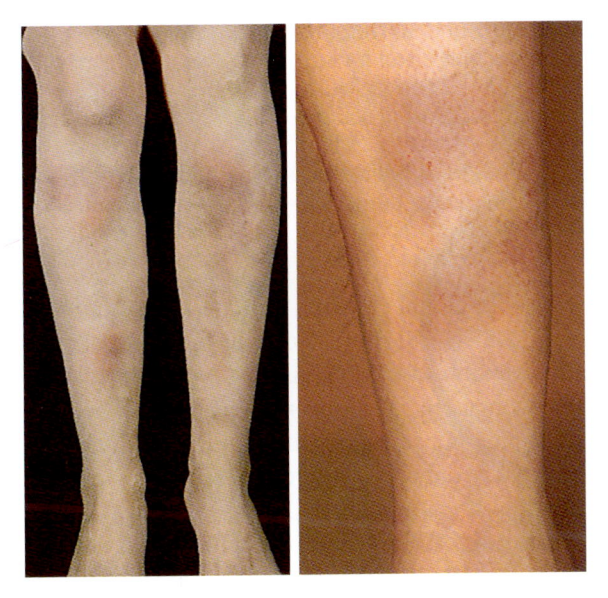

*Fig. 2.* Pretibial myxedema.

probably expressed in orbital tissues, there is no direct proof for it to be the responsible autoantigen, although it remains the most reasonable candidate. Development of new animal models of Graves' disease is needed in order to finally address this issue.

## Are There Any Other Extrathyroidal Manifestations of Graves' Disease Apart from Graves' Orbitopathy?

The two extrathyroidal manifestations are localised myxedema and thyroid acropachy [15].

*Localised Myxedema*
Also called pretibial myxedema because of its usual location, this condition is characterised by skin thickening and is often asymptomatic but may be associated with pruritus and occasional pain. The lesion, which is a raised yellow brown area, is usually localised to the pretibial area but has been seen on the feet, toes and upper extremities as well as the forehead and ear (fig. 2). About 90% of patients with pretibial myxedema have a history of hyperthyroidism but it is observed in patients with GO who have never had hyperthyroidism. Approximately 4% of patients with clinical GO will have pretibial

myxedema with an incidence of up to 12% in severe GO. Occasionally, the dermopathy occurs in the absence of clinical ophthalmopathy. Histological and biochemical examination of the lesion shows that the main constituent is an accumulation of glycosaminoglycans in the dermis. There is only minimal lymphocyte infiltration. The excess glycosaminoglycans are thought to cause dermal edema which will compress lymphatics thereby aggravating the edema.

*Thyroid Acropachy*

Thyroid acropachy presents with digital clubbing of fingers (but not toes) and swelling of digits and toes together with a periosteal reaction of extremity bones. It is rare, occurring in approximately 1% of patients with Graves' disease. It is probably more common in females and may postdate hyperthyroidism, ophthalmopathy and dermopathy in that order. Similar to ophthalmopathy, it may occur in euthyroid or hypothyroid patients. A review of 178 patients with dermopathy showed that more than one fifth had acropachy and that this condition is an indicator of the severity of ophthalmopathy and dermopathy. Like dermopathy, it is nearly always associated with high titres of thyroid hormone receptor-stimulating antibodies.

## References

1. Means JH: Hyperophthalmic Graves' disease. Ann Intern Med 1945;23:779–789.
2. Wiersinga WM, Smit T, Van der Gaag R, Koornneef L: Temporal relationship between onset of Graves' ophthalmopathy and onset of thyroidal Graves' disease. J Endocr Invest 1988;11:615–619.
3. Marcocci C, Bartalena L, Bogazzi F, Panicucci M, Pinchera A: Studies on the occurrence of ophthalmopathy in Graves' disease. Acta Endocrinol (Copenh) 1989;120:473–478.
4. Burch HB, Wartofsky L: Graves' ophthalmopathy: current concepts regarding pathogenesis and management. Endocr Rev 1993;14:747–793.
5. Gleeson H, Kelly W, Toft A, Dickinson J, Kendall Taylor P, Fleck B, Perros P: Severe thyroid eye disease associated with primary hypothyroidism and thyroid-associated dermopathy. Thyroid 1999;11:1115–1118.
6. Gamblin GT, Harper DG, Galentine P, Buck DR, Chernow B, Eil C: Prevalence of increased intraocular pressure in Graves' disease: evidence of frequent subclinical ophthalmopathy. N Engl J Med 1983;308:420–424.
7. Enzmann DR, Donaldson SS, Kriss JP: Appearance of Graves' disease on orbital computed tomography. J Comp Assist Tomogr 1970;3:815–819.
8. Prabhakar BS, Bahn RS, Smith TJ: Current perspective on the pathogenesis of Graves' disease and ophthalmopathy. Endocr Rev 2003;24:802–835.
9. Bahn RS: TSH receptor expression in orbital tissue and its role in the pathogenesis of Graves' ophthalmopathy. J Endocrinol Invest 2004;27:216–220.
10. Agretti P, Chiovato L, De Marco G, Marcocci C, Mazzi B, Sellari-Franceschini S, Vitti P, Pinchera A, Tonacchera M: Real-time PCR provides evidence for thyrotropin receptor mRNA expression in orbital as well as in extraorbital tissues. Eur J Endocrinol 2002;147:733–739.
11. Agretti P, De Marco G, De Servi M, Marcocci C, Vitti P, Pinchera A, Tonacchera M: Evidence for protein and mRNA TSHr expression in fibroblasts from patients with thyroid-associated ophthalmopathy (TAO) after adipocytic differentiation. Eur J Endocrinol 2005;152:777–784.

12 Many MC, Costagliola S, Detrait M, Denef F, Vassart G, Ludgate MC: Development of an animal model of autoimmune thyroid eye disease. J Immunol 1999;162:4966–4974.
13 Baker G, Mazziotti G, von Ruhland C, Ludgate M: Reevaluating thyrotropin receptor-induced mouse models of Graves' disease and ophthalmopathy. Endocrinology 2005;146:835–844.
14 Eckstein AK, Plicht M, Lax H, Neuhauser M, Mann K, Lederbogen S, Heckmann C, Esser J, Morgenthaler NG: Thyrotropin receptor autoantibodies are independent risk factors for Graves' ophthalmopathy and help to predict severity and outcome of the disease. J Clin Endocrinol Metab 2006;91:3464–3470.
15 Fatourechi V. Localized myxedema and thyroid acropachy; in Braverman LE, Utiger RD (eds): The Thyroid: A Fundamental and Clinical Text, ed 9. New York, Lippincott Williams & Wilkins, 2005, pp 488–499.

Prof. J.H. Lazarus
Centre for Endocrine and Diabetes Sciences, Cardiff University
Cardiff CF14 4XN, Wales (UK)
Tel. +44 29 2071 6900, Fax +44 29 2071 2045, E-Mail Lazarus@cf.ac.uk

# Epidemiology

C. Daumerie[a], R. Kalmann[b]

[a]Department of Endocrinology, Université catholique de Louvain, Brussels, Belgium;
[b]Department of Ophthalmology, University Medical Center Utrecht, Utrecht, The Netherlands

## What Is the Present Estimated Prevalence of Graves' Orbitopathy? Has It Changed over the Last Decade?

Estimates of the prevalence of Graves' orbitopathy (GO) are influenced by several variables, including the sensitivity of the detection method.

Graves' ophthalmopathy is clinically relevant in approximately 25% of unselected patients with Graves' disease if eyelid signs are excluded, and 40% if eyelid changes are included. Subclinical abnormalities can be shown in the majority of them by computed tomography or magnetic resonance imaging or by measurement of intraocular pressure. Severe forms of GO account for no more than 3–5% of the cases [1, 2]. The estimated incidence of Graves' ophthalmopathy in the general population is 16 women and 3 men per 100,000 population per year [3].

The prevalence of GO seems to have declined in recent years, as well as that of the more severe expression of eye disease. Review of the clinical records of the first consecutive patients diagnosed at the same eye clinic in 1960 and 1990 showed a significant decrease of clinically relevant ophthalmopathy from 57% in 1960 to 37% in 1990 [4]. This trend might be related to both an earlier diagnosis (facilitated by the introduction of sensitive assays of TSH in the late 1980s) and treatment by the endocrinologists as well as an enhanced attention of the ophthalmologists to the link between the initial ocular manifestations and thyroid dysfunction. Alternatively, smoking behaviour might be involved. In an international survey on the current management of GO, most respondents from Western European countries thought that the prevalence of GO has declined over the last decade, in line with the decreased prevalence of smoking.

Conversely, respondents who considered that the prevalence of GO increased originated from countries such as Poland and Hungary, where the prevalence of smoking had increased since 1989 [5].

## Is the Age and Sex Distribution of Graves' Orbitopathy Similar to that of Graves' Disease?

GO patients are older than patients with Graves' hyperthyroidism, with a mean age of 46.4 years for patients with GO and Graves' hyperthyroidism, but 40.0 years for patients with Graves' hypothyroidism only [4, 6]. In 152 newly referred GO patients from 8 EUGOGO centers, the mean age of GO patients was 49 years [7].

Graves' ophthalmopathy, like Graves' hyperthyroidism, is more common in women than in men. The female to male ratio was 9.3 in patients with mild ophthalmopathy, 3.2 in those with moderate ophthalmopathy, and 1.4 with severe ophthalmopathy [1–4].

A sex-related difference in the severity of GO has been noted, with men comprising a relatively greater proportion of cases of severe ophthalmopathy. Eye disease tends to be more severe in older patients and in men. The reason for this effect of gender is not clear but the higher prevalence of smoking among men likely plays a role.

## Are There Ethnic Differences?

Europeans have a substantially greater risk of developing GO than Asians, with a prevalence of 42% compared to 7.7% in Asians [8].

The reasons for this difference are not clear. Recent genetic studies suggest that the common $-318$ C/T polymorphism in the promoter region of CTLA4 gene is associated with a reduced risk of ophthalmopathy in Chinese Graves' patients [9]. However, extended analyses with large sample sizes should be carried out in patients of different ethnic origin to verify this association. Environmental or anatomic factors are more likely to be involved. Adequate adjustments of normal and abnormal values of exophthalmos are important for a correct diagnosis of TAO [10].

## What Are the Risk Factors for the Occurrence of Graves' Orbitopathy?

Several factors may increase the risk of ophthalmopathy in patients with Graves' disease, namely tobacco, gender, genetics, type of treatment for hyperthyroidism, TSH receptor antibodies, drugs, advanced age and stress.

The evidence for a genetic component to the pathogenesis of Graves' disease may apply also to GO. However, no evidence of a distinct genetic risk for eye disease has actually been confirmed.

Graves' ophthalmopathy, like hyperthyroidism, is more common in women than men. However, men who have GO are more likely to have an increase in severity during follow-up [1–4].

TSH-R autoantibodies (TRAB) might be involved in the disease process of GO and their detection may be of clinical benefit. In a euthyroid Caucasian population, GO activity and proptosis were mainly associated with the TRAb fraction binding inhibitory antibodies (TBII). TBII levels were significantly higher in patients with a severe course of GO compared with patients with a mild course, and it is a risk factor independent of age and smoking. However, this observational study must be confirmed by a prospective study [11].

The type of treatment given for Graves' disease may be a risk factor for GO. Subtotal thyroidectomy and antithyroid drugs do not appear to have a negative influence on the course of GO. In comparison, most but not all studies suggest that radioiodine treatment might lead to the development or worsening of GO [1, 12].

Other possible risk factors for GO include advanced age, stress [13], neck irradiation for Hodgkin disease [14], and drugs such as lithium [15] or interferon-α [16].

## Is Tobacco Bad for Graves' Orbitopathy?

Cigarette smoking is the strongest modifiable risk factor for developing GO. Despite various limitations and difficulties in comparing available studies, there is strong evidence for a causal association between smoking and development of GO [17–19].

A positive association between smoking and GO is found in four case-control studies when compared with control patients with Graves' disease but no ophthalmopathy (OR 1.94–10.1) and in seven case-control studies in which control subjects did not have thyroid disease (OR 1.22–20.2) [19].

According to the EUGOGO study, 40% of GO patients are smokers [7]. Among patients with ophthalmopathy, smokers were more likely to have severe disease than nonsmokers. The severity of GO is related to the number of cigarettes smoked per day. The volume of intra-orbital connective tissue also correlates well with cumulative smoking [20]. Current smokers were also more likely to experience disease progression or poorer outcome of treatment [1, 2]. The effect of medical treatment of GO may be attenuated in cigarette smokers. Among patients with mild GO, eye disease progression after radioiodine treatment seems to be significantly higher in smokers than nonsmokers.

### Is Ocular Co-Morbidity Relevant for Graves' Orbitopathy?

Cataract and age-related macular degeneration should be excluded as a cause of decreased vision in patients with suspected dysthyroid optic neuropathy (DON). Bio-microscopy, fundoscopy, visual field examination and visual-evoked potential testing can distinguish between DON and the mentioned ophthalmological conditions.

Preexistent strabological disorders may complicate the orthoptic assessment in patients with GO and ocular motility disorders. Patients who do not have binocular vision because of congenital eso- or exotropia will not complain of diplopia. Strabismus surgery can be performed for cosmetic rehabilitative reasons in those patients.

Diagnosis of primary open angle glaucoma (POAG) and measurement of ocular pressure should be made with special care.

### Is Elevated Intraocular Pressure Relevant in Graves' Orbitopathy?

The intraocular pressure (IOP) is determined by aqueous humor production by the ciliary body, the resistance to aqueous outflow across the trabecular meshwork, and the level of episcleral venous pressure. Primary open angle glaucoma (POAG) is characterized by an IOP over 21 mm Hg, an open angle and visual field defects with optic disc cupping. In POAG, the rise in IOP is caused by increased resistance in the drainage channels. Risk factors in the development of glaucomatous optic nerve damage are high IOP, increasing age, family history of glaucoma, and black race [21, 22].

Patients with IOP over 21 mm Hg but normal visual field and cup-disc ratio are classified as having ocular hypertension (OH). These patients are usually managed by observation alone. In cases at increased risk, treatment is considered after carefully weighing up the advantages and disadvantages of therapy. Since POAG is a chronic and progressive disease, the diagnosis has serious implications for the patient.

In patients with GO, an absolute increase of IOP of 1–15 mm upon upgaze is a common finding (60–100%) [23]. This phenomenon is explained by the inelasticity of the inferior rectus muscle as a result of fibrosis and thus the incapacity to relax on the globe when the antagonist pulls the eye upwards causes compression and therefore increase episcleral venous pressure and orbital congestion. If an elevated IOP is measured in a patient with GO, the question will arise whether the elevated IOP is just a sign of GO or if glaucoma should be considered. In other words, should all patients with elevated IOP and GO be treated?

In a retrospective study of 482 patients with GO, 23 patients (4.8%) had elevated IOPs as measured in primary gaze. They were all using glaucoma medication at referral. Four patients (0.8%) turned out to have real POAG [24]. This prevalence of POAG in the population of GO patients corresponds to the 1.1% prevalence in the Dutch population [25]. That means that although IOP is elevated on upgaze in the majority of GO patients, it does not lead to glaucomatic injury more often than in the normal population. Nineteen patients (3.9%) had elevated IOPs without visual field defects and with normal optic discs [24]. This prevalence of ocular hypertension is higher than the 1.9% prevalence of OH in the normal Dutch population [25]. This difference is probably caused by the fact that normally when using the applanation tonometer, the eyes are in mild upgaze, giving rise to a slight elevation in IOP in patients with GO. It is important that when measuring the IOP in patients with GO, the position of the eyes is checked.

Diagnostic confusion may occur in patients with elevated IOP, visual field defects and severe GO. In the above-mentioned study [24], 4 patients were considered to have glaucoma because of elevated IOP and visual field defects. After treatment of their optic neuropathy (orbital decompression and/or steroids intravenously), the visual field defects disappeared. Looking back, the absence of glaucomatous cupping of the optic disc could have been decisive.

The diagnosis of POAG in patients with GO should be made with special care. Increase in IOP when looking up is common in patients with GO, but does not cause glaucoma more often than in the normal population. An increased IOP might be the result of a slight elevation of the eyes during applanation tonometry. Precise assessment of the optic disc can prevent false diagnosis of PAOG in patients with GO and visual field defects.

## Is There Significant Non-Ocular Co-Morbidity (Like Diabetes) which Is Relevant for Graves' Orbitopathy?

In the EUGOGO study, 9% of the 152 new consecutively included patients had diabetes [7]. The prevalence of type 1 diabetes mellitus (DM) or insulin-dependent diabetes mellitus (IDDM) is higher in patients with GO than in the normal population. In a Dutch study, of 482 patients with GO, 3.1% also had diabetes mellitus: 8 (1.7%) had type 1 diabetes, and 7 (1.4%) had type 2 diabetes [26].

Patients with GO and DM seem to have a higher incidence of DON. Several studies show a higher incidence of DON (15–35%) in GO patients with DM compared to GO patients without DM (3–4%) [26, 27]. The higher incidence of DON in patients with GO and DM could be explained by a marginal oxygenation of the optic nerve in diabetic patients, due to the vasculopathy; this makes the optic nerve more suitable to pressure of the enlarged extraocular muscles. Patients with DON and DM also have worse recovery of visual acuity after treatment. Mourits et al. [28] showed that 67% of the patients with DON who did not respond to orbital decompression were diabetics. In one study, 33% of the diabetics developed DON with 50% improvement of visual acuity after treatment, whereas in the whole population of 482 GO patients, 19 had DON (3.9%) showing 69.4% improvement of vision after treatment [26].

Patients with GO and DM have also a higher risk of bleeding during or after surgery because of a generalized vasculopathy and platelet disorder.

Myasthenia gravis (MG) is another auto-immune disease which may complicate the diagnosis and course of GO. MG is 50 times more common in patients with GO when compared to the normal population. While GO is a restrictive myopathy, with the inferior and medial rectus muscle involved most frequently, in MG a paresis of the extraocular muscles can be present, with no special pattern. In GO, retraction of the upper eyelids is almost pathognomonic, whereas in MG ptosis is worsening during the day [29]. Therefore, in patients with GO who have ptosis and/or atypical ocular motility, concomitant MG should be suspected. The diagnosis of MG can be established by clinical and serological testing (anticholinesterase antibodies). Forced duction test of the eye muscles can distinguish between restriction and paresis. In patients with GO and MG, prediction of strabismus surgery will be more complicated. Deterioration of diplopia after initial success of strabismus surgery is a common problem in patients with GO and MG.

## References

1 Bartalena L, Pinchera A, Marcocci C: Management of Graves' ophthalmopathy: reality and perspectives. Endocr Rev 2000;21:168–199.
2 Wiersinga WM, Bartalena L: Epidemiology and prevention of Graves' ophthalmopathy. Thyroid 2002;12:855–860.
3 Bartley GB, Fatourechi V, Kadrmas EF, Jacobsen SJ, Ilstrup DM, Garrity JA, Gorman CA: The incidence of Graves' ophthalmopathy in Olmsted County, Minnesota. Am J Ophthalmol 1995;120: 511–517.
4 Perros P, Kendall-Taylor P: Natural history of thyroid eye disease. Thyroid 1998;8:423–425.
5 Weetman AP, Wiersinga WM: Current management of thyroid-associated opthalmopathy in Europe: results of an international survey. Clin Endocrinol 1998;49:21–28.
6 Prummel MF, Wiersinga WM: Smoking and risk of Graves' disease. JAMA 1993;269:479–482.
7 Prummel MF, Bakker A, Wiersinga WM, Baldeschi L, Mourits MP, Kendall-Taylor P, Perros P, Neoh C, Dickinson AJ, Lazarus JH, Lane CM, Heufelder AE, Kahaly GJ, Pitz S, Orgiazzi J, Hullo A, Pinchera A, Marcocci C, Sartini MS, Rocchi R, Nardi M, Krassas GE, Halkias A: Multi-Center study on the characteristics and treatment strategies of patients with Graves' orbitopathy: the first European Group on Graves' Orbitopathy experience. Eur J Endocrinol 2003;148:491–495.
8 Teller M, Cooper J, Edmonds C: Graves' ophthalmopathy in relation to cigarette smoking and ethnic origin. Clin Endocrinol 1992;36:291–294.
9 Han S, Zhang S, Zhang W, Li R, Li Y, Wang Z, Xie Y, Mao Y: CTLA4 polymorphisms and ophthalmopathy in Graves' disease patients: association study and meta-analysis. Hum Immunol 2006;67:618–626.

10 Tsai CC, Kau HC, Kao SC, Hsu WM: Exophthalmos of patients with Graves' disease in Chinese of Taiwan. Eye 2006;20:569–577.
11 Eckstein AK, Plicht M, Lax H, Neuhauser M, Mann K, Lederbogen S, Heckmann C, Esser J, Morgenthaler NG: Thyrotropin receptor autoantibodies are independent risk factors for Graves' ophthalmopathy and help to predict severity and outcome of the disease. J Clin Endocrinol Metab 2006;91:3464–3470.
12 Tallstedt L, Lundell G, Torring O, Wallin G, Ljunggren JG, Blomgren H, Taube A: Occurrence of ophthalmopathy after treatment for Graves' hyperthyroidism. The Thyroid Study Group. N Engl J Med 1992;326:1733–1738.
13 Salvi M, Zhang Zg, Haegert D, Wall J: Patients with endocrine ophthalmopathy not associated with overt thyroid disease have multiple thyroid immunological abnormalities. J Clin Endocrinol Metab 1990;70:89.
14 Jackson R, Rosenberg C, Kleinmann R, Vagenakis AG, Braverman LE: Ophthalmopathy after neck irradiation therapy for Hodgkin's disease. Cancer Treat Rep 1979;63:1393–1395.
15 Byrne AP, Delaney WJ: Regression of thyrotoxic ophthalmopathy following lithium withdrawal. Can J Psychiatry 1993;38:635–637.
16 Villanueva RB, Brau N: Graves' ophthalmopathy associated with interferon-alpha treatment for hepatitis C. Thyroid 2002;12:737–738.
17 Hägg E, Asplund K: Is endocrine ophthalmopathy related to smoking? Br Med J 1987;295:634–635.
18 Shine B, Fells P, Edwards OM, Weetman AP: Association between Graves' ophthalmopathy and smoking. Lancet 1990;335:1261–1264.
19 Thornton J, Kelly SP, Harrison RA, Edwards R: Cigarette smoking and thyroid eye disease: a systematic review. Eye 2006;15:1–11.
20 Szurks-Farkas Z, Toth J, Kollar J, Galuska L, Burman KD, Boda J, Leovey A, Varga J, Ujhelyi B, Szabo J, Berta A, Nagy EV: Volume changes in intra- and extraorbital compartments in patients with Graves' ophthalmopathy: effect of smoking. Thyroid 2005;15:146–151.
21 Lyons DE: Postural changes in IOP in dysthyroid exophthalmos. Trans Ophthalmol Soc 1971;91: 799–803.
22 Gamblin GT, Harper DG, Galentine P, Bruck DR, Chemow B, Eil C: Prevalence of increased intraocular pressure in Graves' disease-evidence of frequent subclinical ophthalmopathy. N Engl J Med 1983;308:420–424.
23 Fishman DR, Benes SC: Upgaze intraocular pressure changes and strabismus in Graves' ophthalmopathy. J Clin Neuro-ophthamol 1991;11:162–165.
24 Kalmann R, Mourits MP: Prevalence and management of elevated intraocular pressure in patients with Graves'orbitopathy. Br J Ophthalmol 1998;82:754–775.
25 Dielemans I, Vingerling JR, Wolfs RC, Hofman A, Grobbee DE, de Jong PT: The prevalence of glaucoma in a population-based study in the Netherlands: the Rotterdam Study. Ophthalmology 1994;101:1851–1855.
26 Kalmann R, Mourits MP: Diabetes mellitus: a risk factor in patients with Graves' orbitopathy. Br J Ophthalmol 1999;83:463–465.
27 Neigel JM, Rootman J, Belkin RI, Nugent RA, Drance SM, Beattie CW, Spinelli JA: Dysthyroid optic neuropathy: the crowded orbital apex syndrome. Ophthalmology 1988;95:1513–1521.
28 Mourits P, Koornneef L, Wiersinga WM, Prummel MF, Bergout A, van der Gaag R: Orbital decompression for Graves' ophthalmopathy by inferomedial, inferomedial plus lateral, and by coronal approach. Ophthalmology 1990;97:636–641.
29 Drachman DB: Myasthenia Gravis. N Engl J Med 1994;330:1797.

Dr. Chantal Daumerie
Service d'Endocrinologie et Nutrition
Université catholique de Louvain, Cliniques Universitaires St Luc
Avenue Hippocrate 54, UCL 54.74
BE–1200 Brussels (Belgium)
Tel. +32 2 764 54 75, Fax +32 2 764 54 18, E-Mail daumerie@diab.ucl.ac.be

# Pathogenesis

*Jacques Orgiazzi*

Service d'Endocrinologie-Diabétologie, Université Claude-Bernard-Lyon 1 et Hospices Civils de Lyon, Groupe Hospitalier Sud, Pierre-Bénite, France

## What Are the Pathological Changes in Orbital Tissue of Graves' Orbitopathy?

The pathological processes within the orbit include:
- inflammation;
- expansion of adipose tissue within the connective tissue of the muscle endomysium and perimysium and the fatty connective tissue which surrounds the muscles, and
- excess production by orbital fibroblasts of glycosaminoglycans (GAG), which lead, on the whole, to an increase in the volume of extraocular muscles and orbital fat/connective tissue (fig. 1).

Orbit imaging shows a variable balance among patients between muscle enlargement, the more frequent abnormality observed, and expansion of orbital fat/connective tissue (fig. 2). Enlarged muscles may reach 2–3 times the normal volume, sometimes at the expense of the orbital fat tissue volume [1]. The inferior rectus is predominantly affected followed by the medial rectus, the other muscles being less often involved. Only the belly part of the muscles is affected, tendons remaining unchanged, which differentiates Graves' orbitopathy (GO) from extraocular myositis. In any case, swelling of tissues contained within the inextensible bony orbital cavity leads to an increase in intra-orbit pressure. This has mechanical consequences which account for most of the signs and symptoms of GO.

In the retrobulbar region extraocular muscles and connective/adipose tissue are closely intertwined. Tenon's capsule which connects the capsules of

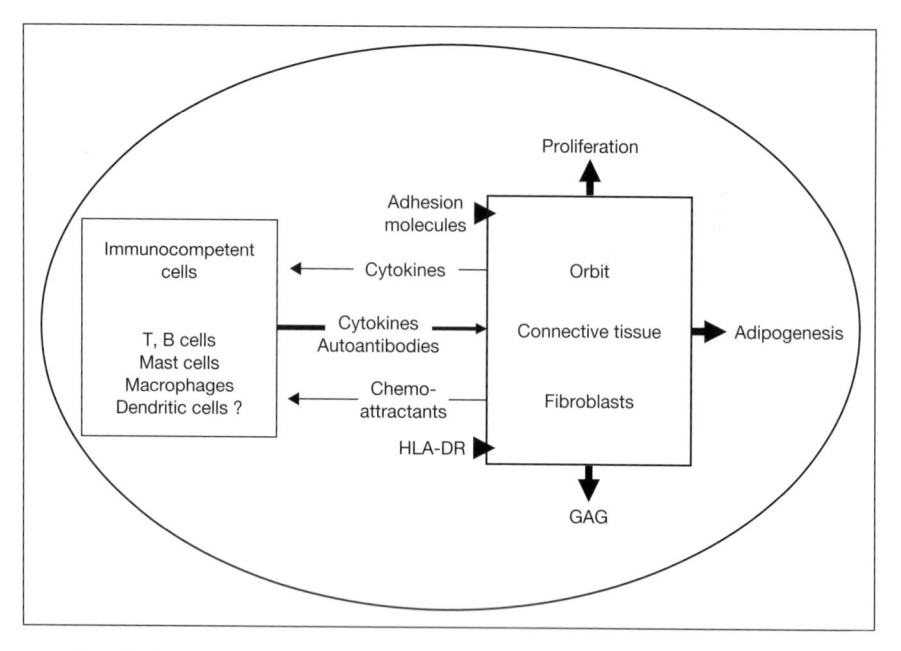

**Fig. 1.** Overview of the interactions which take place, within the orbit, between the immune/inflammatory cells and the orbit fibroblasts, and their functional consequences. The fibroblast is the central actor responsible for the deleterious effects of the up-regulation of many of its functions. 'Autoantibodies' refers to anti-TSH receptor and anti-IGF-1 receptor antibodies. The figure does not define the potential role of the TSH receptor as the autoantigen responsible for the initiation of the process because of persisting uncertainties.

each of the rectus muscles extending from the eyeball to the apex of the orbit delimits extra- and intraconal compartments. The intraconal compartment, centred by the optic nerve, contains arteries, veins, lymphatic and nerves.

*Early Inflammatory Changes.* These are characterized by sparse mononuclear cell infiltrates, both focal and diffuse, within the muscle endomysium and the fatty connective tissue [2]. The majority of cells are T lymphocytes, CD4+ or CD8+, as well as CD45RO+ and CD45RB+. B lymphocytes are only occasionally observed. A few mast cells are present with a perivascular distribution. Macrophages are increased in early disease and less so in late disease. HLA-DR expression by interstitial cells including fibroblasts, but not muscle fibres, is observed in both early and late stages. As lymphocytes, plasma cells and macrophages increase in number, fibroblasts within the interstitium enlarge and proliferate producing collagen and mucopolysaccharides. Muscles become enlarged, firm and rubbery. Microscopically, they appear as edematous and

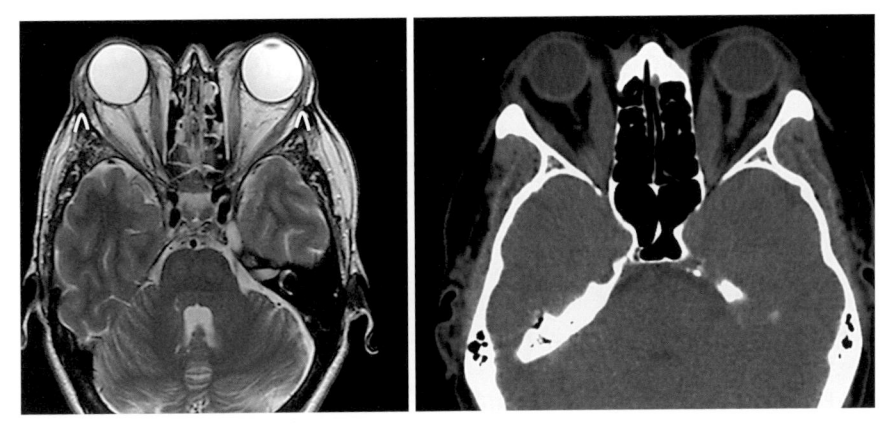

*Fig. 2.* Opposite contribution of muscle (right, TDM imaging) and extramuscular tissue (left, NMR) to the swelling of the retrobulbar compartment. Notice that exophthalmos is even more marked in the patient with the mildest muscle hypertrophy. The external orbit rims, on the NMR slice, are marked.

fibrous with an increase in fat content, mucin and water. Proliferation of fibroblasts within the perimysium may lead subsequently to a scarring process with muscle atrophy, fibrosis and sclerosis. It is noticeable that muscle fibres are relatively spared in GO, the changes affecting mainly the connective tissue between the fibres.

*De novo Adipogenesis.* Orbital fibroblasts include a subpopulation of cells (preadipocytes) which may differentiate into adipocytes [3, 4]. De novo adipogenesis in orbital adipose/connective tissue is demonstrated by an increase in the mRNA of 'adipocyte-related immediate early genes', including the angiogenic inducer, followed by increased expression of PPAR gamma, preadipocyte factor 1, adiponectin, leptin and stearyl-CoA-desaturase [5]. In vitro, orbital fibroblasts differentiate into mature adipocytes when treated with the PPAR-γ receptor agonist rosiglitazone, a finding in keeping with the clinical observations of GO progression in 1 patient [6], and of a mild increase in eye protrusion in a group of patients [7] after treatment with pioglitazone for type 2 diabetes.

*Increased Production of GAG.* Orbit connective/adipose tissue as well as extraocular muscles are particularly rich in GAG, mainly chondroitin sulphate and hyaluronan, an especially hydrophilic molecule. Hyaluronan synthases are strongly expressed by orbital fibroblasts and upregulated in the presence of various cytokines, notably IL-1β. Enlargement of intra-orbital tissues is largely accounted for by the accumulation of GAG and edema within the connective tissue both within and outside the muscles.

## How Do the Pathological Changes Give Rise to the Clinical Manifestations?

Most of the signs and symptoms of GO result from the local mechanical constraints imposed by the increased volume of intra-orbital tissues. This is in keeping with the cat model of ligation of the superior ophthalmic vein [8].

Lid retraction, the most common ocular sign, may result from excessive sympathetic activity within Muller's muscle. It may follow, also, some degree of retraction of the levator.

Proptosis results from the forward push of the globus. The degree of proptosis is correlated with muscle enlargement. However, proptosis is also conditioned by the resiliency of the orbital fibrous tissue, mainly the sclera. Restriction of the forward displacement of the globus may limit the release of the intra-orbital excess pressure and favour compression of the optic nerve with the risk of ischaemia and optic neuropathy. Chemosis and peri-orbital edema result mainly from decreased venous drainage within the orbit. It is less easy to explain the abnormalities in the eye movements. In many but not all cases, restriction in eye ductions appear to grossly parallel the degree of muscle hypertrophy. At late stages, restriction of the eye movements results from the fibrotic changes that affect the extraocular muscles.

These considerations provide no clue to account for unilateral or grossly asymmetrical forms of the disease.

Additional manifestations may worsen the clinical presentation:
- Excessive exposure of the cornea due to lid retraction and/or proptosis with lid lag may lead to keratitis and, if not treated properly, to cornea ulcer or even perforation. The risk is greater when the Charles Bell phenomenon is impaired due to restriction of the upper duction.
- Impairment of vision may result from optic neuropathy. However, visual impairment may have many other causes: keratitis, photophobia, orbital pain, excessive tearing, mild diplopia and severe lid edema which should be recognised as such. Dysthyroid optic neuropathy (DON) results usually from the compression of the optic nerve by the enlarged posterior segment of the rectus extraocular muscles filling the narrow apex of the orbit. Coronal orbit imaging demonstrates the apical crowding resulting from muscle enlargement and the loss of the peri-nerve lining. In these cases, surgical decompression or glucocorticoid usually lead to visual recovery.

But optic neuropathy may also result from stretching of the optic nerve or from ischemia, a mechanism which is difficult to demonstrate.

**What Triggers Graves' Orbitopathy?**

So far, what really triggers GO is unknown.

Minimal symptoms/signs of GO are very common in Graves' disease (GD) as suggested by meticulous clinical examination and orbit imaging as well as the augmented increase in intra-ocular pressure in the upper gaze. However, full-blown GO is present in only 25–50% of the patients with GD. Therefore, there are two questions:
- What triggers GO?
- Why is GO more prominent or severe in some patients than in others?

GO onset is not related to hyperthyroidism per se as it can precede, follow or coincide with installation of Graves' hyperthyroidism. Also, GO can occur in conjunction with autoimmune thyroiditis, whatever the thyroid status.

It is common observation, however, that there is a gross correlation between the risk of GO and the duration of active GD. The fact that in children and adolescents GD is likely to be recognised and treated without delay could account for the usual lack of severity of GO in this age range.

Three situations/factors appear to precipitate the occurrence of GO:
- RAI treatment of GD: Treatment of hyperthyroid GD with $^{131}$I is susceptible to worsen GO in the case of active GO, especially in smokers and in the presence of markedly elevated T3 levels [9]. It is likely that GO deterioration results from the well-known exacerbation of thyroid inflammation/autoimmunity which occurs 3–5 months after $^{131}$I irradiation as evidenced by a rise in blood levels of anti-thyroid antibodies including anti-TSH receptor antibodies. Interestingly enough, however, glucocorticoid treatment is able to prevent GO worsening but not the rise in circulating antibody levels.
- Occurrence of iatrogenic hypothyroidism: Whatever treatment modality, especially after $^{131}$I therapy, iatrogenic hypothyroidism has been recognised as a risk factor for GO, an unexplained side effect [10].
- Smoking (see below).

A fourth potential factor is trauma. By extension, it should be reminded that the other extra-thyroidal manifestation of GD, namely pretibial myxedema, the pathophysiology of which could resemble that of GO, may be triggered or aggravated by a local trauma to the skin. But, what aggression could be considered likely to traumatize the orbital tissues?

No condition that would protect from, or prevent, the occurrence of GO has been identified. However, it is noticeable that in children and adolescents, both the prevalence and the severity of GO are low. In a series of 83 patients, lower lid retraction was present in 38.6%, upper lid retraction in 4.8% and mild proptosis in 12%, and GO scored class 2 or less in 64% of the cases. In this series, the largest reported so far, no factor that could have predisposed to GO was identified [11].

## Is Graves' Orbitopathy Triggered by an Autoimmune Phenomenon? If so, what Is the Nature of the Auto-Antigen?

GO is an autoimmune disease, related to autoimmune thyroid diseases (AITD):
- GO is associated in nearly 100% of the cases with AITD. GO may occur even in those cases of typical full-blown GD observed within the frame of immune reconstitution following highly active antiretroviral therapy for HIV infection or after iatrogenic lymphocyte removal by anti-CD52 monoclonal antibody in multiple sclerosis [12].
- Orbital tissues are infiltrated with inflammatory and immune cells.
- There is some evidence that immunisation of mice against the TSH receptor may induce intra-orbital inflammatory changes mimicking those observed in the human disease, but a bona fide experimental model of immunological GO has yet to be secured.

The question of the antigen(s) involved in GO is still unsolved [13]. Because of the unique association of GO with AITD, it is hypothesized that the thyroid and the orbital tissues should share antigen(s):
- Thyroglobulin (Tg): Ancient literature suggests that Tg could flow from the thyroid to the orbit. Recent studies have demonstrated the presence of Tg in orbital tissues of patients with GO but in fibro-adipose tissue rather than extraocular muscle. However, because of the lack of the apparent concordance of the presence of anti-Tg antibodies and GO and also of the weak binding of Tg to orbital structures, this antigen does not appear as a good candidate to secure the hypothesis.
- The TSH receptor: The TSH receptor is predominantly involved in the pathogenesis of GD. Higher levels of expression of the transcripts of the TSH receptor have been observed in orbital tissues specimen from GO as compared to controls. Functional TSH receptor protein has also been detected in orbital tissues. In vitro, increased expression of the TSH receptor parallels the adipogenic differentiation of orbit preadipocyte fibroblasts, and IL-6 enhances both [4, 14]. However, the level of the expression of the TSH receptor in the orbit is very low even in patients with active disease, despite markedly elevated expression of inflammatory cytokines [15]. In addition, the

TSH receptor is detectable, both at the mRNA and protein levels, in several tissues unrelated to GD and GO. Recently, transfection of orbit preadipocytes with an activating mutant TSH receptor, while stimulating adipocyte differentiation, has been shown to block PPAR-γ-induced adipogenesis [16].
- The IGF-1 receptor: The IGF-1 receptor could be involved in GO. The presence of anti-IGF-1 receptor antibodies has been demonstrated in patients with GO. These antibodies have been considered as potentially pathogenic for the disease. More recently, antibodies able to compete with the binding of IGF-1 to orbital fibroblasts have been identified in patient with GD. Moreover, these antibodies could activate through the IGF-1 receptor expressed by the orbital fibroblasts the production of the chemokines RANTES and IL-16 in addition to that of hyaluronan [17, 18].
- Extraocular muscle antigens: Relevant auto-antigens from extraocular muscles, despite intensive work, have not been clearly identified as potentially involved in GO, yet.

## Why Is the Orbit a Special Target for Thyroid Autoimmunity?

The concept of the shared antigen, i.e. restriction of an antigen expression to both thyroid and orbit, is debated. It might well be that the involvement of orbital tissues results from a combination of factors including the presence within the orbit of (a) antigenic structures recognized by auto reactive T cells involved in thyroid autoimmune diseases, and (b) specific local conditions such as the presence of fibroblasts/preadipocytes with unique functional characteristics including exaggerated responses to pro-inflammatory cytokines [19]. Other factors could contribute to the association of thyroid and orbit pathologies:
- The orbit and the thyroid share draining lymph nodes so that sensitisation to thyroid antigens could theoretically be extended to the orbit by trafficking dendritic cells originating from the thyroid [20].
- Auto-reactive B cells to the TSH receptor could act locally as antigen-presenting cells and support the initiation or the development of local autoimmunity. Auto-reactive B cells can modulate T cell functions as shown in a different setting of a GAD65-specific human B-T cell line cognate system in vitro [21]. Interaction of antigen-presenting cells with T cells is modulated, among other factors, by CTLA-4, the gene polymorphism of which may be involved in the susceptibility to GO (see below). A clue to the role of B cells as antigen-presenting cells is provided by the unexpected favourable effect of anti-CD20 (Rituximab) monoclonal antibody on GO, an agent which deletes pre-B and B cells but not IgG-secreting plasmocytes [22, 23].

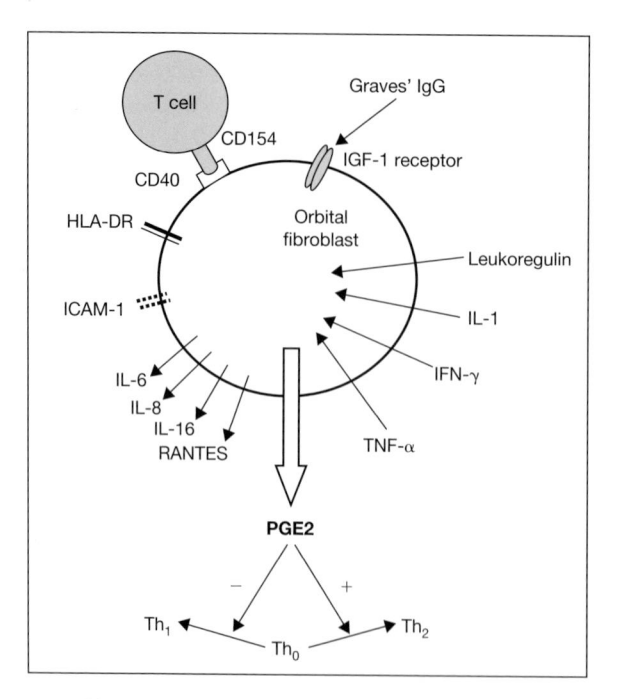

*Fig. 3.* The orbital fibroblast takes part in the activation and perpetuation of the inflammatory process through the expression of HLA-DR and adhesion molecules as well as the production of chemoattractants and cytokines.

## What Kind of Immune Reaction Takes Place within the Orbit?

Inflammatory cells, T and B lymphocytes, macrophages as well as mast cells, infiltrating the orbit interact with orbital fibroblasts through a whole array of cytokines. This interplay amplifies and perpetuates inflammatory/autoimmune reactions and activation of fibroblasts. However, as shown by the Rundle's curve, evolution of GO is monophasic and appears as self-limited and fibrosis ultimately develops, notably in the extraocular muscles.

IL-1, IL-4 and IFN-γ have been detected in orbital connective tissue of patients with GO. T cells obtained from GO orbital tissue appear to elicit a mixed Th1/Th2 pattern. While the Th1 pattern (IL-2, IFN-γ, TNF-α) predominates in recent onset GO, Th2 pattern (IL-4, IL-5, IL-10) might be associated with remission [24]. IL-6 is found in the majority of GO T cell clones. In vitro, cytokines have many stimulatory effects on orbital fibroblasts [19] (figs. 3–5).

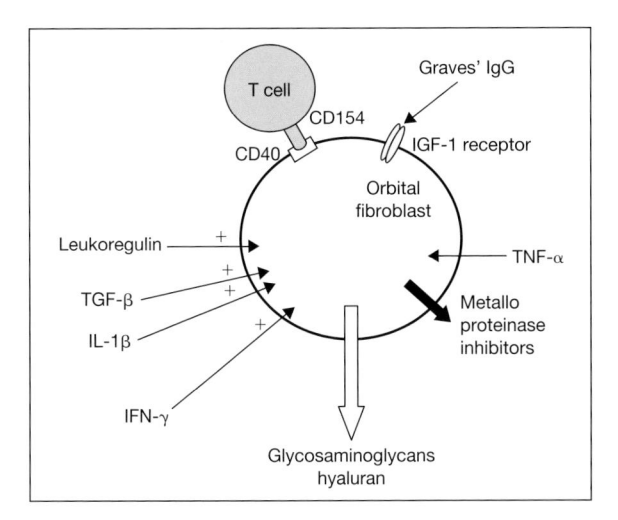

*Fig. 4.* Exacerbation of the production of glycosaminoglycans, notably of hyaluronan, by the fibroblasts is central to the swelling of retro-orbital tissues. Since orbital fibroblasts do not express hyaluronidase, hyaluronan accumulates. Also, the turnover of the extracellular matrix is modified by the increased expression of proteinase inhibitors.

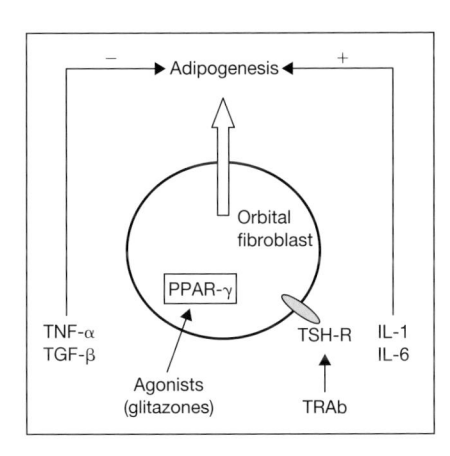

*Fig. 5.* An important feature of the pathogenesis of GO is the differentiation of pre-adipocyte fibroblasts into adipocytes. This evolution is under balanced control by cytokines and activation of PPAR-γ. Central to the pathogenesis of the disease is the possible link between the adipogenic differentiation and the expression at the cell surface of a functional TSH receptor.

They:
- increase the expression of HLA class 2 molecules, heat shock protein 72 (HSP-72) and ICAM-1,
- stimulate the production of prostaglandin E2, a modulator of the immune response,
- stimulate the production of chemoattractants (IL-16, RANTES) as well as of IL-6,

- enhance the synthesis of glycosaminoglycans,
- induce extracellular matrix remodelling activity through modulation of pericellular proteolytic environment [25],
- stimulate adipocyte differentiation: TGF-β, IFN-γ and IL-1, but not IFN-α,
- stimulate adipogenesis, a process on which IFN-α is rather inhibitory [26].

In addition, orbital fibroblasts are upregulated by IFN-γ to express CD40 allowing direct interaction with activated T cells through the CD40 ligand (CD154) which results in fibroblast activation as evidenced by the induction of IL-6 and IL-8 [27].

Finally, IgG from patients with GD can stimulate orbital fibroblasts to produce lymphocyte chemoattractants, an effect possibly mediated by the IGF-1 receptor.

### Do Anti-TSH Receptor Antibodies (TRAb) Play a Role in the Onset or Development of Graves' Orbitopathy?

There is an epidemiological association between GO and TRAb:
- TRAb are detectable in nearly 100% of the patients with GO.
- TRAb are present in the patients in whom GO is associated with autoimmune thyroiditis.
- There is a gross correlation between the presence, or levels, of TRAb and severity of GO [28].

In one study, TBII and TSI levels were closely correlated with clinical activity score of GO. Also, there is a correlation, although weak, between TRAb levels and proptosis [1]. A follow-up study showed that levels and prevalence of TRAb were higher in patients with a more severe course of GO; in 50% of the patients, TRAb appeared to be a significant independent risk factor of GO, independent from age and smoking [29].

However, TRAb are not directly responsible for GO as shown by the absence of GO in hyperthyroid neonates with TRAb-driven hyperthyroidism.

### Is There a Familial Predisposition to Graves' Orbitopathy? Is There a Specific Genetic Background for Graves' Orbitopathy?

Among the non-modifiable risk factors for GO, male gender and age are significant, although more for the severity of the disease than for its occurrence [30].

Genetic predisposition to GD is demonstrated by familial clustering and twin studies. However, as far as GO is concerned, no clear familial aggregation has been observed in 114 consecutive patients with severe GO. Only 3/114 had a family history of GO and all 3 were second-degree relatives [31].

GD appears to be inherited as a complex multigenic disorder and candidate gene studies (HLA on chromosome 6p21, *CTLA4* on chromosome 2q33, *LYP* on chromosome 1p13 and *TSHR* on chromosome 14) are promising. The *CTLA4* gene is associated with susceptibility to GO. The G allele at exon 1 *CTLA4*(49)A/G polymorphism is associated with GO (OR: 1.65). More importantly, G allele frequency is correlated with severity of GO. The T allele at intron 1 *CTLA4*(1822)C/T, but not the *CTLA4*(−318)C/T polymorphism in the promoter region, has also showed an association with GO (OR: 1.70). Moreover, exon 1 and intron 1 polymorphisms are in linkage disequilibrium with each other [32]. These findings are in line with the fact that, for several other autoimmune disorders, exon polymorphism of *CTLA4* is associated with more severe forms. As to *TSHR*, recent work using single nucleotide polymorphisms has identified an association of the *TSHR* region with GD but not autoimmune thyroiditis. However, no data concerning GO have been reported in this work [33].

## Smoking Increases the Risk of Graves' Orbitopathy and Its Severity: What Is the Mechanism for It?

Smoking is the strongest modifiable risk factor for GO [34].

Smoking increases the incidence and the severity of GO. Smoking confers a current risk: former smokers have a lower risk than current smokers to develop GO, even for comparable life-time tobacco consumption. Smoking influences the course of GO: the response to treatment is poorer and delayed in smokers. Also, smoking increases the risk of progression of GO after radioiodine treatment. GD patients who smoke have 5 times more risk to develop GO than those who do not. The effect of smoking is dose-dependent: the relative risk of diplopia or proptosis has been reported to be 1.8 at 1–10 cigarettes/day, 3.8 for 11–20 cigarettes/day and 7.0 for more that 20 cigarettes/day. In ex-smokers, the risk is no longer significant even at >20 cigarettes/day. This suggests a direct and immediate effect of smoking. Serum levels of cytokines do not differ in smoker and non-smoker patients with GO. Finally, stopping smoking is the only GO preventive measure.

How smoking affects GO is conjectural. Several mechanisms have been discussed:

- superoxide radicals generated by smoking can induce orbital fibroblasts to proliferate,
- hypoxia also can stimulate orbital fibroblasts to proliferate and produce GAG,
- nicotine and tar can increase class II HLA molecules expression by orbital fibroblasts in the presence of IFN-$\gamma$, and
- total cigarette smoke extract increases in vitro GAG production by orbital fibroblasts as well as adipogenesis [35].

The adipogenic effect of cigarette smoke extract is synergistic with that of IL-1. However, relevant compounds within cigarette smoke extract have not been identified, yet. It is important to note that in the absence of thyroid disease, smoking does not appear to alter orbit content. This suggests that smoking has mainly a potentiating effect. Cigarette smoke extract does not increase ICAM expression which suggests that it does not stimulate the release of cytokine IL-1, TNF-$\alpha$, IFN-$\gamma$ by orbital fibroblasts.

## How May the Observations Described Above and the Current Understanding of the Disease Lead to More Effective Treatment of Graves' Orbitopathy?

Current understanding of the pathophysiology of GO sets the orbital fibroblast as the main target of the autoimmune process. On stimulation by pro-inflammatory cytokines, orbital fibroblasts are induced to interact with activated auto-reactive immune cells present within orbital tissues. As a consequence, they produce an excess of GAG, proliferate and can differentiate into adipocytes, and secrete cytokines, chemoattractants and an excess of PGE2.

Current therapeutic approaches are based on non-specific immunosuppression by glucocorticoids and orbit radiotherapy. For years, more specific immunomodulatory treatments have been considered and some tested [36, 37]. Among the classical immunosuppressants, only ciclosporine has shown some efficacy in combination with glucocorticoids. Somatostatin analogs, if assimilated to immunosuppressive agents because of the expression of somatostatin receptors by activated lymphocytes, have not proved to be of significant efficacy.

At this point, several possible therapeutic routes could theoretically be explored:
- Interfering with up-regulated functions of orbital fibroblasts: While glucocorticoids interfere with the production of both GAG and PGE, more

specific agents could be considered, for instance cyclo-oxygenase inhibitors and non-steroidal anti-inflammatory drugs. Due to its central role in adipogenesis, the use of antagonists of PPAR-γ or of selective PPAR-γ modulators represents a logical route to be considered. However, because of the pleiotropic effects of PPAR-γ on metabolism, inflammation, fibrosis, cell cycle regulation, etc. preliminary studies using reliable experimental models of GO are mandatory.

– Inhibition of cytokine actions: GO appears as a cytokine-driven disease, therefore anti-cytokine approaches could be considered as in other autoimmune/inflammatory affections such as rheumatoid arthritis and Crohn's disease. Anti-TNF-α (etanercept, TNF-α receptor ectodomain fusion protein antagonist), which neutralises the expression of other pro-inflammatory cytokines, has been tested in a small open-label trial in 10 patients with some improvement of CAS from moderate to marked in 60% of the patients [38]; tolerance was satisfactory. Controlled trials are obviously needed. The use of anti-IL-1 and anti-IL-6 could also be considered. A trial of pentoxifylline, a non-specific cytokine antagonist, is currently tested in a controlled trial within the EUGOGO consortium.

– Deletion or downregulation of activated autoreactive lymphocytes: Several approaches are possible. The CTLA-4 agonist (abatacept), a potent inhibitor of T cell proliferation, has been tested in psoriasis and rheumatoid arthritis. A non-mitogenic humanised anti-CD3 monoclonal antibody, the effect of which is to induce CD8+ and CD4+CD25+ T regulator cells, has been beneficial in 2 large controlled trials in type 1 diabetes. In GO, two reports have recently shown the potential beneficial effect of B cell depletion by anti-CD20 monoclonal antibody (rituximab) [22, 23]. As in other diseases such as rheumatoid arthritis, systemic lupus erythematosus and idiopathic thrombopenia, rituximab has proved efficient. This observation was unexpected and points out to B cell playing an important role in the pathogenesis of autoimmune diseases not only in producing antibodies but also as antigen-presenting cells, as mentioned above, and in secreting cytokines. Other B cell-depleting pathways are available through blockade of ligands from the TNF family such as BAFF and APRIL.

However, a word of caution is necessary. Indeed, not only is the pathogenic antigenic system of GO still uncertain but it is obvious that modulation of the cytokine network as well as that of the number and functional state of T or B cells might induce deleterious consequences disproportionate with the usual morbidity of GO. The availability of in vitro or, rather, in vivo models of GO is therefore badly needed.

# References

1 Kvetny J, Puhakka KB, Rohl L: Magnetic resonance imaging determination of extraocular eye muscle volume in patients with thyroid-associated ophthalmopathy and proptosis. Acta Ophthalmol Scand 2006;84:419–423.
2 Heufelder AE, Bahn RS: Elevated expression in situ of selectin and immunoglobulin superfamily type adhesion molecules in retroocular connective tissues from patients with Graves' ophthalmopathy. Clin Exp Immunol 1993;91:381–389.
3 Sorisky A, Pardasani D, Gagnon A, Smith TJ: Evidence of adipocyte differentiation in human orbital fibroblasts in primary culture. J Clin Endocrinol Metab 1996;81:3428–3431.
4 Valyasevi RW, Erickson DZ, Harteneck DA, Dutton CM, Heufelder AE, Jyonouchi SC, Bahn RS: Differentiation of human orbital preadipocyte fibroblasts induces expression of functional thyrotropin receptor. J Clin Endocrinol Metab 1999;84:2557–2562.
5 Lantz M, Vondrichova T, Parikh H, Frenander C, Ridderstrale M, Asman P, Aberg M, Groop L, Hallengren B: Overexpression of immediate early genes in active Graves' ophthalmopathy. J Clin Endocrinol Metab 2005;90:4784–4791.
6 Starkey K, Heufelder A, Baker G, Joba W, Evans M, Davies S, Ludgate M: Peroxisome proliferator-activated receptor-gamma in thyroid eye disease: contraindication for thiazolidinedione use? J Clin Endocrinol Metab 2003;88:55–59.
7 Dorkhan M, Lantz M, Frid A, Groop L, Hallengren B: Treatment with a thiazolidinedione increases eye protrusion in a subgroup of patients with type 2 diabetes. Clin Endocrinol (Oxf) 2006;65:35–39.
8 Saber E, McDonnell J, Zimmermann KM, Yugar JE, Feldon SE: Extraocular muscle changes in experimental orbital venous stasis: some similarities to Graves' orbitopathy. Graefes Arch Clin Exp Ophthalmol 1996;234:331–336.
9 Tallstedt L, Lundell G, Torring O, Wallin G, Ljunggren JG, Blomgren H, Taube A: Occurrence of ophthalmopathy after treatment for Graves' hyperthyroidism. N Engl J Med 1992;326:1733–1738.
10 Tallstedt L, Lundell G, Blomgren H, Bring J: Does early administration of thyroxine reduce the development of Graves' ophthalmopathy after radioiodine treatment? Eur J Endocrinol 1994;130:494–497.
11 Chan W, Wong GW, Fan DS, Cheng AC, Lam DS, Ng JS: Ophthalmopathy in childhood Graves' disease. Br J Ophthalmol 2002;86:740–742.
12 Chen F, Day SL, Metcalfe RA, Sethi G, Kapembwa MS, Brook MG, Churchill D, de Ruiter A, Robinson S, Lacey CJ, Weetman AP: Characteristics of autoimmune thyroid disease occurring as a late complication of immune reconstitution in patients with advanced human immunodeficiency virus (HIV) disease. Medicine (Baltimore) 2005;84:98–106.
13 Bartalena L, Wiersinga WM, Pinchera A: Graves' ophthalmopathy: state of the art and perspectives. J Endocrinol Invest 2004;27:295–301.
14 Valyasevi RW, Harteneck DA, Dutton CM, Bahn RS: Stimulation of adipogenesis, peroxisome proliferator-activated receptor-gamma (PPARgamma), and thyrotropin receptor by PPARgamma agonist in human orbital preadipocyte fibroblasts. J Clin Endocrinol Metab 2002;87:2352–2358.
15 Wakelkamp IM, Bakker O, Baldeschi L, Wiersinga WM, Prummel MF: TSH-R expression and cytokine profile in orbital tissue of active vs. inactive Graves' ophthalmopathy patients. Clin Endocrinol (Oxf) 2003;58:280–287.
16 Zhang L, Baker G, Janus D, Paddon CA, Fuhrer D, Ludgate M: Biological effects of thyrotropin receptor activation on human orbital preadipocytes. Invest Ophthalmol Vis Sci 2006;47:5197–5203.
17 Pritchard J, Han R, Horst N, Cruikshank WW, Smith TJ: Immunoglobulin activation of T cell chemoattractant expression in fibroblasts from patients with Graves' disease is mediated through the insulin-like growth factor I receptor pathway. J Immunol 2003;170:6348–6354.
18 Smith TJ, Hoa N: Immunoglobulins from patients with Graves' disease induce hyaluronan synthesis in their orbital fibroblasts through the self-antigen, insulin-like growth factor-I receptor. J Clin Endocrinol Metab 2004;89:5076–5080.

19 Prabhakar BS, Bahn RS, Smith TJ: Current perspective on the pathogenesis of Graves' disease and ophthalmopathy. Endocr Rev 2003;24:802–835.
20 Drexhage HA: Are there more than antibodies to the thyroid-stimulating hormone receptor that meet the eye in Graves' disease? Endocrinology 2006;147:9–12.
21 Banga JP, Moore JK, Duhindan N, Madec AM, van Endert PM, Orgiazzi J, Endl J: Modulation of antigen presentation by autoreactive B cell clones specific for GAD65 from a type I diabetic patient. Clin Exp Immunol 2004;135:74–84.
22 El Fassi D, Nielsen CH, Hasselbalch HC, Hegedus L: The rationale for B lymphocyte depletion in Graves' disease: monoclonal anti-CD20 antibody therapy as a novel treatment option. Eur J Endocrinol 2006;154:623–632.
23 Salvi M, Vannucchi G, Campi I, Rossi S, Bonara P, Sbrozzi F, Guastella C, Avignone S, Pirola G, Ratiglia R, Beck-Peccoz P: Efficacy of rituximab treatment for thyroid-associated ophthalmopathy as a result of intraorbital B-cell depletion in one patient unresponsive to steroid immunosuppression. Eur J Endocrinol 2006;154:511–517.
24 Pappa A, Lawson JM, Calder V, Fells P, Lightman S: T cells and fibroblasts in affected extraocular muscles in early and late thyroid associated ophthalmopathy. Br J Ophthalmol 2000;8: 517–522.
25 Han R, Smith TJ: Induction by IL-1 beta of tissue inhibitor of metalloproteinase-1 in human orbital fibroblasts: modulation of gene promoter activity by IL-4 and IFN-gamma. J Immunol 2005;174:3072–3079.
26 Cawood TJ, Moriarty P, O'Farrelly C, O'Shea D: The effects of tumour necrosis factor-alpha and interleukin-1 on an in vitro model of thyroid-associated ophthalmopathy: contrasting effects on adipogenesis. Eur J Endocrinol 2006;155:395–403.
27 Kazim M, Goldberg RA, Smith TJ: Insights into the pathogenesis of thyroid-associated orbitopathy: evolving rationale for therapy. Arch Ophthalmol 2002;120:380–386.
28 Gerding MN, van der Meer JW, Broenink M, Bakker O, Wiersinga WM, Prummel MF: Association of thyrotrophin receptor antibodies with the clinical features of Graves' ophthalmopathy. Clin Endocrinol (Oxf) 2000;52:267–271.
29 Eckstein AK, Plicht M, Lax H, Neuhauser M, Mann K, Lederbogen S, Heckmann C, Esser J, Morgenthaler NG: Thyrotropin receptor autoantibodies are independent risk factors for Graves' ophthalmopathy and help to predict severity and outcome of the disease. J Clin Endocrinol Metab 2006;91:3464–3470.
30 Manji N, Carr-Smith JD, Boelaert K, Allahabadia A, Armitage M, Chatterjee VK, Lazarus JH, Pearce SH, Vaidya B, Gough SC, Franklyn JA: Influences of age, gender, smoking, and family history on autoimmune thyroid disease phenotype. J Clin Endocrinol Metab 2006;9: 4873–4880.
31 Villanueva R, Inzerillo AM, Tomer Y, Barbesino G, Meltzer M, Concepcion ES, Greenberg DA, MacLaren N, Sun ZS, Zhang DM, Tucci S, Davies TF: Limited genetic susceptibility to severe Graves' ophthalmopathy: no role for CTLA-4 but evidence for an environmental etiology. Thyroid 2000;10:791–798.
32 Vaidya B, Oakes EJ, Imrie H, Dickinson AJ, Perros P, Kendall-Taylor P, Pearce SH: CTLA4 gene and Graves' disease: association of Graves' disease with the CTLA4 exon 1 and intron 1 polymorphisms, but not with the promoter polymorphism. Clin Endocrinol (Oxf) 2003;58: 732–735.
33 Dechairo BM, Zabaneh D, Collins J, Brand O, Dawson GJ, Green AP, Mackay I, Franklyn JA, Connell JM, Wass JA, Wiersinga WM, Hegedus L, Brix T, Robinson BG, Hunt PJ, Weetman AP, Carey AH, Gough SC: Association of the TSHR gene with Graves' disease: the first disease specific locus. Eur J Hum Genet 2005;13:1223–1230.
34 Krassas GE, Wiersinga W: Smoking and autoimmune thyroid disease: the plot thickens. Eur J Endocrinol 2006;154:777–780.
35 Cawood TJ, Moriarty P, O'Farrelly C, O'Shea D: Smoking and thyroid-associated ophthalmopathy: a novel explanation of the biological link. J Clin Endocrinol Metab 2007;92:59–64.
36 Krassas GE, Heufelder AE: Immunosuppressive therapy in patients with thyroid eye disease: an overview of current concepts. Eur J Endocrinol 2001;14:311–318.

37 Bahn RS: Pathophysiology of Graves' ophthalmopathy: the cycle of disease. J Clin Endocrinol Metab 2003;88:1939–1946.
38 Paridaens D, van den Bosch WA, van der Loos TL, Krenning EP, van Hagen PM: The effect of etanercept on Graves' ophthalmopathy: a pilot study. Eye 2005;19:1286–1289.

Prof. Jacques Orgiazzi
Service d'Endocrinologie-Diabétologie, Université Claude-Bernard-Lyon 1 et Hospices
Civils de Lyon, Groupe Hospitalier Sud
165, chemin du Grand Revoyet
FR–69495 Pierre-Bénite (France)
Tel. +33 4 78 86 14 88, Fax +33 4 78 86 65 93, E-Mail jacques.orgiazzi@chu-lyon.fr

# Orbital Imaging

*Susanne Pitz*

Neuroophthalmology and Orbital Unit, Department of Ophthalmology, Johannes Gutenberg-University, Mainz, Germany

### Is Orbital Imaging Always Necessary?

The clear answer to this question is 'no'. In a typical clinical case, featuring subjective complaints such as retrobulbar pain and gritty sensation as well as objective signs such as lid swelling, lid retraction, motility impairment and proptosis, it is rather unlikely that a therapeutic decision would be substantially influenced by additional information obtained by any imaging technique. If, however, it comes to a very asymmetrical clinical picture (20% of Graves' orbitopathy [GO] patients are characterized by an asymmetrical orbital involvement), inflammatory orbital disorders of non-thyroidal aetiology or orbital tumours have to be ruled out. A second situation which will prompt orbital imaging is the clinical suspicion of optic nerve involvement in GO. This is known to be bilateral in about 2/3 of cases, otherwise reliable clinical signs such as a relative afferent pupillary deficit (RAPD) or colour desaturation may not be present. Under these circumstances, orbital imaging is most useful in making the clinical decision of optic nerve compression.

### What Are the Relative Benefits of Orbital CT and MRI?

Orbital CT is a quick (approx. 20 min), largely available and rather cheap investigation technique providing detailed imaging of the orbital anatomy and the typical imaging characteristics of GO (figs. 1, 2). Modern CT techniques even do not require neck flexion of the patient's head for obtaining coronal sections. If a quick overview of all orbital tissue structures is needed, then orbital

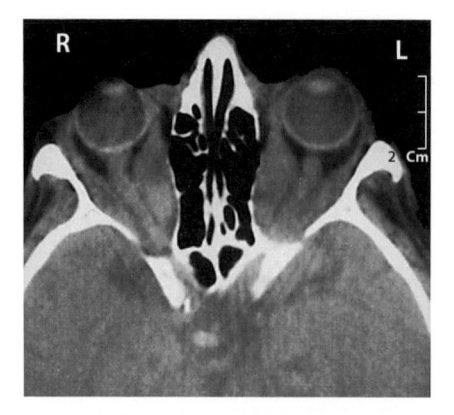

*Fig. 1.* Axial CT scan with marked horizontal muscle enlargement, apical crowding, and 'spontaneous decompression' of both laminae papyraceae ('coca cola sign').

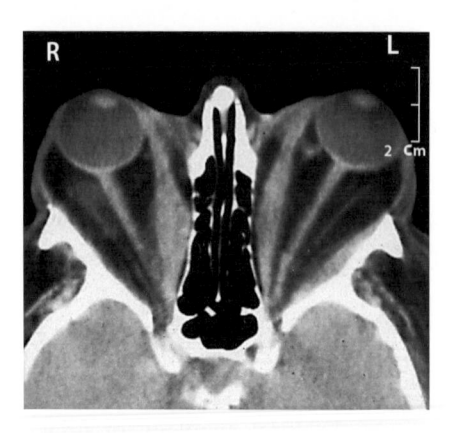

*Fig. 2.* Axial CT scan exhibiting proptosis, marked optic nerve stretching, increased volume of orbital fat and deformation of the medial orbital wall due to medial rectus enlargement.

CT is the technique of choice. The good simultaneous visualization of both bony structures and soft tissues is one of the reasons why most orbital surgeons would require a CT scan prior to bony decompression. Additionally, CT is more sensitive in identifying enlarged extraocular muscles than is MRI [1]. Its quick performance may be extremely valuable for the very young and elderly patients. However, one has to keep in mind the high radiation burden for the human lens, rendering orbital CT problematic for repeated follow-up investigations in children.

MRI, on the contrary, gives a better resolution of orbital soft tissues, making it superior to CT in the work-up of suspected non-GO orbital inflammation or orbital tumours (fig. 3). Besides, it is free of any radiation burden. However, MRI is costly and lengthy in comparison to CT, and is not as broadly available. In the context of GO, MRI offers the advantage to add information regarding

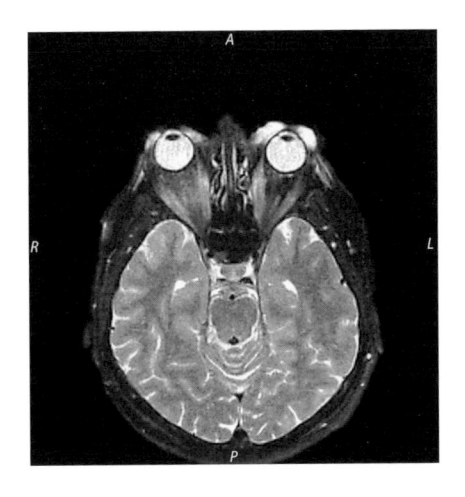

*Fig. 3.* Axial T$_2$-weighted MRI scan exhibiting inhomogeneous signalling in both medial – and to a lesser extent – lateral rectus muscles, corresponding to inflammatory edema.

disease activity: the amount of inflammatory edema within the extraocular muscles can be assessed by measuring the T2 relaxation time [2–6]. The prolonged T2 relaxation time – reflecting an increased content of protons and thus edema – correlates to a better response to anti-inflammatory treatment. However, T2 relaxation time is more reliable to detect the inactive stage of GO than the inflammatory, edematous phase [4, 5]. Therefore, the information drawn from MRI scanning should be interpreted together with other clinical data allowing a comprehensive assessment of disease activity.

The good imaging quality of both CT as well as MRI scans have revealed that the muscle tendon of the extraocular muscles – formerly believed not to be involved in GO – may show a thickening in up to 6.4% of GO patients [7].

Both CT and MRI allow the assessment of orbital tissue volumes. While it seems reasonable to expect such quantifiable parameters to give good correlation to different stages of GO, there are technical obstacles preventing a routine application. Measurement errors range at 3.5%; a volume change of at least 6–17% is required to demonstrate a significant difference. Because of the time required and the complexity of the measurements, extraocular muscle volume measurement is as yet only suitable for research purposes [8].

## What Is Apical Crowding?

The term apical crowding or 'crowded orbital apex syndrome' originates from a 1988 CT study describing 58 patients suffering from dysthyroid optic neuropathy (DON) [9]. These, in comparison to a control group of GO patients, were

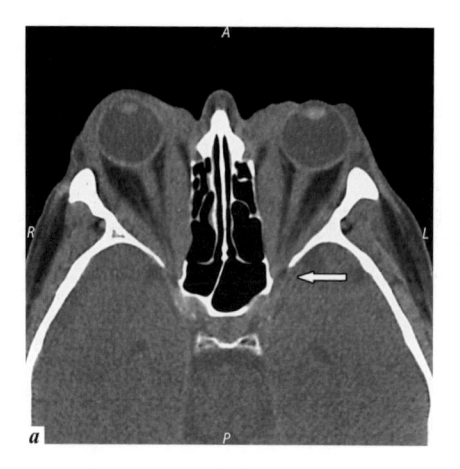

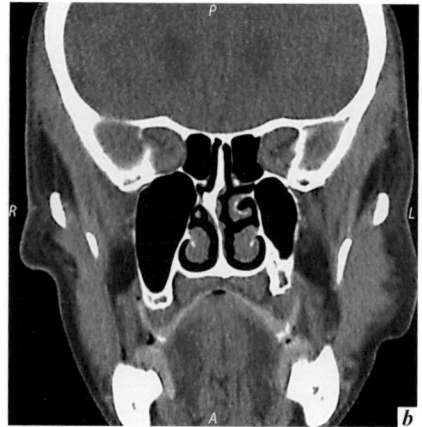

*Fig. 4. a* Axial CT scan with marked enlargement of both medial rectus muscles as well as prolapse of orbital fat via the left superior orbital fissure (arrow). *b* Coronal CT scan of the same patient demonstrating a crowded orbital apex with an almost complete effacement of the perineural orbital fat.

older at the time of examination (58 vs. 49 years) and were more likely to be male (female to male ratio of 1.6:1 vs. 3.3:1 in the non-DON group). Bilateral DON was seen in 78% of patients. Clinically, the most important clinical signs to identify DON were pathological visual-evoked potentials (VEP) and impaired colour vision. Imaging characteristics of the crowded orbital apex syndrome (fig. 4a) were increased extraocular muscle diameter, apical crowding, optic nerve flattening at the orbital apex, proptosis, superior ophthalmic vein enlargement and anterior displacement of the lacrimal gland. Profound apical crowding was defined as an obliteration of fat planes surrounding the optic nerve at the apex of the orbit consisting in a perineural fat effacement of >25% of the optic nerve circumference (fig. 4b). Despite this multitude of imaging characteristics, the diagnosis of optic nerve compression in the majority of cases can be founded on additional clinical evidence. Subsequent data have pointed to the fact that there is no consensus on which level of extraocular muscle enlargement inevitably leads to optic nerve compression. Likewise, the positive predictive value of features like proptosis, lacrimal gland displacement of superior ophthalmic vein enlargement is low [10]. A more reliable imaging hallmark of DON is the intracranial prolapse of orbital fat via the superior ophthalmic fissure (fig. 4a, b) [11].

In summary, the diagnosis of DON is virtually always based on clinical as well as radiological findings, and imaging alone will rarely be the only indicator of this complication of GO. The usefulness of imaging in this setting is rather to complete clinical data, which may be equivocal in cases of bilateral

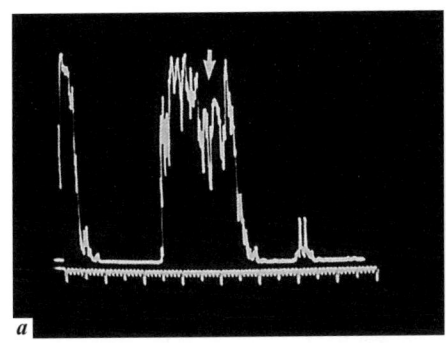

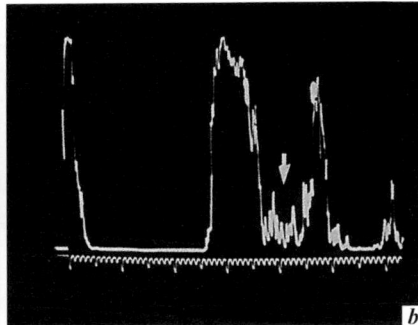

*Fig. 5.* Characteristic example of the A-mode ultrasonographic pattern of the orbital contents in a patient with inactive (*a*) and active GO (*b*): high and irregular reflectivity pattern of external eye muscle (arrow) in patient A, and low reflectivity of the eye muscle in patient B. With permission from [12].

optic nerve involvement. The other main application of imaging is the assessment of anatomy prior to surgical decompression.

### What Is the Place of Orbital Ultrasound?

Ultrasound has a long history as an ancillary test in GO. Its major advance is its non-invasiveness, allowing assessment of muscle thickness and reflectivity (fig. 5a, b). Orbital ultrasound is an ideal technique to detect pathologies of the globe and the anterior 2/3 of the orbit. However, it does not allow visualization of the orbital apex.

Though muscle reflectivity seems to correlate with disease activity, its low inter-observer reproducibility renders the reliability of orbital ultrasound questionable [12]. Recently, Fledelius et al. [13] pointed out that neither reflectivity nor thickness of the rectus muscles are paralleling the clinical course and thus should be judged with caution. Another difficulty arises from problems to reproducibly investigate the rectus muscles at identical planes on follow-up. This especially holds true for the inferior rectus – which, on the other hand, is the muscle most often involved in GO.

The configuration of an enlarged extraocular muscle belly on imaging studies has traditionally been used to differentiate GO from other inflammatory processes such as orbital myositis, as the tendon is typically spared in GO. Though this sign undoubtedly is helpful in sonographic evaluation of a patient with suspected GO, one has to keep in mind that Ben Simon et al. [7] demonstrated an involvement of the muscle tendon on axial CT or MRI in 6.4% of their GO patients.

Given these problems, orbital ultrasound obviously has its place, but this seems to be a limited one. It serves to detect muscle enlargement and, in consequence, might save some CT or MRI scans. Volpe et al. [14] identified about 26% of patients out of a group with unexplained ocular misalignment otherwise without clinical signs of GO as having occult thyroid eye disease. On the other hand, ultrasound is not adequate to rule out optic nerve involvement, and the assessment of muscle reflectivity does not seem to be superior to the evaluation of T2 relaxation time obtained by MRI.

## What Lessons Can We Learn from Orbital Octreoscan?

Somatostatin receptors are expressed on orbital fibroblasts. As their expression is enhanced on fibroblasts derived from GO patients in comparison to controls [15], this finding provides the rationale for applying octreotide scintigraphy in GO patients. There is a broad consensus that the orbital uptake of octreotide is higher in active GO than in inactive stages of the disorder (fig. 6a, b) [16–18]. Gerding et al. [19] demonstrated a good correlation of octreotide uptake and treatment response to orbital radiotherapy. However, there are a number of limitations to this technology: octreoscan is expensive. It requires meticulous standardization in order to correct for background radioactivity. The radiation burden is by no means negligible. Attempts to lower radiation burden and costs have been made by performing octreotide scintigraphy using $^{99m}$Tc-P829 as a tracer [20].

Probably most problematic, however, is the fact that octreoscan turned out to be rather unspecific, as labelling is found in diverse orbital inflammatory disorders, orbital lymphoma and even meningioma [18]. Thus, especially in cases of unclear differential diagnosis or suspected optic nerve compression, CT and/or MRI imaging will still be necessary. In summary, octreoscan might have its role in identifying patients who will benefit from an anti-inflammatory therapy, and in whom this therapeutic decision cannot be made on clinical grounds alone. It does, however, not play a significant role in the routine work-up of the majority of GO patients.

## What Other Imaging Techniques May Be Useful?

Colour Doppler ultrasonography is widely applied to investigate blood flow characteristics in diverse ocular conditions. Several investigations have demonstrated a reduced blood flow in the superior ophthalmic vein [21–24]. This supports animal studies in which a ligation of the venous outflow of the orbit results in the clinical picture of proptosis and enlarged extraocular muscles in cats [25].

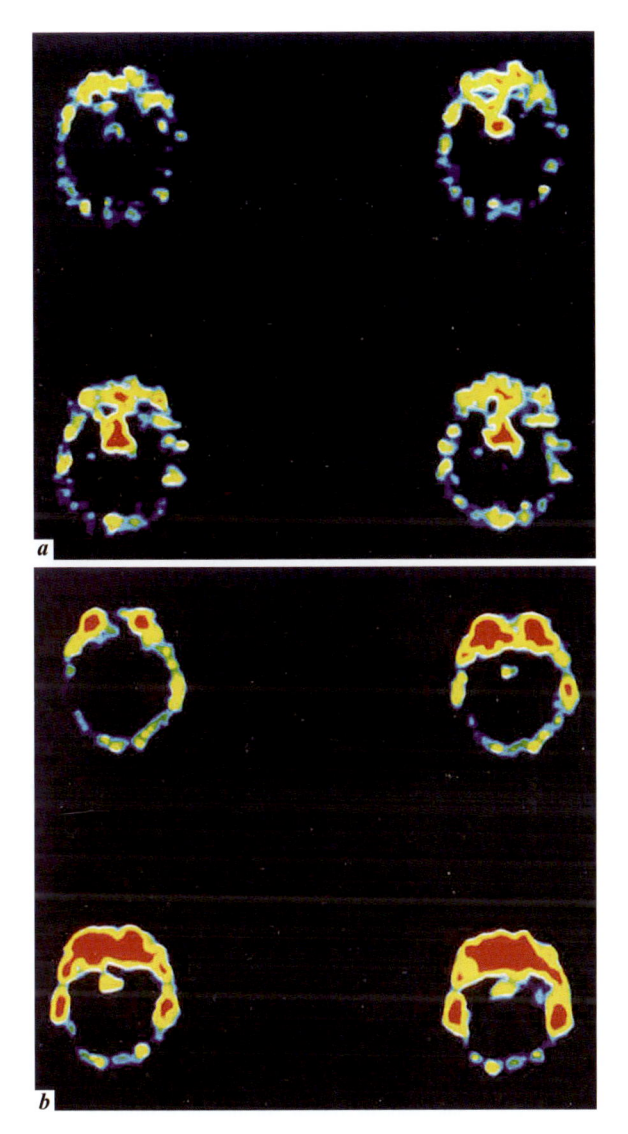

*Fig. 6. a, b.* Octreoscan. *a* Scan of a patient with inactive GO, showing enhancement in the hypophysis, but no relevant signal within both orbits. *b* Pronounced signalling of both orbits in a case of active GO.

While these data shed an interesting light on the pathogenetic mechanisms in GO, they do not add substantially to the routine evaluation of GO patients, as the detection of reduced flow in the superior ophthalmic vein has only a low positive predictive value in terms of detection of optic nerve compression.

Kuo et al. [26] recently described a case of recent onset GO in whom 2-deoxy-2-[$^{18}$F]fluoro-D-glucose positron emission tomography/computed tomography (FDG-PET/CT) revealed eye muscle involvement not evident on MRI scanning. FDG-PET is used to monitor diverse inflammatory processes, ranging from osteomyelitis to brain abscesses. The authors suggest that this technique might be useful in early/subclinical stages of the disease. Other scintigraphic techniques are under development hopefully enabling the prediction of response to anti-inflammatory therapy. One example for such techniques is gallium-67 scintigraphy, which has been reported to have a 91% positive predictive value to predict treatment response. This compares favourably to the clinical activity score (CAS) and is about equal to the above-mentioned indium-octreotide scan as well as the T2 relaxation time on MRI [27].

Another sector where future developments are to be awaited is modification of actual MRI protocols. One of these is the use of STIR (short tau inversion recovery sequence), in which the analysis of so-called 'hot spots' – sites of extensive inflammation within the extraocular muscles – might be useful in determining disease activity and possible response to treatment [3, 28].

## Acknowledgments

CT and MRI scans: courtesy of Prof. W. Müller-Forell, Institute for Neuroradiology, University Hospital, Mainz; octreoscan: courtesy of Prof. G. J. Kahaly.

## References

1 Polito E, Leccisotti A: MRI in Graves' ophthalmopathy: recognition of enlarged muscles and prediction of steroid response. Ophthalmologica 1995;209:182–186.
2 Hosten N, Sander V, Cordes M, et al: Graves' ophthalmopathy: MR imaging of the orbits. Radiology 1989;172:759–762.
3 Hiromatsu Y, Kojima K, Ishisaka N, et al: Role of magnetic resonance imaging in thyroid-associated ophthalmopathy: its predictive value for therapeutic outcome on immunosuppressive therapy. Thyroid 1992;2:299–305.
4 Just M, Kahaly G, Higer HP, et al: Graves' ophthalmopathy: role of MR imaging in radiation therapy. Radiology 1991;179:187–190.
5 Ohnishi T, Noguchi S, Murakami N, et al: Extraocular muscles in Graves' ophthalmopathy: usefulness of T2 relaxation time measurements. Radiology 1994;190:857–862.
6 Silaire I, Ravel A, Dalens H, et al: Graves' ophthalmopathy: usefulness of T2 weighted muscle signal intensity. J Radiol 2003;84:130–142.
7 Ben Simon GJ, Syed HM, Douglas R, et al: Extraocular muscle enlargement with tendon involvement in thyroid-associated orbitopathy. Am J Ophthalmol 2004;137:1145–1147.
8 Bijlsma WR, Mourits MP: Radiologic measurement of extraocular muscle volumes in patients with Graves' orbitopathy: a review and guideline. Orbit 2006;25:83–91.
9 Neigel JM, Rootman J, Belkin RI, et al: Dysthyroid optic neuropathy: the crowded orbital apex syndrome. Ophthalmology 1988;95:1515–1521.

10 Nugent RA, Belkin RI, Neigel JM, et al: Graves' orbitopathy: correlation of CT and clinical findings. Radiology 1990;177:675–682.
11 Birchall D, Goodall KL, Noble JL, Jackson A: Graves' ophthalmopathy: intracranial fat prolapse on CT images as an indicator of optic nerve compression. Radiology 1996;20:123–127.
12 Prummel MF, Suttorp-Schulten MSA, Wiersinga WM, et al: A new ultrasonographic method to detect disease activity and predict response to immunosuppressive treatment in Graves' ophthalmopathy. Ophthalmology 1993;100:556–561.
13 Fledelius HC, Zimmermann-Belsing T, Feldt-Rasmussen U: Ultrasonically measured horizontal eye muscle thickness in thyroid associated orbitopathy: cross-sectional and longitudinal aspects in a Danish series. Acta Ophthalmol Scand 2003;81:143–150.
14 Volpe NJ, Sbarbaro JA, Livingston KG, et al: Occult thyroid eye disease in patients with unexplained ocular misalignment identified by standardized orbital echography. Am J Ophthalmol 2006;142:75–81.
15 Pasquali D, Vassalo P, Esposito D, et al: Somatostatin receptor gene expression and inhibitory effects of octreotide on primary cultures of orbital fibroblasts from Graves' ophthalmopathy. J Mol Endocrinol 2000;25:63–71.
16 Postema RTE, Krenning EP, Wijngaarde R, et al: [$^{111}$In-DPTA-D-Phe] octreotide scintigraphy in thyroidal and orbital Graves' disease: a parameter for disease activity? J Clin Endocrinol Metabol 1994;79:1845–1851.
17 Kahaly G, Diaz M, Hahn K, et al: Indium-111-pentreotide scintigraphy in Graves' ophthalmopathy. J Nucl Med 1995;36:550–554.
18 Durak I, Durak H, Ergin M, et al: Somatostatin receptors in the orbit. Clin Nucl Med 1995;20:237–242.
19 Gerding MN, van der Zant FM, van Royen EA, et al: Octreotide-scintigraphy is a disease-activity parameter in Graves' ophthalmopathy. Clin Endocrinol 1999;50:373–379.
20 Burggasser G, Hurtl I, Hauff W, et al: Orbital scintigraphy with the somatostatin receptor tracer 99mTc-P829 in patients with Graves' disease. J Nucl Med 2003;44:1547–1555.
21 Nakase Y, Osanai T, Yoshikawa K, Inoue Y: Color Doppler imaging of orbital venous flow in dysthyroid optic neuropathy. Jpn J Ophthalmol 1994;38:80–86.
22 Benning H, Lieb W, Kahaly G, Grehn F: Farbduplexsonographische Befunde bei Patienten mit endokriner Orbitopathie. Ophthalmologe 1994;91:20–25.
23 Alp MN, Ozgen A, Can I, et al: Colour Doppler imaging of the orbital vasculature in Graves' disease with computed tomographic correlation. Br J Ophthalmol 2000;84:1027–1030.
24 Somer D, Özkan SB, Özdemir H, et al: Colour doppler imaging of superior ophthalmic vein in thyroid-associated eye diesease. Jpn J Ophthalmol 2002;46:341–345.
25 Saber E, McDonell J, Zimmermann KM, et al: Extraocular muscle changes in experimental orbital venous stasis: some similarities to Graves' orbitopathy. Graefe's Arch Clin Exp Ophthalmol 1996;234:331–336.
26 Kuo PH, Monchamp T, Deol P: Imaging of inflammation in Graves' ophthalmopathy by positron emission tomography/computed tomography. Thyroid 2006;16:419–420.
27 Konuk O, Atasever T, Unal M, et al: Orbital gallium-67 scintigraphy in Graves' ophthalmopathy: a disease activity parameter that predicts the therapeutic response to immunosuppressive treatment. Thyroid 2005;15:358–363.
28 Mayer EJ, Fox DL, Herdman G, et al: Signal intensity, clinical activity and cross-sectional areas on MRI scans in thyroid eye disease. Eur J Radiol 2005;56:20–24.

Dr. Susanne Pitz
Neuroophthalmology and Orbital Unit, Department of Ophthalmology
Johannes Gutenberg-University
Langenbeckstrasse 1
DE–55101 Mainz (Germany)
Tel. +49 6131 176762, Fax +49 6131 173455, E-Mail pitz@augen.klinik.uni-mainz.de

Wiersinga WM, Kahaly GJ (eds): Graves' Orbitopathy: A Multidisciplinary Approach.
Basel, Karger, 2007, pp 66–77

# Diagnosis and Differential Diagnosis of Graves' Orbitopathy

*Maarten P. Mourits*

Department of Ophthalmology, Academic Medical Center – AMC,
University of Amsterdam, Amsterdam, The Netherlands

### Can You Give an Overall Scheme for the Diagnosis of Graves' Orbitopathy?

The diagnosis of Graves' orbitopathy (GO) is based on (1) the presence of eye signs and symptoms, (2) the presence of thyroid auto-immunity, and (3) the exclusion of an alternative diagnosis. None of the eye signs are specific for GO. It is the bilateral symmetric nature of the orbitopathy in a patient known to have Graves' hyperthyroidism which makes the diagnosis straightforward in most patients. However, GO may precede the onset of Graves' hyperthyroidism. In those patients, laboratory evidence of existing thyroid auto-immunity might favour GO as the cause of the eye changes. Euthyroidism does not exclude GO and the same holds true for (predominantly) unilateral eye changes occurring in as much as 15% [1] of all GO patients. Indeed, GO is the most frequent cause of unilateral proptosis. In such cases, it is prudent to perform orbital imaging to exclude other diseases.

### Which Clinical Findings Are Helpful in Making a Diagnosis of Graves' Orbitopathy?

Clinical symptoms found in GO are eyelid swelling, eyelid retraction, proptosis, eye muscle restriction, corneal staining and decreased visual acuity. During the active state of the disease additional symptoms are redness of the

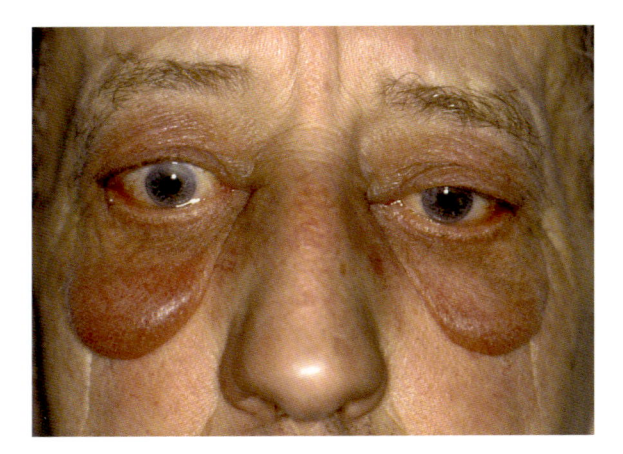

*Fig. 1.* Patient with lower lid swelling due to GO.

*Table 1.* Differential diagnosis of soft eyelid swelling

1 Infection of dermis (impetigo, erysipelas) or adnexae (chalazion)
2 Toxic (chemical or bacterial toxins)
3 Auto-immune disease (Graves' orbitopathy, dermatomyositis)
4 Allergic (urticaria, angioneurotic, eczematous, contact allergy, medicine-induced, bites)
5 Static (orbital tumor, heartfailure)
6 Metabolic (myxedema, nephrotic syndrome)
7 Miscellaneous (blepharochalazis syndrome, haemorrhage)

lids and conjunctiva, chemosis and caruncula swelling. GO is at least 3 times more common in females than in males [2].

*Eyelid swelling* (fig. 1) is a very common finding in patients with GO, but it is often hard to say if and to what extent the swelling is caused by the orbitopathy and what is the contribution of age, smoking habits, general condition, etc. Moreover, eyelid swelling may fluctuate over the day. Strict criteria for a definition of eyelid swelling do not exist and therefore the prevalence of eyelid swelling in GO is unknown. Eyelid swelling in GO is caused by edema and fat increase and is thus easily distinguishable by palpation from swelling by firm lesions. However, differentiation from other forms of soft eyelid swelling may be difficult (table 1). The von Graefe's sign (1864), a dissociation of the movements of the eyelid and the globe showing sclera above the cornea in downgaze, can be considered a precursor of frank retraction and can be used to track down GO.

In the absence of other symptoms, eyelid swelling may be overlooked as an initial sign of GO and surgery to correct the eyelid swelling (e.g. blepharoplasty)

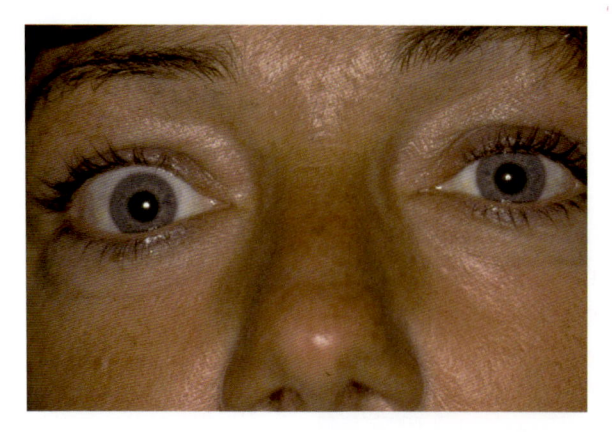

*Fig. 2.* Patient with unilateral upper lid retraction in mild GO.

*Table 2.* Differential diagnosis of eyelid retraction

| | |
|---|---|
| 1 | Physiological in newborns |
| 2 | Some degree of retraction might be physiological in adults |
| 3 | Thyrotoxicosis (by pure sympathetic stimulation) |
| 4 | Graves' orbitopathy (by a combination of factors) |
| 5 | Scarring after inflammation, trauma or surgery (e.g. after blepharoplasty) |
| 6 | In case of unilateral ptosis of the other eye (Hering's law) |
| 7 | Marcus-Gunn phenomenon |
| 8 | Parinaud's syndrome and midbrain disease |
| 9 | Myostatic paresis of Parkinsonism (by muscular rigidity) |
| 10 | Hepatic cirrhosis (also by muscular rigidity) |
| 11 | Sympathomimetic drugs |

may then easily result into a undesired situation such as an inability to close the eyes. An attempt has been made to monitor eyelid swelling by repeated photographs taken under standardized circumstances [3].

In most individuals with their heads in the primary position, the upper eyelids cover the cornea at the 12 o'clock position for 0–1.5 mm, whereas the lower lids just touch the corneal limbus at the 6 o'clock position [4].

*Eyelid retraction* (fig. 2) is present when, in the absence of staring, these criteria are not fulfilled and a band of white sclera between limbus and eyelid margin is visible [5]. In contrast to what is often thought, not proptosis, but eyelid retraction is the most frequent symptom assessed in GO (occurring in up to 70%) [6], but it is certainly not pathognomonic for GO. Eye lid retraction is seen in many other conditions (table 2).

*Table 3.* Differential diagnosis of proptosis

| | |
|---|---|
| 1 | Inflammatory diseases |
| 2 | Vascular lesions |
| 3 | Neoplasia |
| 4 | Structural lesions (such as cysts) |

*Proptosis* (=exophthalmos) is present when the distance between the vortex of the cornea and the anterior surface of the bony lateral orbital rim is above the upper limit of normal found in a healthy population. Exophthalmometry values are race and gender dependent and show a wide range in healthy individuals. Attempts have been made to define pathologic exophthalmometry values [7, 8]. In GO, proptosis is caused by an increase of extraocular muscle (EOM) size and of orbital fat. Moreover, in contrast to some other causes of proptosis, such as for instance swelling of the lacrimal gland, the proptosis is axial in nature. However, the list of conditions causing axial proptosis is long (table 3) and the presence of axial proptosis alone is therefore insufficient to make a diagnosis of GO. Nevertheless, it is important to realise that the most common cause of both unilateral and bilateral proptosis is GO [2]. The prevalence of proptosis in patients with GO in our series is 60% [1]. Proptosis may be absent in patients with GO and especially in those with dysthyroid optic nerve compression, in whom spontaneous orbital decompression resulting in forward displacement of the globe did not occur.

Pseudoproptosis refers to appearance of proptosis in the absence of axial displacement of the globe. Well-known pitfalls are high myopia, buphthalmos, eyelid retraction, and contralateral enophthalmos.

*Eyeball motility restriction*, sometimes causing diplopia, in GO is caused by tethering of the inflamed EOMs. Because the inferior and medial rectus muscles are often involved, elevation and less often abduction limitation results. In more severe cases these restrictions may lead to frank hypo- or esotropia. Attempts to elevate the eyes in GO may cause an aqueous outflow restriction by compression of the globe by the opposing inelastic EOMs resulting in a transient intraocular pressure rise [9]. This phenomenon can be used to assess even mild forms of GO. Enlarged, restrictive EOMs are also found in patients with orbital myositis or metastasis to EOM's.

*Corneal stippling* or ulceration is seen in any condition, in which there is inability to close or to moisten the cornea. In GO, this phenomenon is now considered a secondary one due to proptosis and eyelid retraction.

*Decreased visual acuity* in GO is found in patients with corneal involvement and/or compression of the optic nerve. Its prevalence is 5% of untreated GO patients.

The above clearly shows that no single symptom or sign is pathognomonic for GO. However, the combination of eyelid retraction and proptosis must raise a high suspicion for GO. One should realize, however, that the absence of proptosis and retraction does not exclude GO and that eyelid swelling and/or acquired diplopia warrants an investigation for GO.

## Can One Make a Diagnosis of Graves' Orbitopathy Based on Medical History and Clinical Picture Alone?

There is a close temporal relationship between the onset of GO and of Graves' thyroid disease (GTD). In almost 80% of patients, GO and GTD develop concomitantly, that is within a period of 18 months [10, 11]. GO sometimes precedes GTD, more often manifests shortly after GTD. GO can be present in the absence of thyroidal disease and is then called ophthalmic or euthyroid Graves' disease [12, 13], although more sensitive tools show that in almost all patients orbitopathy and thyroid disease co-exist. GO is an auto-immune disorder and thus occurs often in patients with other auto-immune disorders such as myasthenia and impetigo. Apart from these general aspects of the medical history, eye complaints can help to make a diagnosis of GO. GO patients may complain about changed looks (swollen eyelids, popping eyes), retrobulbar discomfort, tearing, grittiness, double and blurred vision.

Combining elements of the medical history with the clinical picture leads to a diagnosis of GO in the majority of cases. However, carefulness is required, because for instance a 50-year-old woman with hyperthyroidism and popping eyes might suffer from hyperthyroidism plus bilateral orbital non-Hodgkin lymphoma. Therefore, before a diagnosis of GO can be made, mimicking diseases have to be excluded.

## Do We Always Need to Order Thyroid Autoantibodies and Thyroid Function Tests?

At present, no definitive laboratory tests to demonstrate GO exist. However, elevated serum concentrations of TBII (TSH-binding inhibitory immunoglobulins) and TPO (thyroperoxidase) antibodies are commonly elevated in GO. Depending on the assay used elevated TBII are seen in more than 95% of patients with Graves' disease [14]. Especially in euthyroid patients, TPO antibodies and TBII are important to make a diagnosis of GO. TBII are found elevated in more than 90% of patients with euthyroid GO. TBII are found to correlate with disease severity and activity of GO [15, 16] and have prognostic significance for the course of GO [17]. The course of GO is influenced by the thyroid status. Normalization of hyper- or hypothyroidism ameliorates the orbitopathy to a certain extent [18]. Therefore, it is our opinion that TSH and free T4 [to assess hyper- or (subclinical) hypothyroidism], in some cases T3 (to assess subclinical hyperthyroidism or T3 toxicosis) and TBII plus TPO antibodies should be known of each patient in whom GO is suspected.

## Which Imaging Technique Is Best to Make a Diagnosis of Graves' Orbitopathy and Is Imaging Always Requested?

Among orbitologists around the world there is no doubt that the best way to detect GO by imaging is making a coronal (for assessment of EOM swelling) and axial CT scan (for assessment of apical crowding) of the orbits and paranasal sinuses. CT scanning is fast, only few 1.5 mm slices are required and no contrast enhancing is needed. Orbital CT scans clearly show the globe, the optic nerve, the EOMs, the lacrimal gland, the paranasal sinuses and the bony structures. Enlarged superior ophthalmic veins and abnormal structures can also be seen easily. The irradiation burden of a series of orbital CT scans is no more than 30 mGy. In contrast, MRI scans require considerable scanning time and show bony structures less clearly, which is a disadvantage when used for possible orbital decompression planning. Echography of the orbital contents is a fast method, but cannot be used to demonstrate swelling of the superior rectus muscle and deep orbital structures. Both CT and MRI scans show enlargement of the EOMs, apical crowding and stretching of the optic nerve and tenting of the posterior globe when present. The presence of fat increase is deducted when there is proptosis in the absence of EOM swelling or a pathological orbital space occupying lesion. More accurate assessment of fat will become available, when orbital volumes can be measured and compared to standard values [19]. In GO, the inferior rectus muscle is involved most frequently (fig. 3), followed by the medial rectus and the superior rectus/levator complex. The lateral rectus and superior oblique participate only in more severe forms. Swelling of the lateral rectus in the absence of swelling of the other EOMs points to other diseases than GO such as orbital myositis [see below, Which are the most frequent conditions mimicking Graves' orbitopathy?]. Scans are not only made to demonstrate eye muscle enlargement, but also to exclude other pathologies causing axial proptosis such as benign and malignant tumors (e.g. intraconal cavernous haemangioma and non-Hodgkin lymphoma).

Imaging in GO is not always necessary. In patients with mild orbitopathy in whom the diagnosis is straightforward, there is no need for scanning. Apart from for academic purposes (e.g. follow-up after immunomodulatory

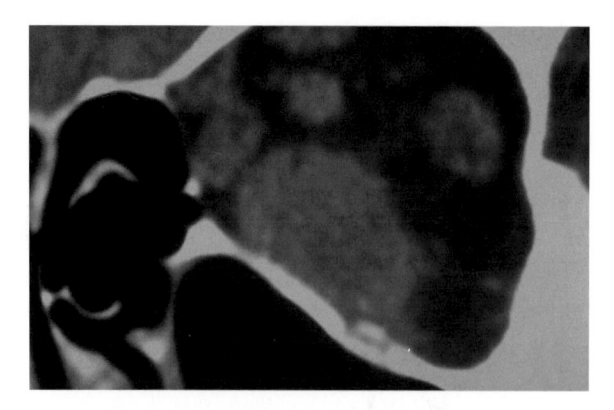

*Fig. 3.* Enlarged inferior rectus muscle in a patient with GO shown on coronal CT scan.

interventions), imaging is required in doubtful cases to exclude any other pathology and/or to plan orbital decompression.

## Which Are the Most Frequent Conditions Mimicking Graves' Orbitopathy?

The most frequent diseases mimicking GO are orbital meningioma, orbital myositis, caroticocavernous fistula and non-Hodgkin lymphoma, which will be discussed briefly.

*Orbital Meningioma*
Orbital meningioma occurs frequently in middle aged women. There are two common forms:
(1) Sphenoid wing meningioma, causing hyperostosis of the larger sphenoid wing resulting in axial protrusion of the globe.
(2) Optic nerve sheath meningioma, causing visual obscurations prior to reduced visual acuity and axial proptosis.

In addition to their proptosis, these patients usually have some degree of ptosis in stead of retraction. Diagnosis is based on CT scan or better on contrast enhanced MRI scans (fig. 4a–c).

*Orbital Myositis and 'Pseudotumour Orbitae'*
Orbital myositis (fig. 5) is an idiopathic non-infectious inflammation of one or more EOMs belonging to the group of aspecific acute or subacute inflammatory orbital diseases, which were called pseudotumour in the past.

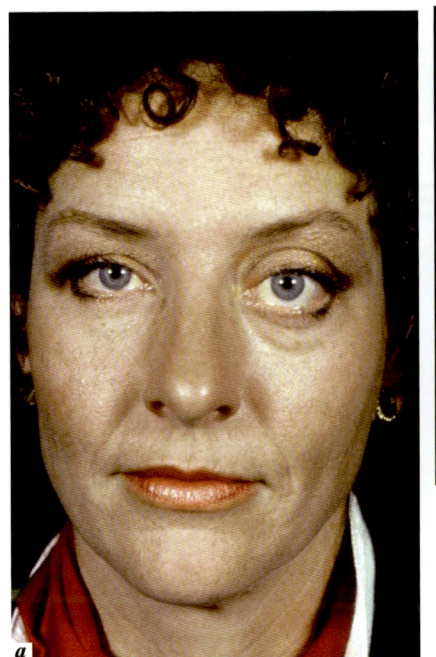

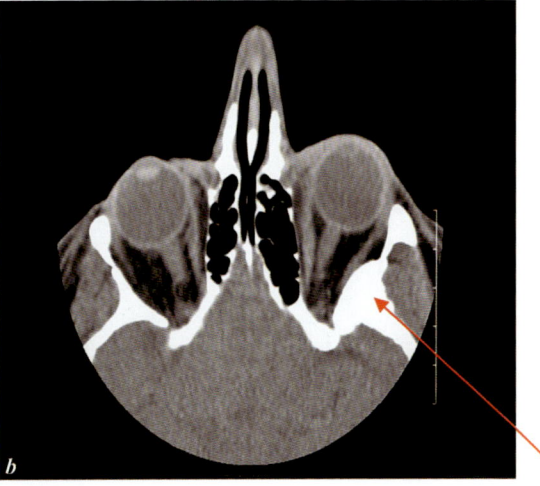

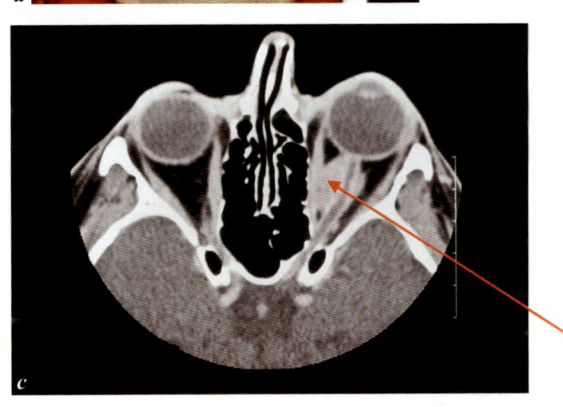

*Fig. 4a–c.* Clinical presentation of a patient with an orbital meningioma, and CT scans of patients with sphenoid wing and optic nerve sheet meningioma. Arrow showing hyperostosis of the greater wing of the sphenoid wing on axial CT scan (*b*). Arrow showing tubular swelling around the optic nerve leaving the optic nerve untouched (tram-track phenomenon), typical presentation of optic nerve sheet meningioma (*c*).

Aspecific inflammatory orbital diseases present as space occupying lesions anywhere in the orbit (fig. 6) and have inflammatory signs as seen in active GO. Unlike in GO, pain is usually the most important reason for the patient to seek doctor's advice. When located within an EOM, the condition is called orbital

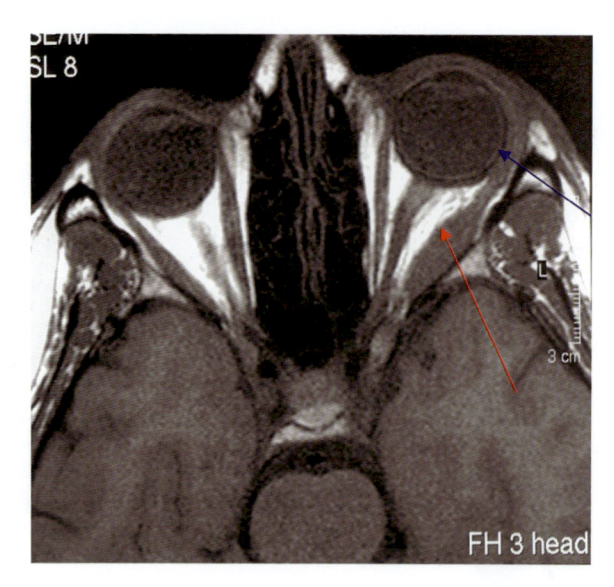

*Fig. 5.* CT scan of a patient with an orbital myositis (red arrow). Note thickened muscle tendon of external rectus (blue arrow).

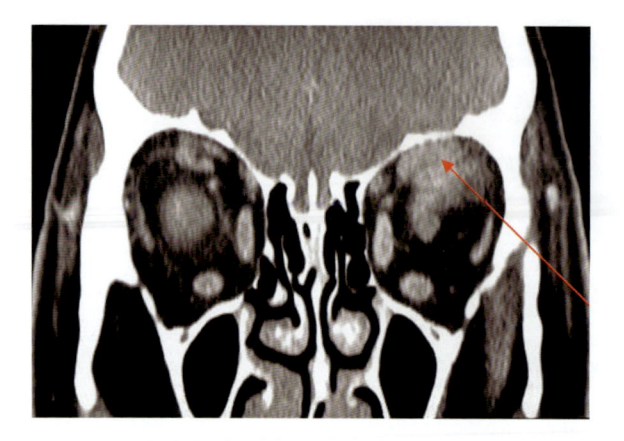

*Fig. 6.* CT scan of an idiopathic inflammatory orbital inflammation (pseudotumor orbitae, red arrow): ill-defined mass near levator/superior rectus complex.

myositis. In contrast to GO, these diseases are seen at all ages and typically respond well to a course of prednisone. Orbital myositis can 'jump' from one muscle to another (in the same or the contralateral orbit). Several clinical and imaging qualities (table 4) distinguish orbital myositis from GO.

*Table 4.* Differentiation between GO and orbital myositis

|  | Graves' orbitopathy | Myositis |
|---|---|---|
| *Clinic* | | |
| Onset | weeks to months | days |
| Pain | mild | severe |
| Eye lid position | retraction frequent | ptosis frequent/retraction rare |
| Steroid response | incomplete and slow | usually complete and fast |
| *Imaging* | | |
| Bilateral | frequently | sometimes |
| Muscle involved | usually > one, ERM seldom | rarely > one, ERM frequent |
| Muscle borders | regular, no fat noise | irregular, fat noise |
| Tendon involved | no | yes |

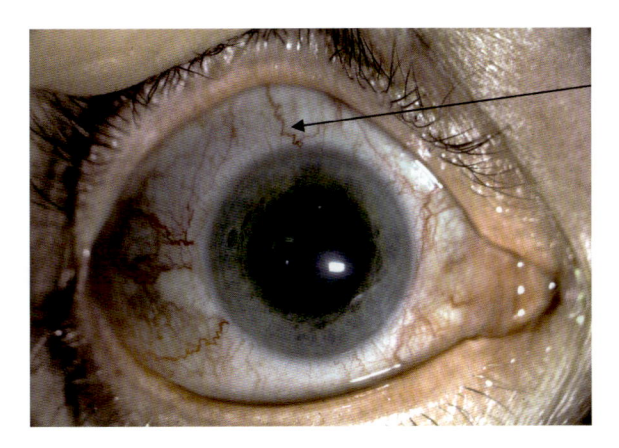

*Fig. 7.* Corkscrew dilated episcleral vessels (arrow) in a patient with an acquired AV fistula.

### Caroticocavernous Fistula

Pathological communications between the arterious and venous systems in the cavernous sinus can cause axial proptosis, so called corkscrew dilated episcleral vessels (fig. 7) and enlargement of all EOMs due to congestion. A traumatic and arteriosclerotic form are distinguished, the latter sometimes hold for GO. The presence of the episcleral vessels and a severely enlarged superior ophthalmic vein seen on orbital scans makes the diagnosis. Localisation of the pathologic communication can be assessed with angiographic investigations.

*Non-Hodgkin Lymphoma*

In elderly people, non-Hodgkin lymphoma is one of the most common malignancies seen in the orbit. The typical presentation is a salmon-coloured elevated lesion of the conjunctiva, but primary intraorbital manifestations account for more than 50% of all cases [20]. Diagnosis is by imaging and consecutive biopsy.

## Conclusion

In most patients the diagnosis of GO is straightforward: lid retraction combined with uni- or bilateral proptosis in a person with a history of hyper- or hypothyroidism. Imaging is done to exclude orbital space occupying lesions other than swelling of one or more EOMs or an increase of orbital fat. GO patients can also present with acquired diplopia and motility impairment. When only eyelid swelling is present, the diagnosis can easily be missed and careful history taking and additional tests are required. Euthyroidism does not exclude GO.

## References

1. Wiersinga WM, Smit T, Schuster-Uittenhoeve ALJ, Van der Gaag R, Koornneef L: Clinical presentation of Graves' ophthalmopathy. Ophthalmic Res 1989;21:73–82.
2. Burch HB, Wartofsky L: Graves' ophthalmopathy: current concepts regarding pathogenesis and management. Endocr Rev 1993;14:747–793.
3. Gerding MN, Prummel MF, Kalmann R, Koornneef L, Wiersinga WM: Colour slides are useful to assess changes in soft-tissue involvement in Graves' ophthalmopathy. J Endocrinol Invest 1998;21:459–462.
4. Mourits MP, Koornneef L: Lid lengthening by sclera interposition for eyelid retraction in Graves' ophthalmopathy. Br J Ophthalmol 1991;75:344–347.
5. Duke-Elder S, MacFaul PA: Motor disorders and deformations of the lids; in: System of Ophthalmology, vol XIII, part I, chap VIII. London, Henry Kimpton, 1974, pp 568–570.
6. Bartley GB, Fatourechi V, Kardmas EF, Jacobsen SJ, Ilstrup DM, Garrity JA, Gorman CA: The incidence of Graves' ophthalmopathy in Olmsted County, Minnesota. Am J Ophthalmol 1995;120:511–517.
7. Werner SC: Classification of the eye changes of Graves' disease. J Clin Endcrinol Metab 1969;29:982–984.
8. Mourits MP, Lombardo SH, van der Sluijs FA, Fenton S: Reliability of exophthalmos measurement and exophthalmometry value distribution in a healthy Dutch population and in Graves' patients: an exploratory study. Orbit 2004;23:161–168.
9. Gamblin GT, Harper DG, Galentine P, Buck DR, Chernow B, Eil C: Prevalence of increased intraocular pressure in Graves' disease: evidence of frequent subclinical ophthalmopathy. N Engl J Med 1983;308:420–424.
10. Gorman CA: The presentation and management of endocrine ophthalmopathy. Clin Endocrinol Metab 1978;7:67–96.
11. Wiersinga WM, Smit T, van der Gaag R, Koornneef L: Temporal relationship between onset of Graves' ophthalmopathy and onset of thyroidal Graves' disease. J. Endocrinolol Invest 1988;11: 615–619.

12   Weetman AP. Thyroid-associated eye disease: pathophysiology. Lancet 1991;338:25–28.
13   Sergott RC, Glaser JS: Graves' ophthalmopathy: a clinical and immunologic review. Surv Ophthalmol 1981;26:1–21.
14   Paunkovic J, Paunkovic N: Does autoantibody-negative Graves' disease exist? A second evaluation of the clinical diagnosis. Horm Metab Res 2006;38:53–56.
15   Morris J, Hay ID, Nelson RE, Jiang Nai S: Clinical utility of thyrotropin receptor antibody assays: comparison of radioreceptor and bioassay methods. Mayo Clin Proc 1988;63:707–712.
16   Gerding MN, vanderMeer JWC, Broenink M, Bakker O, Wiersinga WM, Prummel MF: Association of thyrotropin receptor antibodies with the clinical features of Graves' ophthalmopathy. Clin Endocrinol 2000;52:267–271.
17   Eckstein AK, Plicht M, Lax H, Neuhauser M, Mann K, Lederbogen S, Heckmann C, Esser J, Morgenthaler NG: Thyrotropin receptor autoantibodies are independent risk factors for Graves' ophthalmopathy and help to predict severity and outcome of the disease. J Clin Endocrinol Metab 2006;91:3464–3470.
18   Prummel MF, Wiersinga WM, Mourits MP, Koornneef L, Berghout A, van der Gaag R: Effect of abnormal thyroid function on the severity of Graves' ophthalmopathy. Arch Intern Med 1990;50:1098–1101.
19   Bijlsma WR, Mourits MP: Radiologic measurement of extraocular muscle volumes in patients with Graves' orbitopathy: a review and guideline. Orbit 2006;25:83–91.
20   Plaisier MP, Sie-Go DMDS, Berendschot TTJM, Petersen EJ, Mourits MP: Ocular adnexal lymphoma classified using the WHO classification: not only histology and stage, but also gender is a predictor of outcome. Orbit 2007;2:83–88.

Prof. Dr. M.P. Mourits
Department of Ophthalmology, Academic Medical Center – AMC
University of Amsterdam, Meibergdreef 9
NL–1105 AZ Amsterdam (The Netherlands)
Tel. +31 20 566 3518, Fax +31 20 566 9053, E-Mail m.p.mourits@amc.uva.nl

# Natural History

*Pat Kendall-Taylor*

Department of Endocrinology, University of Newcastle upon Tyne,
Newcastle upon Tyne, UK

## Does Graves' Orbitopathy Occur at the Same Time as Hyperthyroidism?

The onset of Graves' orbitopathy (GO) is closely related to Graves' hyperthyroidism in most patients.

GO may precede or follow the onset of hyperthyroidism, but in many cases the GO comes to light at the same time as the hyperthyroidism (fig. 1). In a study from Pisa, Italy [1], GO was associated with hyperthyroidism in 91.4% of 221 patients; the remaining 8.6% patients had other mild thyroid abnormalities. It is unusual for GO to precede hyperthyroidism by more than 1 year, but it may develop at any time following the onset and treatment of hyperthyroidism.

Although commonly associated with hyperthyroidism, GO may also occur in other types of thyroid dysfunction: for example, in an incidence cohort of 120 cases [2], 90% had hyperthyroidism, 0.8% hypothyroidism, 3.3% Hashimoto's thyroiditis and 5.8% were euthyroid.

The mean age of onset is about 44 years, which is a little older than for hyperthyroidism (mean age of onset about 35 years) reflecting the fact that GO may occur in patients who develop hyperthyroidism at a later age, or may develop some time after treatment of hyperthyroidism [3].

## Does Restoring Euthyroidism Lead to Improvement in Graves' Orbitopathy?

Many studies have looked at the effect on GO of each of the different modalities for treatment of hyperthyroidism. From these there is no good evidence that restoring euthyroidism with antithyroid drugs leads to improvement

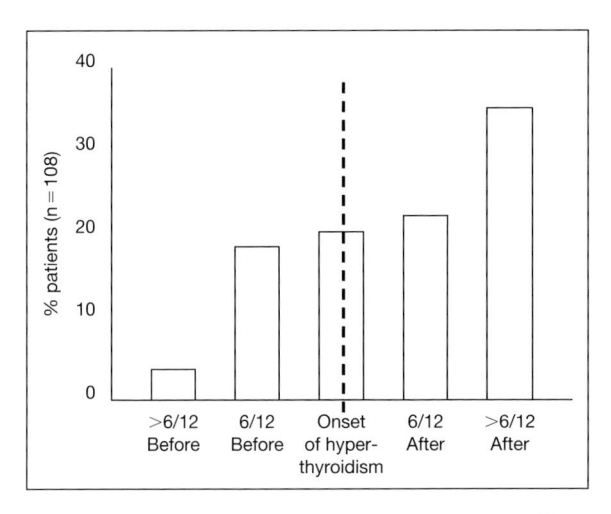

*Fig. 1.* The onset of GO in relation to the onset of hyperthyroidism [from ref. 2].

in GO. Outcome after thyroidectomy is inconsistent with several series showing no effect [4], but a recent prospective study finding a decrease in total eye score [5]; however, this could relate more to an effect on the autoimmune process rather than thyroid status. Two large prospective studies found that in ~15% cases $^{131}$I therapy led to either the de novo development of GO or deterioration in existing mild GO, specially in high-risk cases [6, 7]; this number could be reduced by the administration of early T4, presumably by preempting the development of hypothyroidism.

Thus, restoring euthyroidism in hyperthyroid patients probably does not itself cause improvement in the GO. However, what is reasonably clear is that hypothyroidism leads to deterioration of GO, so avoiding episodes of hypothyroidism and maintaining euthyroidism is an important aspect of treatment.

It is interesting to note that GO has become less prevalent in recent decades [8]; although the reasons for this are not known it seems likely to relate to improved management of thyroid dysfunction and smoother control of thyroid function, made possible by more accurate assays for thyroid function tests.

**What Effect May Hypothyroidism Have?**

This has been discussed briefly in the above paragraph. Although primary hypothyroidism is not often associated with GO, when hypothyroidism occurs in a patient with Graves' disease, usually as a result of treatment, it is commonly associated with worsening of GO [9, 10]. Hypothyroidism after $^{131}$I should be treated with thyroxine replacement as soon as it is suspected or even given

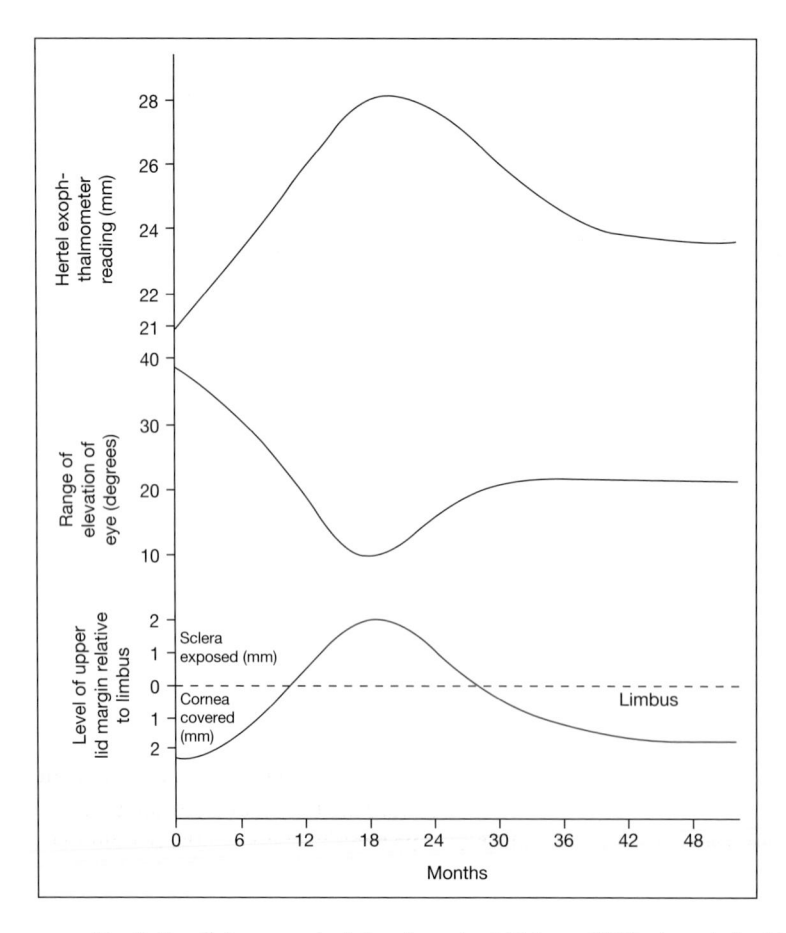

*Fig. 2.* Rundle's curves depicting the natural history of GO, characterized by an initial dynamic phase of deterioration and remission, followed by the static end-phase [from ref. 12].

prophylactically [11]. Every effort must be made to avoid hypothyroidism in a patient with GO.

## What Is the Typical Course of the Disease?

A significant proportion of patients with GO improve spontaneously. The typical course of GO in patients receiving no specific treatment, other than that to control thyroid dysfunction, was first described by Rundle [12] and depicted by him graphically as shown in figure 2 – now known as Rundle's curve. The onset is usually insidious but is occasionally acute. Initially, there is

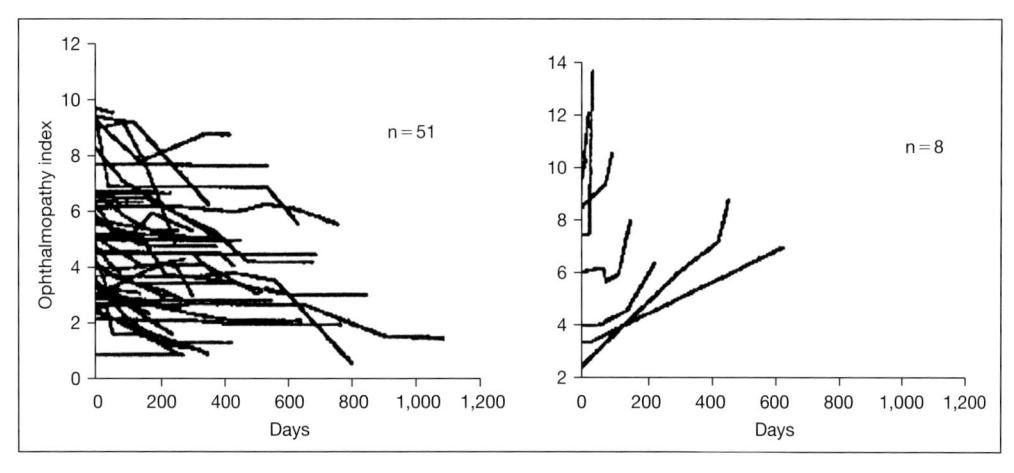

*Fig. 3.* Change with time in 59 patients given no specific treatment [from ref. 14].

progressive deterioration (the 'active progressive phase') which may last several months and reflects the evolution of the autoimmune process – when there is inflammation of retrobulbar tissues, lymphocytic infiltration, production of glycosaminoglycans (GAGs) and edema. As the activity subsides a plateau is reached; this is followed by a phase of spontaneous slow improvement that may last a year or more, after which the condition becomes static; but with regression of the inflammatory process, fibrosis may develop, so that the affected tissues do not return to their previous healthy state and the patient may still have some residual features such as proptosis and chronic dysfunction of extraocular muscles.

In some early studies, GO deteriorated in up to 30% patients in the years following diagnosis [13]. In a more recent study [14], 59 patients with mild/moderate GO, given no specific treatment, were assessed regularly over the course of 1 year, during which time definite improvement was seen in 22%, minor improvement in 42.4%, no change in 22%, and 13.5% deteriorated (fig. 3).

## What Is the Difference between Activity and Severity?

The course of the disease with respect to the activity and severity can now be more accurately depicted, as shown in figure 4 [15].

The *activity* of GO refers to the initial inflammatory phase, when there is progressive development of the disease. This active inflammation resolves, at least partially, but as it does so it tends to give rise to fibrosis of the extraocular muscles. The clinical features of '*activity*' were defined by Mourits et al. [16],

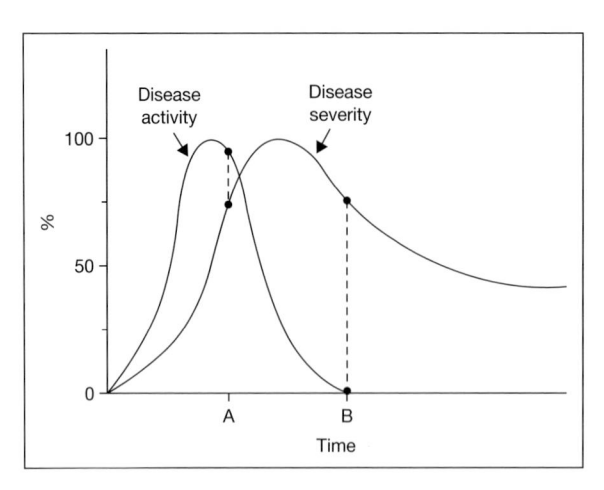

*Fig. 4.* Diagram to illustrate the relationship between disease activity and severity in the natural history of GO. Immunosuppressive treatment, administered to patients with the same level of disease severity, is likely to be successful when GO is very active (time A) but not when GO is inactive (time B) [from ref. 15].

*Table 1.* Clinical activity score [16] (a point is given for each item)

---
Painful, oppressive feeling on or behind the globe
Pain on attempted up-, side- or downgaze
Redness of the eyelids
Diffuse redness of the conjunctiva
Chemosis
Swollen caruncle or plica
Edema of the eyelids
Increase of 2 mm or more in proptosis in the last 1–3 months
Decrease in visual acuity in the last 1–3 months
Decrease in eye movements of 8° or more in the last 1–3 months

---
Some of these features may actually reflect congestion rather than inflammation.

---

based upon the classical signs of inflammation of pain, redness, swelling, and impaired function. They comprise: spontaneous retrobulbar pain, pain on eye movements, eyelid erythema, conjunctival injection, chemosis, swelling of the caruncle, eyelid edema or fullness. A clinical activity score (CAS) can be derived from assessment of these features (table 1).

The concept of *severity* relates to the features that result from the chronic changes in the extraocular muscles and soft tissues. The clinical features of severity include proptosis, which if very severe may lead to secondary exposure keratitis and corneal ulceration or perforation; extraocular muscle dysfunction and the resulting diplopia; and visual loss or impairment secondary to optic neuropathy. The assessment of severity is discussed in detail in the chapter by Dickinson [pp. 1–26].

### How Do You Determine which Phase of the Disease the Patient Is Displaying? [see also chapter by Dickinson, pp. 1–26]

Firstly, a history should be taken, particularly noting how long the patient has been aware of a problem with the eyes, how it has developed over recent weeks or months, as well as the specific symptoms.

If the condition is of relatively recent onset with primarily inflammatory features, then it is in the active phase. The presence of symptoms such as grittiness, watering or pain are usually indicative of activity. On the other hand, if the history is rather long with a paucity of inflammatory features but chief concerns of proptosis or diplopia, then the chronic phase is more likely. To be certain, the features should be documented in detail and repeated (assuming there is no optic neuropathy present) after an interval of about 2 months; if there has been deterioration then the disease is active, if no change activity is less likely.

A convenient way to determine the *activity* of the disease is to estimate the CAS, as shown in table 1. A point is given for each item. If the score is >3 the GO is generally considered to be active. Other methods used to assess activity are A-mode ultrasonography, increased levels of glycosaminoglycan (GAG) in serum or urine, prolonged T2 relaxation time on orbital MRI, and octreoscan.

A comparative atlas [17] enabled these soft tissue inflammatory features to be assessed consistently, and a summary score for soft tissue inflammation (STI) was also derived comprising periorbital edema, conjunctival redness, chemosis, redness of lateral rectus insertion and caruncle.

Severity can be assessed using the time-honoured method of the NOSPECS classification [18]. The patient's own assessment of severity must also be taken into account and an MRI scan if available (or if not a CT scan) will help define the severity.

### How Does the Phase of the Disease Influence Choice of Treatment?

For the clinician it is helpful to assess the degrees of activity and severity independently; both are important in deciding whether a patient requires treatment and if so which type of treatment is indicated. If the disease is mild no treatment is necessary even though there may be some evidence of activity. If the disease is in the active phase and severity is moderate-to-severe then anti-inflammatory or immunomodulatory treatment (e.g. corticosteroids) or orbital radiotherapy may be indicated.

If the patient has severe orbital involvement, with little evidence of activity there is unlikely to be a response to medical treatment, and then surgical treatment (e.g. orbital decompression or rehabilitative surgery) may be indicated.

Understanding the process of development and the natural trend towards improvement in untreated GO (though in a smaller number deterioration may occur) has important implications for the choice of treatment, as well as for the design of clinical trials. The doctor should try to determine whether the condition is in the steep ascending part of the curve, or at the same level but on the other side of the plateau. What might be interpreted as therapy-induced improvement may be due to spontaneous change; or the apparent absence of response may indicate that progression of the active disease has been delayed.

### Will the Graves' Orbitopathy Eventually Burn Itself Out?

Yes, the GO will eventually burn itself out. However this takes a variable period of time, which may be as long as several years. When this occurs the signs of 'activity', or inflammation, will have resolved; but there is often residual evidence of GO in the form of lid abnormality, proptosis or muscle dysfunction.

### Will the Orbital Changes Return to Normal when the Condition Eventually Resolves?

The orbital changes do not always return to normal when the condition resolves. Mild cases will more or less regress spontaneously, but a patient with more severe disease, even one who responds to treatment, is unlikely to revert to the premorbid state. As indicated above there is often residual evidence of GO in the form of lid abnormality, proptosis or muscle dysfunction. The best chance of reversing the course of the disease in the severely affected case and restoring the orbital changes to 'normal' is often with a combination of disease-modifying treatment, surgical decompression and corrective muscle and lid surgery. The outcome is better in patients who have had the diagnosis made early and treatment started promptly [19].

Despite the use of all available surgical and medical treatments, many patients feel that their eyes are still abnormal years later. A long-term follow-up study (median 9.8 years) of 120 patients found that of 92 respondents, 61% felt that their appearance had not returned to its former level, and 52% still thought their eyes appeared abnormal [20].

## How Long Is it Likely to Take before the Disease Becomes Inactive?

It is impossible to answer this question for an individual patient. However, for most patients the time period will be from several months to 1 or 2 years. Most patients with active disease of mild-to-moderate severity will receive some form of treatment such as orbital radiotherapy or corticosteroids. This may shorten the time it takes for the GO to become inactive, although conclusive evidence for this is not available.

## Once the Condition Has Become Inactive (Whether Treated or Untreated) Is it Likely to Flare Up Again?

Once the GO has become inactive it is very unlikely to flare up again. However, it does occasionally happen, particularly if the patient becomes hypothyroid or develops recurrent Graves' hyperthyroidism. Perhaps in some of these instances the condition had been wrongly assumed to have become inactive. However, in one report [21] late reactivation, defined as active orbitopathy occurring after more than 5 years of quiescent disease, was found in 8 (5%) of 193 cases, with a mean time interval of 12 years (range 6–30 years).

## Are There Any Other Factors, Additional to Thyroid Status, which May Influence the Course of the Disease?

There is evidence that the severity of GO is related to the severity of the thyroid autoimmunity, in that the clinical features of GO [9, 22] correlate with TSH-R antibody (Ab) levels. The course of GO was also found in a recent study to correlate with TSHRAb level (as measured by TBII); furthermore, the TBII data could be used in at least some patients to indicate prognosis [23].

Cigarette smoking markedly increases the risk of developing GO [24]; it also increases the severity of the GO [19, 25]. Smokers appear to respond less well to treatment with steroids or radiotherapy than non-smokers [19]. The mechanism for these effects of cigarette smoking are as yet unknown, but it is clear that smoking influences the risk, the severity and the response to treatment.

Gender and age both influence the severity of GO. Patients over the age of 60, particularly males, are at risk of developing severe disease and being male itself confers an increased risk [26].

Although there are as yet no direct data demonstrating genetic effects on the course of GO, it appears that the disease severity may be increased in association with certain genetic factors. The CTLA-4 gene is a susceptibility locus for Graves' disease, and there appears to be a particularly strong association in patients who also have GO [27]; however, much more work is needed to clarify the role of genetic factors in GO.

## References

1 Marcocci C, Bartalena L, Bogazzi F, Panicucci M, Pinchera A: Studies on the occurrence of ophthalmopathy in Graves' disease. Acta Endocrinol (Copenh) 1989;129:473–478.
2 Bartley GB, Fatourechi V, Kadrmas EF, Jacobsen SJ, Ilstrup DM, Garrity JA, Gorman C: Clinical features of Graves' ophthalmopathy in an incidence cohort. Am J Ophthalmol 1996;121:284–290.
3 Kendler DL, Lippa J, Rootman J: The initial clinical characteristics of Graves' orbitopathy with age and sex. Arch Ophthalmol 1993;111:197–201.
4 Marcocci C, Bruni-Bossio G, Manetti L, Tanda ML, Miccoli P, Iacconi P, Bartolomei MP, Nardi M, Pinchera A, Bartalena L: The course of Graves' ophthalmopathy is not influenced by near total thyroidectomy: a case-control study. Clin Endocrinol (Oxf) 1999;51:503–508.
5 Järhult J, Rudberg C, Larsson E, Selvander H, Sjövall K, Winsa B, Rastad J, Karlsson FA, the TEO Study Group: Graves' disease with moderate-severe endocrine ophthalmopathy: long term results of a prospective, randomized study of total or subtotal thyroid resection. Thyroid 2005;15: 1157–1164.
6 Tallstedt L, Lundell G, Torring O, Wallin G, Ljunggren JG, Blomgren H, Taube A: Occurrence of ophthalmopathy after treatment for Graves' hyperthyroidism. The Thyroid Study Group. N Engl J Med 1992;326:1733–1738.
7 Bartalena L, Marcocci C, Bogazzi F, Manetti L, Tanda ML, Dell'Unto E, Bruno-Bossio G, Nardi M, Bartolomei MP, Lepri A, Rossi G, Martino E, Pinchera A: Relation between therapy for hyperthyroidism and the course of Graves' ophthalmopathy. N Engl J Med 1998;338:73–78.
8 Perros P, Anwar A, Toft AD: Evidence for a decline in the incidence and severity of thyroid-associated ophthalmopathy: twenty years experience of a large thyroid clinic. J Endocrinol 1996;148 (suppl):253.
9 Karlsson AF, Westermark K, Dahlberg PA, Jansson R, Enoksson P: Ophthalmopathy and thyroid stimulation. Lancet 1989;ii:691.
10 Prummel MF, Wiersinga WM, Mourits MP, Koornneef L, Berghout A, van der Gaag R: Effect of abnormal thyroid function on the severity of Graves' ophthalmopathy. Arch Intern Med 1990;150:1098–1101.
11 Tallstedt L, Lundell G, Blomgren H, Bring J: Does early administration of thyroxine reduce the development of Graves' ophthalmopathy after radioiodine treatment? Eur J Endocrinol 1994;130: 494–497.
12 Rundle FF: Management of exophthalmos and related ocular changes in Graves' disease. Metabolism 1957;6:36–47.
13 Hales IB, Rundle FF: Ocular changes in Graves' disease. Quart J Med 1960;29:113–126.
14 Perros P, Crombie AL, Kendall-Taylor P: Natural history of thyroid associated ophthalmopathy. Clin Endocrinol 1995;42:45–50.

15  Wiersinga WM, Prummel MF: Therapeutic controversies: retrobulbar radiation in Graves' ophthalmopathy. J Clin Endocrinol Metab 1995;80:345–347.
16  Mourits MP, Koornneef L, Wiersinga WM, Prummel MF, Berghout A, van der Gaag R: Clinical criteria for the assessment of disease activity in Graves' ophthalmopathy: a novel approach. Br J Ophthalmol 1989;73:639–644.
17  Dickinson AJ, Perros P: Controversies in the clinical evaluation of active thyroid-associated orbitopathy: use of a detailed protocol with comparative photographs for objective assessment. Clin Endocrinol (Oxf) 2001;55:283–303.
18  Werner SC: Modification of the classification of the eye changes in Graves' disease: recommendations of the ad hoc committee of the American Thyroid Association. J Clin Endocrinol Metab 1977;44:203–209.
19  Bartalena L, Pinchera A, Marcocci C: Management of Graves' ophthalmopathy: reality and perspectives. Endocr Rev 2000;21:168–199.
20  Bartley GB, Fatourechi V, Kadrmas EF, Jacobsen SJ, Ilstrup DM, Garrity JA, Gorman CA: Long term follow-up of Graves' ophthalmopathy in an incidence cohort. Ophthalmology 1996;103:958–962.
21  Selva D, Chen C, King G: Late reactivation of thyroid orbitopathy. Clin Exp Ophthalmol 2004;32:46–50.
22  Gerding MN, van der Meer JW, Broenink M, Bakker O, Wiersinga WM, Prummel MF: Association of thyrotrophin receptor antibodies with the clinical features of Graves' ophthalmopathy. Clin Endocrinol (Oxf) 2000;52:267–271.
23  Eckstein AK, Plicht M, Lax H, Neuhäuser M, Mann K, Lederbogen S, Heckmann C, Esser J, Morgenthaler N: Thyrotropin receptor autoantibodies are independent risk factors for Graves' ophthalmopathy and help to predict severity and outcome of the disease. J Clin Endocrinol Metab 2006;91:3464–3470.
24  Hagg E, Asplund K: Is endocrine opthalmopathy related to smoking? Br Med J 1987;295:634–635.
25  Mann K: Risk of smoking in thyroid-associated orbitopathy. Exp Clin Endocrinol Diabetes 1999;107(suppl 5):S164–S167.
26  Perros P, Crombie AL, Matthews JN, Kendall-Taylor P: Age and gender influence the severity of thyroid-associated ophthalmopathy: a study of 101 patients attending a combined thyroid-eye clinic. Clin Endocrinol (Oxf) 1993;38:367–372.
27  Vaidya B, Kendall-Taylor P, Pearce SH: The genetics of autoimmune thyroid disease. J Clin Endocrinol Metab 2002;87:5385–5397.

Dr. Pat Kendall-Taylor
The Barn
Newton
Northumberland
NE43 7UL (UK)

# Management

Wiersinga WM, Kahaly GJ (eds): Graves' Orbitopathy: A Multidisciplinary Approach.
Basel, Karger, 2007, pp 88–95

# General Management Plan

K. Boboridis[a], P. Perros[b]

[a]Panagia General Hospital, Thessaloniki, Greece; [b]Department of Endocrinology, Freeman Hospital, Newcastle upon Tyne, UK

## What Are the Priorities when Faced with a New Presentation of Graves' Orbitopathy?

When confronted with a new patient with Graves' orbitopathy (GO), two initial questions need to be addressed:
(a) Is the diagnosis of GO correct?
(b) Does the patient have sight-threatening orbitopathy?

The diagnosis is usually clinically obvious in patients with a history of Graves' hyperthyroidism and typical clinical eye features (lid retraction, periorbital edema, proptosis). However, patients with Graves' hyperthytoidism are as prone to other ocular pathologies as anyone else. If there are unusual features (for example, unilateral disease, or no background of thyroid autoimmunity, unusual extraocular muscle group involvement like lateral or superior recti being affected), other important diagnoses need to be excluded, and this usually means imaging by CT or MRI.

Dysthyroid optic neuropathy and severe corneal ulceration constitute sight-threatening orbitopathy and can be recognised by their symptoms and signs as described in the chapter by Dickinson [pp. 1–26]. A further rare potential cause of sight-threatening GO is globe subluxation [see chapter by von Arx, pp. 212–220]. Recognition of sight-threatening GO should prompt urgent referral to an ophthalmologist, preferably in a multidisciplinary setting [1].

The next step is damage limitation, i.e. avoidance of factors that can aggravate the condition. Smoking is a hugely important issue and patients who are smokers should receive counselling and help to give up the habit (table 1). Both hypo- and hyperthyroidism can make GO worse and one of the objectives is stability of thyroid status. Radioiodine should be avoided in the active phase of the

*Table 1.* Available ways of helping patients stop smoking and effectiveness

| Method | Success rate, % |
| --- | --- |
| Brief opportunistic advice from a doctor | 2 |
| Face-to-face intensive behavioural support from a specialist | 7 |
| Proactive telephone counseling | 2 |
| Written self-help leaflets | 1 |
| Nicotine replacement therapy (NRT) | 5–12 |
| Bupropion | 9 |
| Intensive behavioural support plus NRT or bupropion | 13–19 |

disease (or if alternative treatment modalities cannot be used, it should be combined with a short course of oral steroids).

Before considering immunosuppressive treatments, orbital radiotherapy or surgery, don't forget simple ways of helping patients' symptoms (see below, 'What simple measures can help the eyes?').

## How Good Is the Evidence that Quitting Smoking Helps?

The association between smoking and GO is striking and has been confirmed by many studies. The risk of GO in smokers is increased 7- to 8-fold [2]. Furthermore, there is a dose-response relationship between number of cigarettes consumed per day and severity of the eye disease [3]. Patients who are current smokers have a less favourable response to treatment like radiotherapy or steroids [4, 5]. An association between smoking and progression of GO after radioiodine treatment has also been documented [4]. The risk of worsening GO is reduced drastically in patients who give up smoking [3]. So, although there are no studies that have directly assessed the effect of giving up smoking on GO, the evidence is highly suggestive that giving up smoking reduces the risk of GO becoming worse, and improves the chance of having a good response to treatment [6].

## Does Thyroid Status Affect the Eyes?

Observational studies have found an association between severity of GO and both hypothyroidism and hyperthyroidism [7–10]. Hypothyroidism following radioiodine is associated with a risk of deterioration or emergence of new GO [11], and this effect can be at least partially prevented by maintaining

*Table 2.* Simple measures that may help patients with GO

| | |
|---|---|
| Artificial tears | help surface symptoms |
| Lubricant ointments | help protect the corneae during sleep |
| Taping of lids at night | help protect the corneae during sleep |
| Sunglasses | help patients with photophobia and excess lachrymation in response to wind when outdoors; also comforting for some patients who are self-conscious of their appearance |
| Prisms | improve diplopia |
| Achieve and maintain euthyroidism | increases the chance of spontaneous improvement reduces the chance of deterioration |
| Smoking cessation | increases the chance of spontaneous improvement reduces the chance of deterioration increases the chance of a better response to treatment |
| Counselling | reduces anxiety and may provide reassurance may help develop better coping strategies |

euthyroidism [11, 12]. There is therefore convincing, albeit circumstantial, evidence that dysthyroidism is detrimental to the eyes.

## What Simple Measures Can Help the Eyes?

Clinicians often forget that simple solutions can have a significant impact on symptoms (table 2).

Artificial tear drops or gels (administered 4–6 times daily) can alleviate the ocular surface symptoms (such as grittiness, excessive watering, photophobia) from reduced tear production and corneal exposure, which are both common features in patients with GO [13, 14].

Lubricant ointments prior to sleeping can help, particularly if surface symptoms are prominent on waking up. Taping the lids at night to prevent exposure keratopathy from lagophthalmos may also be an effective temporary measure, though if the orbitopathy is severe enough to require such measures, surgery needs to be considered.

A short course of weak corticosteroid (fluorometholone) or non-steroidal anti-inflammatory (ketorolac) eye drops can reduce the ocular symptoms and inflammatory signs especially when combined with intensive lubrication. The use of preservative free eye drops can help to avoid the allergic reactions, epithelial toxicity and chronic conjunctival inflammation produced by the preservatives and particularly benzalkonium chloride.

Several adrenergic blocking agents have been used topically and systemically to control eyelid retraction caused by increased sympathetic tone affecting Muller's muscle. Topical guanethidine 2% has been found to control upper eyelid retraction in the majority of patients [15]. Unpredictable response, limited long-term effect, conjunctival hyperaemia, miosis and epithelial toxicity are the most frequently encountered complications responsible for the limited acceptability of this approach.

Spectacle correction of the induced refractive changes can improve visual acuity and sunglasses likewise can protect and minimise surface symptoms in response to wind or sunlight, and help some patients feel less self-conscious.

Patients with troublesome diplopia in the active stage should be considered for prisms before surgical correction can be applied. Monitoring and lowering intraocular pressure can reduce the chances of progression to glaucoma in some of those patients [16].

Diuretics and raising the head of the bed have been advocated as means of reducing the amount of periorbital edema, but objective evidence in favour of these measures is lacking and in the authors' experience the former is ineffective and the latter poorly tolerated.

A sympathetic approach by the clinician and explanation of the various aspects of the disease and its treatment is appreciated by many patients. All patients can be reassured that with optimal management blindness (a dreaded fear by most patients with GO) is highly unlikely. The clinician should also encourage patients to be positive towards the disease. These basic strategies help to reduce the anxiety that many patients experience, and make life more tolerable, especially in the early days after diagnosis. Patient-led self-help groups also have an important role.

### Is There a Place for Botulinum Toxin?

Botulinum toxin type A has been used to reduce lid retraction by injecting it into the levator complex of the upper lid through the skin or conjunctiva in both the active and inactive stage of the disease [17]. Similarly, it can be used to reduce the amount of diplopia by injecting into the appropriate extraocular muscles which also has a significant lowering effect on intraocular pressure [18]. The relief is temporary lasting for less than 12 weeks but often appreciated by patients and has a role until the eye disease is sufficiently inactive for lid and eye muscle surgery. Botulinum toxin has been successfully used for chemical denervation of the overactive corrugator supercilii and treatment of glabellar lines in patients with GO [19]. This was the first FDA-approved cosmetic application of botulinum toxin.

## How Do You Define Mild, Moderately Severe, and Very Severe Graves' Orbitopathy?

Although different clinicians with experience in managing GO are likely to classify the severity of individual patients similarly, agreeing on a definition that may be applicable to all patients is difficult [20]. This is because GO manifests in many different ways and in the same individual some features may be mild while others are severe. Furthermore, the symptoms experienced by patients of similar disease severity may be vastly different. Nonetheless, classifying patients into different categories of disease severity is useful and a guide to whether treatments are justified or not.

Patients with 'mild' disease are usually defined as those with minimal lid changes, little or no proptosis, absent or intermittent diplopia and no impairment of optic nerve function. Such cases usually do not require immunosuppressive or surgical treatment as the potential risks of such currently available therapies outweigh the benefits.

Sight-threatening disease refers to cases where there is evidence of DON and/or corneal breakdown and urgent treatment is required to prevent blindness.

'Moderate to severe' GO are cases that fall between the mild and sight-threatening severe categories. Such cases may benefit from immunosuppressive therapies and/or surgery.

## Can You Give a Simplified Overall Management Scheme?

Patients with mild disease should be managed initially conservatively, focusing on simple measures, addressing their smoking habit and maintaining euthyroidism (fig. 1). The majority of such cases (about 2/3) will improve spontaneously over the following 3–6 months [21]. In special circumstances specific treatment may be justified, although the benefits will be marginal. If no specific treatment is administered, such patients should be monitored every few months to ensure that the disease does not deteriorate. Once the disease has reached its inactive stage, rehabilitative surgery may need to be considered.

Sight-threatening disease needs to be treated urgently. If sight is not threatened, treatment is not mandatory, but should be given serious consideration. Deciding whether to treat and with what modality depends on assessment of disease activity [22, 23]. During the active phase of GO, immunosuppression with steroids, orbital irradiation, or the combination of the two, are likely to be beneficial. If the disease is inactive rehabilitative reconstructive surgery has a major role. In the most severe of cases multiple treatments are required. These need to be planned carefully and in an appropriate sequence. For best results,

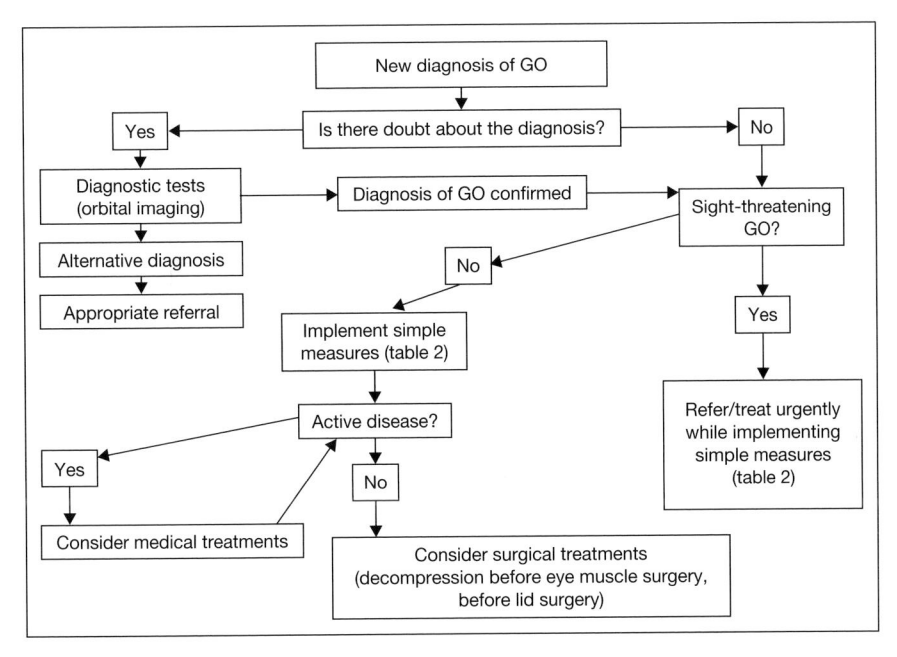

*Fig. 1.* Overall management plan for patients with GO.

steroid therapy with or without orbital irradiation is administered until the disease becomes inactive. If medical treatment does not reverse the features of dysthyroid optic neuropathy, or is poorly tolerated, surgical orbital decompression must be considered sooner rather than later. The presence of significant proptosis which is unacceptable to the patient or troublesome corneal exposure due to proptosis are also indications for surgical decompression. Eye muscle surgery to correct diplopia should follow orbital decompression as new strabismus can occur after surgical decompression [24]. The final stage is lid lengthening to correct retraction followed by cosmetic blepharoplasty [25, 26].

## References

1 Wiersinga WM, Perros P, Kahaly GJ, Mourits MP, Baldeschi L, Boboridis K, Boschi A, Dickinson AJ, Kendall-Taylor P, Krassas GE, Lane CM, Lazarus JH, Marcocci C, Marino M, Nardi M, Neoh C, Orgiazzi J, Pinchera A, Pitz S, Prummel MF, Sartini MS, Stahl M, von Arx G: Clinical assessment of patients with Graves' orbitopathy: the European Group on Graves' Orbitopathy recommendations to generalists, specialists and clinical researchers. Eur J Endocrinol 2006;155: 387–389.
2 Prummel MF, Wiersinga WM: Smoking and risk of Graves' disease. J Am Med Assoc 1993;269: 479–482.

3 Pfeilschifter J, Ziegler R: Smoking and endocrine ophthalmopathy: impact of smoking severity and current vs. lifetime cigarette consumption. Clin Endocrinol (Oxf) 1996;45:477–481.
4 Bartalena L, Marcocci C, Tanda ML, Manetti L, Dell'Unto E, Bartolomei MP, Nardi M, Martino E, Pinchera A: Cigarette smoking and treatment outcomes in Graves' ophthalmopathy. Ann Intern Med 1998;129:632–635.
5 Eckstein A, Quadbeck B, Mueller G, Rettenmeier AW, Hoermann R, Mann K, Steuhl P, Esser J: Impact of smoking on the response to treatment of thyroid associated ophthalmopathy. Br J Ophthalmol 2003;87:773–776.
6 Krassas GE, Wiersinga W: Smoking and autoimmune thyroid disease: the plot thickens. Eur J Endocrinol 2006;154:777–780.
7 Prummel MF, Wiersinga WM, Mourits MP, Koornneef L, Berghout A, van der Gaag R: Amelioration of eye changes of Graves' ophthalmopathy by achieving euthyroidism. Acta Endocrinol (Copenh) 1989;121(suppl 2):185–189.
8 Prummel MF, Wiersinga WM, Mourits MP, Koornneef L, Berghout A, van der Gaag R: Effect of abnormal thyroid function on the severity of Graves' ophthalmopathy. Arch Intern Med 1990;150: 1098–1101.
9 Kim JM, LaBree L, Levin L, Feldon SE: The relation of Graves' ophthalmopathy to circulating thyroid hormone status. Br J Ophthalmol 2004;88:72–74.
10 Karlsson F, Westermark K, Dahlberg PA, Jansson R, Enoksson P: Ophthalmopathy and thyroid stimulation. Lancet 1989;ii:691.
11 Tallstedt L, Lundell G, Blomgren H, Bring J: Does early administration of thyroxine reduce the development of Graves' ophthalmopathy after radioiodine treatment? Eur J Endocrinol 1994;130: 494–497.
12 Perros P, Kendall-Taylor P, Neoh C, Frewin S, Dickinson J: A prospective study of the effects of radioiodine therapy for hyperthyroidism in patients with minimally active Graves' ophthalmopathy. J Clin Endocrinol Metab 2005;90:5321–5323.
13 Eckstein AK, Finkenrath A, Heiligenhaus A, Renzing-Kohler K, Esser J, Kruger C, Quadbeck B, Steuhl KP, Gieseler RK: Dry eye syndrome in thyroid-associated ophthalmopathy: lacrimal expression of TSH receptor suggests involvement of TSHR-specific autoantibodies. Acta Ophthalmol Scand 2004;82:291–297.
14 Gilbard JP, Farris RL: Ocular surface drying and tear film osmolarity in thyroid eye disease. Acta Ophthalmol (Copenh) 1983;61:108–116.
15 Haddad HM: Lid retraction therapy with a guanethidine solution. Arch Ophthalmol 1989;107:169.
16 Cockerham KP, Pal C, Jani B, Wolter A, Kennerdell JS: The prevalence and implications of ocular hypertension and glaucoma in thyroid-associated orbitopathy. Ophthalmology 1997;104: 914–917.
17 Uddin JM, Davies PD: Treatment of upper eyelid retraction associated with thyroid eye disease with subconjunctival botulinum toxin injection. Ophthalmology 2002;109:1183–1187.
18 Kikkawa DO, Cruz RC Jr, Christian WK, Rikkers S, Weinreb RN, Levi L, Granet DB: Botulinum A toxin injection for restrictive myopathy of thyroid-related orbitopathy: effects on intraocular pressure. Am J Ophthalmol 2003;135:427–431.
19 Carruthers JA, Lowe NJ, Menter MA, Gibson J, Nordquist M, Mordaunt J, Walker P, Eadie N: A multicenter, double-blind, randomized, placebo-controlled study of the efficacy and safety of botulinum toxin type A in the treatment of glabellar lines. J Am Acad Dermatol 2002;46: 840–849.
20 Bartalena L, Pinchera A, Marcocci C: Management of Graves' ophthalmopathy: reality and perspectives. Endocr Rev 2000;21:168–199.
21 Perros P, Crombie AL, Kendall-Taylor P: Natural history of thyroid associated ophthalmopathy. Clin Endocrinol (Oxf) 1995;42:45–50.
22 Wiersinga WM, Prummel MF: Graves' ophthalmopathy: a rational approach to treatment. Trends Endocrinol Metab 2002;13:280–287.
23 Bartalena L, Marcocci C, Tanda ML, Piantanida E, Lai A, Marino M, Pinchera A: An update on medical management of Graves' ophthalmopathy. J Endocrinol Invest 2005;28:469–478.

24 Abramoff MD, Kalmann R, de Graaf ME, Stilma JS, Mourits MP: Rectus extraocular muscle paths and decompression surgery for Graves orbitopathy: mechanism of motility disturbances. Invest Ophthalmol Vis Sci 2002;43:300–307.
25 Fenton S, Kemp EG: A review of the outcome of upper lid lowering for eyelid retraction and complications of spacers at a single unit over five years. Orbit 2002;21:289–294.
26 Shorr N, Seiff SR: The four stages of surgical rehabilitation of the patient with dysthyroid ophthalmopathy. Ophthalmology 1986;93:476–483.
27 West R, McNeill A, Raw M: Smoking cessation guidelines for health professionals: an update. Health Education Authority. Thorax 2000;55:987–999.

Dr. P. Perros
Department of Endocrinology, Level 6, Freeman Hospital
Freeman Road
Newcastle upon Tyne NE7 7DN (UK)
Tel. +44 191 213 7245, Ext. 26245, Fax +44 191 2231249, E-Mail petros.perros@ncl.ac.uk

# Combined Thyroid-Eye Clinics

*Wilmar M. Wiersinga*

Department of Endocrinology and Metabolism, Academic Medical Center,
University of Amsterdam, Amsterdam, The Netherlands

## What Are Combined Thyroid-Eye Clinics?

The diagnosis of Graves' orbitopathy (GO) is very easy in patients with already known Graves' hyperthyroidism in whom bilateral symmetric ophthalmopathy develops. The diagnosis is more difficult when the ophthalmopathy occurs in euthyroid patients, which happens in about 10% of all GO patients, and can be even more challenging in case of unilateral eye changes. In many cases there is a large doctor's delay in arriving at the diagnosis of GO. This is not too surprising in view of the low age-adjusted annual incidence rate of 16 and of 2.9 per 100,000 females and males, respectively [1]. General internists and ophthalmologists and especially family physicians will see GO patients infrequently, and may not be familiar with the wide variety in the clinical presentation. Working together in a team of ophthalmologists/orbital surgeons and internists/endocrinologists who see a large number of GO patients, is very helpful in becoming acquainted with the diverse manifestations of GO.

We now know that it matters for the eyes whether or not the patient is euthyroid, and how the patient is rendered euthyroid. We have also learned that the efficacy of immunosuppression is high in the active inflammatory stage of the eye disease, but low when applied in the late inactive 'burnt-out' stage with predominant fibrosis; along the same lines, rehabilitative surgery is best done in the inactive stage [2].

It is clear that in the management of GO there must be a fine-tuning between the endocrinologic and ophthalmologic treatment options, tailored to the individual patient's need. This is accomplished most successfully if the endocrinologist and the ophthalmologist are looking simultaneously at the same patient sitting in front of them, assessing together the current thyroid state and the severity and activity of the eye disease, and then, in close consultation with the patient, delineating

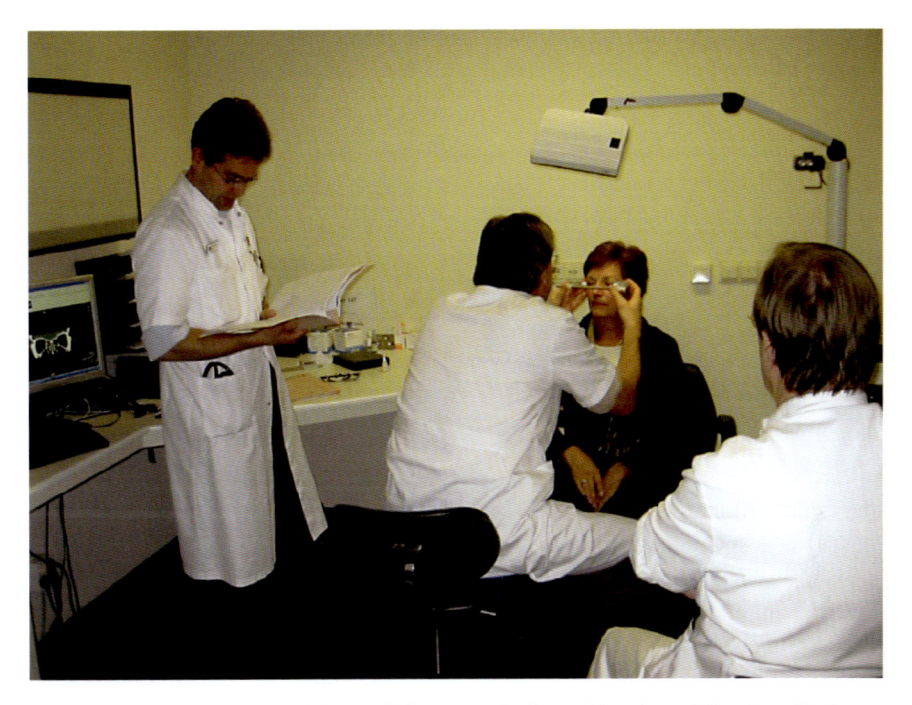

*Fig. 1.* Combined thyroid-eye clinics at work: the resident in training (standing) presents the patient to the consultants in endocrinology and ophthalmology (both seen at the back); results of all laboratory tests, ophthalmological measurements and orbital CT scans can be viewed at the screen of the computer connected to the hospital patients' database.

the most appropriate management plan. This requires combined thyroid-eye clinics of the two specialties (fig. 1). According to patient load, the combined clinics can be organized once weekly, every fortnight, or every month.

### Why Is a Multidisciplinary Approach Recommended?

Accurate diagnosis and appropriate management of GO requires the combined expertise of endocrinologist and ophthalmologist. Although the expertise of the clinicians is critical and the setting perhaps less so, evidence from other clinical disciplines would suggest that a dedicated multidisciplinary clinic results in better outcomes [3, 4]. The European Group on Graves' Orbitopathy (EUGOGO) therefore recommends that patients with GO should be managed in combined thyroid-eye clinics with input from endocrinologists and ophthalmologists [5]. EUGOGO strongly believes that multidisciplinary groups enhance

*Table 1.* High-speed track for patients with GO, operative in the Academic Medical Center, Amsterdam

| | |
|---|---|
| 08.00 h | Venipuncture for TSH, FT4, TPO-Ab and TSH; R-Ab assays in serum, and routine clinical chemistry |
| 08.30 h | Consultation with internist/endocrinologist |
| 10.00 h | Orthoptic examination |
| 11.00 h | Visual fields |
| 12.00 h | Orbital imaging (CT scan) |
| 14.00 h | Consultation with ophthalmologist/orbital surgeon |
| 16.00 h | Patient-support group |
| 16.30 h | All test results are known; consultation in combined thyroid-eye clinics |
| 17.00 h | Patient leaves hospital with diagnosis and management plan |

the quality of care delivered to GO patients. Many patients with GO in Europe never reach specialist centres or are referred too late to benefit from treatments, which results in suboptimal outcomes [6]. It is therefore encouraging to notice that the number of combined thyroid-eye clinics all over Europe is steadily increasing over the last few years.

### Can Patients-Support Groups Be Helpful?

Involvement of patients with GO in the combined thyroid-eye clinics can be very helpful. One may ask representatives of patient support groups to be present in a separate room, simultaneously with the combined thyroid-eye clinics. Patients may wish to get into immediate contact with fellow patients, who as experts by experience may share how it feels to be affected by GO and undergoing specific procedures. It may reduce anxiety for what is coming and offer a realistic view of what is to be expected in terms of outcome. Talking to fellow patients add a dimension not readily provided by the attending physicians. Patient support groups usually distribute very informative brochures on GO.

### I Have Heard of a Fast-Track Clinic for Graves' Orbitopathy Patients: What Is That?

When the patient attends the combined thyroid-eye clinic, he or she has already been seen separately by the ophthalmologist and the endocrinologist, and the results of specific laboratory investigations ordered by these two specialists are known. It means that the patient has already visited the hospital on average 4–6 times for consultations with both specialists, with the orthoptist, the radiology department and the laboratory. To reduce the number of visits, a 'high-speed track' for GO patients can be organized, in which all investigations are being performed on the same day (table 1). The results are in at the end of the afternoon, and can be viewed in the consultation room on the monitor of the computer connected to the large hospital patients' database. The patient is then seen simultaneously by both consultants, and a final diagnosis and management plan can be reached in almost all instances. The logistics of such a high-speed track should not be underestimated, but once it is operative it is very gratifying for doctors and patients alike. Our high-speed track accommodates two new referrals of GO patients every Tuesday [7].

## References

1. Bartley GB, Fatourechi V, Kadmas EF, Jacobson SJ, Ilstrup DM, Garrity JA, Gorman CA: The incidence of Graves' ophthalmopathy in Olmsted Country, Minnesota. Am J Ophthalmol 1995;120:511–517.
2. Wiersinga WM, Prummel MF: Graves' ophthalmopathy: a rational approach to treatment. Trends Endocrinol Metab 2002;13:280–287.
3. Ducharme A, Doyon O, White M, Rouleau JL, Brophy JM: Impact of care at a multidisciplinary congestive heart failure clinic: a randomized clinical trial. Cancer Med Ass J 2005;173:40–43.
4. Sperk-Hillen JM, O'Connor PJ: Factors driving diabetes care improvement in a large medical group: 10 years of progress. Am J Management Care 2005;5:S177–S185.
5. The European Group on Graves' Orbitopathy (EUGOGO): Clinical assessment of patients with Graves' orbitopathy: the European Group on Graves' Orbitopathy recommendations to generalists, specialists and clinical researchers. Eur J Endocrinol 2006;155:387–389.
6. Perros P, Baldeschi L, Boboridis K, Dickinson AJ, Hullo A, Kahaly GJ, Kendall-Taylor P, Krassas GE, Lane CM, Lazarus JH, Marcocci C, Marino M, Mourits MP, Nardi M, Orgiazzi J, Pinchera A, Pitz S, Prummel MF, Wiersinga WM: A questionnaire survey on the management of Graves' orbitopathy in Europe. Eur J Endocrinol 2006;155:207–211.
7. Wiersinga WM: The philosophy of Graves' ophthalmopathy. Orbit 2005;24:165–171.

Prof. Wilmar M. Wiersinga
Department of Endocrinology and Metabolism, Academic Medical Center, Room F5-171
University of Amsterdam
Meibergdreef 9
NL–1105 AZ Amsterdam (The Netherlands)
Tel. +31 20 566 6071, Fax +31 20 691 7682, E-Mail w.m.wiersinga@amc.uva.nl

# Thyroid Treatment

*Claudio Marcocci, Aldo Pinchera*

Department of Endocrinology and Metabolism, University of Pisa, Pisa, Italy

## Does It Matter for the Eyes How the Patient Is Rendered Euthyroid?

Graves' orbitopathy (GO) occurs in about 50% of patients with Graves' disease [1] and may develop before, concomitantly, or even after the onset of hyperthyroidism [2]. In the latter situation, one wonders whether treatment of hyperthyroidism may influence GO course. Information on different treatments often is conflicting because of retrospective and uncontrolled features of most studies and the lack of standardized methods for evaluation of eye changes [3]. Moreover, it may be difficult to ascertain whether changes in ocular conditions reflect the natural history of eye disease [4] or are attributable to the effect of the treatments undertaken to control hyperthyroidism. The latter point is clearly demonstrated in the patient shown in figure 1, in whom lid retraction which was present when hyperthyroid disappeared when the patient was rendered euthyroid (methimazole and thyroidectomy).

### Thionamides

Antithyroid drug (ATD) treatment effectively controls thyroid hyperfunction and is the most common treatment for Graves' hyperthyroidism in Europe and Japan [5]. Improvement of ocular conditions often follows ATD administration [3, 6]; this initial beneficial effect appears to be related to restoration of euthyroidism rather than to a direct ATD effect on GO [6]. In the long term, ATD treatment does not substantially affect the course of GO; accordingly, it is not a disease-modifying treatment [7]. A major limitation of ATD therapy is the high rate of relapsing hyperthyroidism after treatment withdrawal [8]. Recurrence causes reactivation of thyroid autoimmune phenomena, with an increase in

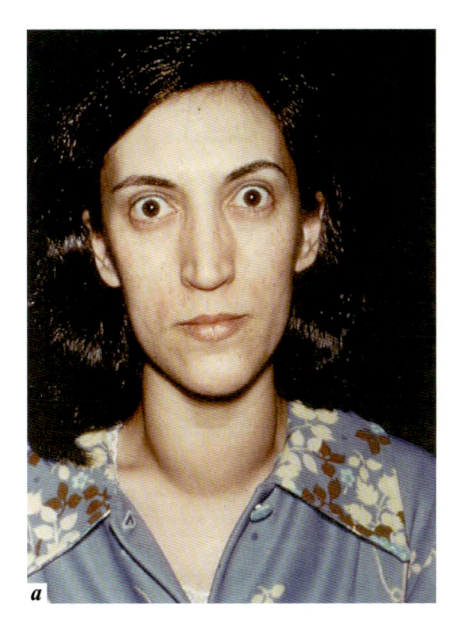

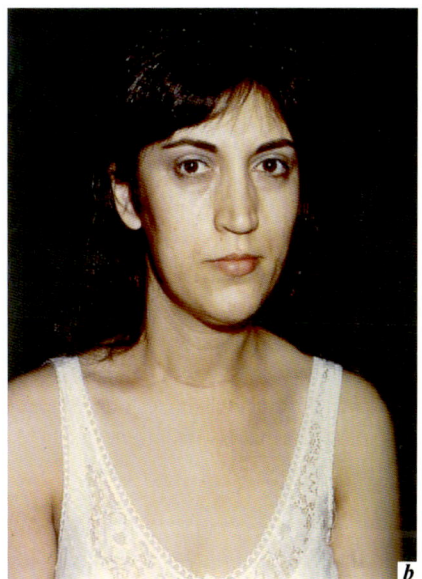

*Fig. 1.* Disappearance of lid retraction in a hyperthyroid patient (*a*) rendered euthyroid with methimazole + thyroidectomy (*b*).

serum TSH-receptor autoantibody (TRAb) and other thyroid autoantibodies levels [1, 3]. Although the pathogenic link between thyroid and orbit autoimmune phenomena remains to be definitely proven, flare up of autoimmune reactions against antigen(s) share by thyroid and orbit might cause GO progression. This is one of the arguments used to advocate permanent control of hyperthyroidism by either radioiodine therapy or thyroidectomy in Graves' patients with GO [9].

*Radioiodine*

Radioiodine therapy is the first-line treatment of Graves' hyperthyroidism in the USA [5]. Opinions on its effects on GO are controversial [1, 10–12], but results of the few available randomized studies are more concordant, because they show GO progression after radioiodine therapy in 15–37% of patients [13–15] (fig. 2). GO exacerbation is more likely in patients who had GO prior to radioiodine therapy, and can be prevented by a concomitant course of oral glucocorticoids [see below, 'Should the presence of Graves' orbitopathy limit the use of radioiodine therapy?'], which also contribute to improve pre-existing eye manifestations [13, 15]. If radioiodine is given to patients with absent or minimally active/inactive GO, progression of the eye disease is unlikely, if other risk factors [see below, 'Is there any risk factor which may predict worsening of Graves' orbitopathy after radioiodine?'] are absent [16, 17].

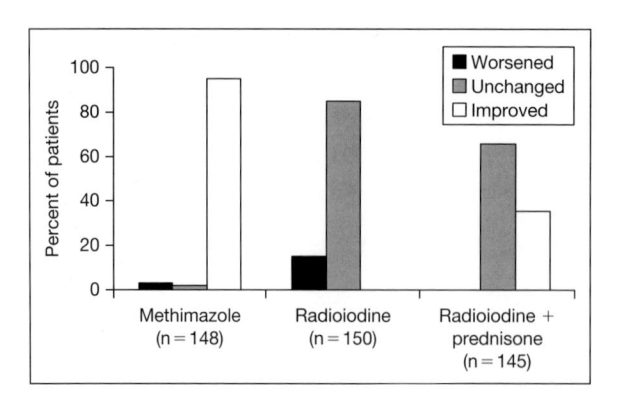

*Fig. 2.* Outcome of GO after treatment of hyperthyroidism with methimazole, radioiodine or radioiodine + prednisone in a randomized clinical trial [15].

The pathogenic mechanism responsible for radioiodine-associated progression of GO is probably related to the release of thyroid antigens after radiation injury, which might trigger or exacerbate autoimmune responses towards antigens shared by thyroid and orbit [1, 3], and/or to a transient phase of hypothyroidism associated with TSH receptor (TSHR) stimulation by TSH [18].

Although in the short-term radioiodine may be detrimental for GO, in the long-term it may have beneficial effects owing to antigen deprivation and removal of thyroid autoreactive T lymphocytes [19, 20].

*Thyroidectomy*

The issue of whether thyroidectomy affects the course of GO is also unsettled [1, 3, 7]. However, results of recent studies support the concept that thyroidectomy is not a disease-modifying treatment and does not influence the natural history of GO [1, 3, 7]. Accordingly, glucocorticoids are not needed after thyroidectomy for Graves' disease [21].

Since thyroidectomy also causes leakage of thyroid antigens, why it is not followed, as in the case of radioiodine therapy, by GO progression? This is probably due to the different temporal modality of thyroid injury (long lasting after radioiodine therapy and short lasting after surgery) and to the consequent modification of the thyroid autoimmune response [21]. Moreover, at variance with radioiodine, the initiation of levothyroxine treatment shortly after surgery may protect surgical patients from the occurrence of hypothyroidism, which, as mentioned above, may adversely affect GO [21].

In summary, thionamides and thyroidectomy do not substantially affect the course of GO, whereas radioiodine therapy is associated with GO progression

*Table 1.* Advantages and disadvantages of different treatment of hyperthyroidism

| Thyroid treatment | Advantages | Disadvantages |
|---|---|---|
| Thionamides | no effects of GO | fluctuation of thyroid function may be detrimental for GO[1] recurrence of hyperthyroidism and possible worsening of GO |
| Radioiodine | depletion of autoreactive T lymphocytes antigen deprivation | possible worsening of GO[2] |
| Thyroidectomy | depletion of autoreactive T lymphocytes antigen deprivation | surgical risk |

[1]This can be avoided by using the block-replace regimen.
[2]Worsening can be prevented by protective glucocorticoid therapy (0.5 mg/kg body weight for 1 month, gradually withdrawn over 2 months) [13, 15].

in a minority of patients. Glucocorticoid coverage should be given in at-risk patients treated with radioiodine (table 1).

### Are There Any Specific Criteria to Prefer One of the Treatment Modalities for Hyperthyroidism in Graves' Orbitopathy?

Any hyperthyroid patient with GO, independent of its severity, should receive prompt treatment with thionamides in order to restore euthyroidism. The issue discussed herein is whether the choice of subsequent treatment of hyperthyroidism in patients with GO should be made, in addition to established criteria (goitre size, age, first episode *vs.* recurrence of hyperthyroidism, etc.), on the basis of other features related to the presence of GO. In any case, a coordinated approach to the treatment of Graves' hyperthyroidism and orbitopathy should be taken.

The presence of active GO has generated two lines of thought in the last 20–30 years. The first suggests that when GO is active, it may be preferable to continue ATD treatment and, if needed, associate immunosuppression (glucocorticoids and/orbital irradiation) or orbital decompression as appropriate. The use of radioiodine or surgery would be delayed until the eye disease is burnt-out [22]. The second approach favours, in view of the pathogenic link between thyroid and orbit, definitive therapy of hyperthyroidism (radioiodine or surgery) and concomitant treatment for GO as appropriate [10]. No controlled studies are available to establish whether either approach is better.

The first approach is reasonable in mild cases of GO not requiring specific therapeutic measures (except for the local treatments) in that it allows the eye disease to run its natural course. In moderate-to-severe GO cases, the second approach might be preferred, because radioiodine or surgery might have, in the long run, a beneficial effect on GO following removal of shared thyroid antigens and autoreactive T lymphocytes [19, 20].

The identification of risk factors which are associated with an increased risk of GO worsening after radioiodine therapy should prompt to select thionamides (or thyroidectomy, when appropriate) as the treatment of choice for hyperthyroidism, or to associate glucocorticoids with radioiodine therapy.

## Is There Any Risk Factor which May Predict Worsening of Graves' Orbitopathy after Radioiodine?

GO progression after radioiodine therapy occurs only in a minority of patients (~15%). Therefore, other risk factors must contribute to this outcome. Some of these factors have been identified, including the following:

(1) Pre-existing orbitopathy (especially if active): In one study GO worsened in 17 of 72 (24%) patients with pre-existing orbitopathy and appeared only in 6 of 68 (8%) patients without eye involvement prior to radioiodine therapy [15];

(2) Severity of hyperthyroidism prior to radioiodine therapy: GO aggravation of was more likely in patients with higher serum thyroid hormone concentrations before treatment (T3 level ≥5 nmo/l) [14];

(3) High serum TSH or TSHR antibodies levels: Circumstantial evidence suggests that high serum TSH [18] or TSHR antibodies [23, 24] may also play a role in the exacerbation of GO after radioiodine;

(4) Cigarette smoking: Worsening or de novo appearance of GO is quite rare in non-smokers (4 of 68 patients, 6%), but much more frequent in smokers (19 of 82 patients, 23%) [25].

It is therefore important to collect adequate information regarding the above issues before using radioiodine therapy. In fact, identification of risk factors allows the identification of patients in whom GO is more likely to progress. In these patients, concomitant glucocorticoid therapy should be given after radioiodine therapy, since it avoids progression of eye disease [10, 13, 15, 17] [see below, 'Should the presence of Graves' orbitopathy limit the use of radioiodine therapy?'].

In addition to factors predicting the worsening of ophthalmopathy, it is very important to avoid late correction of hypothyroidism [26] [see below, 'Does transient hypothyroidism following therapy influence the course of Graves' orbitopathy?'].

## Should the Presence of Graves' Orbitopathy Limit the Use of Radioiodine Therapy?

As previously discussed [see above, 'Does it matter for the eyes how the patient is rendered euthyroid?')], radioiodine therapy carries a small but definite risk of causing progression of GO [1, 7, 13–15]. However, progression is usually observed in patients in whom other risk factors are present [see above, 'Is there any risk factor which may predict worsening of Graves' orbitopathy after radioiodine'] and can be prevented by protective glucocorticoid therapy (0.5 mg/kg body weight for 1 month, gradually withdrawn over 2 months) [13, 15]. Glucocorticoid can be safely administered after radioiodine since it does not affect the outcome of radioiodine therapy for hyperthyroidism [27]. The possible side effects of glucocorticoids and the need to complete the 2-month treatment once radioiodine has been given should be discussed with the patient before radioiodine is chosen as the treatment for hyperthyroidism.

A survey among European endocrinologists showed that the possible untoward effects of radioiodine on GO influenced their willingness to use it in GO patients with recurrent hyperthyroidism [28]. We do not share the view that radioiodine therapy should be avoided in GO patients [1, 9, 10]. Radioiodine is an effective procedure for permanent control of hyperthyroidism and can be safely used in patients with GO following the appropriate guidelines (table 2). In patients with no signs or symptoms of GO or when orbitopathy is inactive, concomitant glucocorticoid therapy may not be necessary, because a new appearance of GO is very rarely observed. Nevertheless, glucocorticoids may certainly be considered, especially if other risk factors (especially cigarette smoking) are present [7] [see above, 'Is there any risk factor which may predict worsening of Graves' orbitopathy after radioiodine?']. In any case, patients given radioiodine should be informed of the low risk of developing GO and glucocorticoids should be offered. In patients with mild and active eye disease, a 2-month course of oral glucocorticoid is recommended [10, 17]. In patients with moderate-to-severe and active GO, radioiodine therapy should be promptly followed by appropriate treatments for GO, such as high-dose intravenous glucocorticoids and/or orbital radiotherapy [1].

## Does Transient Hypothyroidism following Therapy Influence the Course of Graves' Orbitopathy?

Maintenance of stable euthyroidism during therapy with thionamides and prompt restoration of normal thyroid status after radioiodine therapy or thyroidectomy is strongly recommended. Indeed, occurrence of a transient phase

*Table 2.* Guidelines for radioiodine therapy in patients with GO

*All patients*
Restore euthyroidism with antithyroid drugs
Identify possible risk factors for worsening of GO after radioiodine (pre-existing ophthalmopathy, especially if active; severe hyperthyroidism, high serum TSH, high serum TSHR antibody levels, cigarette smoking)
Stop smoking
Start thyroxine treatment 2 weeks after radioiodine to avoid hypothyroidism

*GO absent*
Glucocorticoid coverage
　Yes (presence of risk factors, choice of the patient upon information)
　No (absence of risk factors, choice of the patient upon information)

*GO present*
Mild orbitopathy
　Glucocorticoid coverage
　　Yes (active orbitopathy and/or presence of risk factors, choice of the patient upon information)
　　No (inactive orbitopathy, absence of risk factors, choice of the patient upon information)
Moderate-severe orbitopathy
　Active
　　High-dose intravenous glucocorticoids ± orbital radiotherapy
　Inactive
　　Glucocorticoid coverage in the presence of risk factors

of hypothyroidism has been found by Karlsson et al. [23] in 6 of 15 patients developing severe eye disease after radioiodine therapy. The mechanism whereby hypothyroidism would worsen orbitopathy might involve stimulation of thyroid cells through activation of the TSH receptor by increased serum TSH levels leading to over-expression of thyroid antigens. In addition, binding of TSH to orbital TSHRs might also worsen orbitopathy.

Early administration of levothyroxine after radioiodine (starting 2 weeks after therapy) as compared with its initiation when serum TSH and/or T4 indicated hypothyroidism reduced the rate of deterioration or new occurrence of orbitopathy (18% *vs.* 11%, respectively) [26]. Thus, if patients with GO are treated with radioiodine, it is recommended to start levothyroxine therapy 2 weeks after radioiodine therapy, to carefully monitor serum thyroid hormone and TSH levels, and promptly adjust the levothyroxine dose, when needed.

Prevention of a transient hypothyroidism in GO patients submitted to thyroidectomy by the initiation of levothyroxine treatment shortly after surgery may account, at least in part, for the lack of worsening or appearance of orbitopathy in patients treated surgically [21].

## Has Total Thyroid Ablation a Role in the Management of Hyperthyroidism in Graves' Orbitopathy?

GO is generally believed to be caused by autoimmune reactions against autoantigen(s) shared by thyroid and orbital tissues sustained by intrathyroidal autoreactive T lymphocytes infiltrating the orbit. According to this hypothesis, removal of thyroid antigens and autoreactive T lymphocytes may be beneficial for GO. A recent study in patients with differentiated thyroid cancer and serum thyroid autoantibodies [29] has shown that total ablation of thyroid tissue, achieved by near-total thyroidectomy followed radioiodine administration, is associated with the disappearance of serum thyroglobulin and thyroid peroxidase antibodies within 3–5 years, indicating that removal of thyroid antigens is indeed followed by an attenuation of the autoimmune response.

The idea that total thyroid ablation might be beneficial for GO was originally introduced by Catz and Perzik [30] in the 1960s, although it was soon disputed by others [31]. In 1996, De Groot and Benjasuratwong [32], by retrospective evaluation of a relatively small series of GO patients, concluded that total thyroid ablation may be beneficial for GO. More recently, another retrospective study in a slightly larger number of patients also supported a potential beneficial effect of total thyroid ablation [33]. On the other hand, Järhult et al. [34] in a randomized clinical trial have shown that total thyroidectomy has no advantage over subtotal thyroidectomy on the course of orbitopathy but had a higher complication rate. We have recently completed a prospective, single-blind, randomized study in which 60 patients with mild-to-moderate and active GO were randomized to near-total thyroidectomy (TX) or near-total thyroidectomy + $^{131}$I (total thyroid ablati TTA), and then treated with intravenous glucocorticoids (IVGC) [35]. A significantly (p = 0.0014) better outcome of GO was observed at 9 months in TTA than in TX patients (fig. 3). Radioiodine uptake test and thyroglobulin assay showed complete ablation of thyroid tissue in the majority of TTA, but not of TX patients. Thus, compared with TX alone, TTA is followed by a better short-term outcome of GO in patients given IVGC. Whether TTA maintains this advantage in the long term remains to be established. Our results suggest that total thyroid ablation may be useful in any Graves' patient with clinically relevant GO in whom thyroid surgery is indicated on the basis of standardized criteria. The difference between our results and those of Järhult et al. [34] might be related to the possibility that in the latter study a true total thyroid ablation was not achieved.

In patients with long-standing GO, the orbital autoimmune process is probably maintained by mechanisms which are independent of the evolution of thyroid autoimmunity. In these patients, total thyroid ablation will probably be unable to improve the evolution of GO.

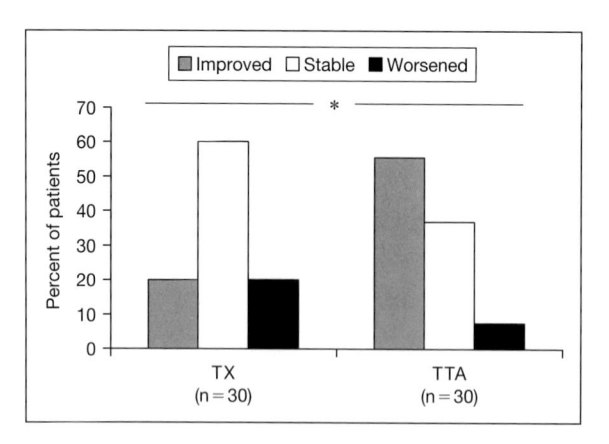

*Fig. 3.* Overall outcome of GO after treatment of hyperthyroidism with near-total thyroidectomy (TX) or near-total thyroidectomy + $^{131}$I therapy (total thyroid ablation; TTA) in patients also given intravenous glucocorticoids in a randomized clinical trial [35]. *p = 0.0014.

## References

1 Bartalena L, Pinchera A, Marcocci C: Management of Graves' ophthalmopathy: reality and perspectives. Endocr Rev 2000;21:168–199.
2 Marcocci C, Bartalena L, Bogazzi F, Panicucci M, Pinchera A: Studies on the occurrence of ophthalmopathy in Graves' disease. Acta Endocrinol (Copenh) 1989;120:473–478.
3 Marcocci C, Bartalena L, Bogazzi F, Bruno-Bossio G, Pinchera A: Relationship between Graves' ophthalmopathy and type of treatment of Graves' hyperthyroidism. Thyroid 1992;2:171–178.
4 Perros P, Crombie AL, Kendall-Taylor P: Natural history of thyroid-associated ophthalmopathy. Clin Endocrinol (Oxf) 1995;42:45–50.
5 Solomon B, Glinoer D, Lagasse R, Wartofsky L: Current trends in the management of Graves' disease. J Clin Endocrinol Metab 1990;70:1518–1524.
6 Prummel MF, Wiersinga WM, Mourits MP, Koornneef L, Berghout A, van der Gaag R: Amelioration of eye changes of Graves' ophthalmopathy by achieving euthyroidism. Acta Endocrinol (Copenh) 1989;121(suppl 2):185–189.
7 Bartalena L, Tanda ML, Piantanida E, Lai A, Pinchera A: Relationship between management of hyperthyroidism and course of the ophthalmopathy. J Endocrinol Invest 2004;27:288–294.
8 Vitti P, Rago T, Chiovato L, Pallini S, Santini F, Fiore E, Rocchi R, Martino E, Pinchera A: Clinical features of patients with Graves' disease undergoing remission after antithyroid drug treatment. Thyroid 1997;7:369–375.
9 Marcocci C, Bartalena L, Pinchera A: Ablative or non-ablative therapy for Graves' hyperthyroidism in patients with ophthalmopathy? J Endocrinol Invest 1998;21:468–471.
10 Pinchera A, Bartalena L, Marcocci C: Radioiodine may be bad for Graves' ophthalmopathy, but.... J Clin Endocrinol Metab 1995;80:342–345.
11 Bonnema SJ, Bartalena L, Toft AD, Hegedüs L: Controversies in radioiodine therapy: relation to ophthalmopathy, the possible radioprotective effect of antithyroid drugs, and the use in large goiters. Eur J Endocrinol 2002;147:1–11.
12 Gorman CA: Radioiodine therapy does not aggravate Graves' ophthalmopathy. J Clin Endocrinol Metab 1995;80:340–342.

13 Bartalena L, Marcocci C, Bogazzi F, Panicucci M, Lepri A, Pinchera A: Use of corticosteroids to prevent progression of Graves' ophthalmopathy after radioiodine therapy for hyperthyroidism. N Engl J Med 1989;321:1349–1352.
14 Tallstedt L, Lundell G, Torring O, Wallin G, Ljunggren J-G, Blomgren H, Taube A, the Thyroid Study Group: Occurrence of ophthalmopathy after treatment for Graves' hyperthyroidism. N Engl J Med 1992;326:1733–1738.
15 Bartalena L, Marcocci C, Bogazzi F, Manetti L, Tanda ML, Dell'Unto E, Bruno-Bossio G, Nardi M, Bartolomei MP, Lepri A, Rossi G, Martino E, Pinchera A: Relation between therapy for hyperthyroidism and the course of Graves' ophthalmopathy. N Engl J Med 1998;338:73–78.
16 Perros P, Kendall-Taylor P, Neoh C, Frewin S, Dickinson J: A prospective study on the effects of radioiodine therapy for hyperthyroidism in patients with minimally active Graves' ophthalmopathy. J Clin Endocrinol Metab 2005;90:5321–5323.
17 Bartalena L: Editorial: Glucocorticoids for Graves' ophthalmopathy: how and when. J Clin Endocrinol Metab 2005;90:5497–5499.
18 Kung AWC, Yau CC, Cheng A: The incidence of ophthalmopathy after radioiodine therapy for Graves' disease: prognostic factors and the role of methimazole. J Clin Endocrinol Metab 1994;79:542–546.
19 Teng W-P, Stark R, Munro AJ, Young SM, Borysiewicz LK, Weetman AP: Peripheral blood T cell activation after radioiodine treatment for Graves' disease. Acta Endocrinol (Copenh) 1990;122:233–240.
20 DeGroot LJ: Radioiodine and the immune system. Thyroid 1997;7:259–264.
21 Marcocci C, Bruno-Bossio G, Manetti L, Tanda ML, Miccoli P, Iacconi P, Bartolomei MP, Nardi M, Pinchera A, Bartalena L: The course of Graves' ophthalmopathy is not influenced by near-total thyroidectomy: a case-control study. Clin Endocrinol (Oxf) 1999;51:503–508.
22 Wiersinga WM: Preventing Graves' ophthalmopathy. N Engl J Med 1998;338:121–122.
23 Karlsson Af, Westermark K, Dahlberg PA, Jansson R, Enoksson P: Ophthalmopathy and thyroid stimulation. Lancet 1989;ii:691.
24 Eckstein AK, Plicht M, Lax H, Neuhäuser M, Mann K, Lederbogen S, Heckmann C, Esser J, Morgenthaler NG: Thyrotropin receptor autoantibodies are independent risk factors for Graves' ophthalmopathy and help to predict severity and outcome of the disease. J Clin Endocrinol Metab 2006;91:3464–3470.
25 Bartalena L, Marcocci C, Tanda ML, Manetti L, Dell'Unto E, Bartolomei MP, Nardi M, Martino E, Pinchera A: Cigarette smoking and treatment outcomes in Graves ophthalmopathy. Ann Intern Med 1998;129:632–635.
26 Tallstedt L, Lundell G, Blomgren H, Bring J: Does early administration of thyroxine reduce the development of Graves' ophthalmopathy after radioiodine treatment? Eur J Endocrinol 1994;130:494–497.
27 Jensen BE, Bonnema SJ, Hegedüs I: Glucocorticoids do no influence the effect of radioiodine therapy in Graves' disease. Eur J Endocrinol 2005;153:15–21.
28 Weetman A, Wiersinga WM: Current management of thyroid associated ophthalmopathy in Europe. Results of an international survey. Clin Endocrinol (Oxf) 1988;49:21–28.
29 Chiovato L, Latrofa F, Braverman LE, Pacini F, Capezzone M, Masserini L, Grasso L, Pinchera A: Disappearance of humoral thyroid autoimmunity after complete removal of thyroid antigens. Ann Intern Med 2003;139:346–351.
30 Catz B, Perzik SL: Total thyroidectomy in the management of thyrotoxic and euthyroid Graves' disease. Am J Surg 1969;118:434–438.
31 Werner SC, Feind CR, Aida M: Graves' disease and total thyroidectomy. Progression of severe eye changes and decrease in serum long-acting thyroid stimulator after operation. N Eng J Med 1967;276:132–138.
32 De Groot LJ, Benjasuratwong Y: Evaluation of thyroid ablative therapy for ophthalmopathy of Graves' disease. Orbit 1996;15:187–196.
33 Moleti M, Mattina F, Salamone I, Violi MA, Numera C, Bardari S, Lo Schiavo MG, Regalbuto C, Trimarchi F, Vermiglio F: Effects of thyroidectomy alone or followed by radioiodine ablation of thyroid remnants on the outcome of Graves' ophthalmopathy. Thyroid 2003;13:653–658.
34 Järhult J, Rudberg C, Larsson E, Selvander H, Sjövall K, Winsa B, Rastad J, Karlsson FA, the TEO Study Group: Graves' disease with moderate-severe endocrine ophthalmopathy: long term results

of a prospective randomized study of total or subtotal thyroid resection. Thyroid 2005;15: 1157–1164.
35   Menconi F, Marinò M, Pinchera A, Rocchi R, Mazzi B, Nardi M, Bartalena L, Marcocci C: Effects of total thyroid ablation vs. total thyroidectomy alone on the short term outcome of mild to moderate Graves' orbitopathy treated with intravenous glucocorticoids. J Clin Endoc Metab 2007;92:1653–1658.

Prof. Claudio Marcocci
Department of Endocrinology and Metabolism, University of Pisa
Via Paradisa 2
IT–56124 Pisa (Italy)
Tel. +39 05099 5001, Fax +39 05099 5078, E-Mail c.marcocci@endoc.med.unipi.it

# Management of Mild Graves' Orbitopathy

*Mario Salvi[a], Nicola Currò[b]*

[a]Endocrine Unit, Departments of Medical Science, and [b]Department of Ophthalmology, University of Milan, Fondazione Ospedale Maggiore Policlinico IRCCS, Milan, Italy

## What Is the Degree of Intra-Orbital Involvement in Mild Graves' Orbitopathy?

Mild GO is usually diagnosed based on the assessment of soft tissue inflammation, in particular eyelid and conjunctival edema and hyperaemia, mild proptosis (<25 mm) and only minor, if any, eye muscle involvement [1] (fig. 1) [see chapter by Dickinson, pp. 1–26]. In a proportion of patients, eye muscles may be significantly involved [2], although motility tests may not reveal the actual degree of inflammation unless orbital imaging is performed [3, 4]. Orbital changes in mild GO are sometimes uniquely limited to eye muscles in the absence of soft tissue inflammation [5]. Recent work has shown that eye muscle enlargement by itself may be more significantly correlated to proptosis than retroocular fat and connective tissue hypertrophy [6].

## Are Mild Forms of Graves' Orbitopathy Likely to Progress to More Severe Graves' Orbitopathy?

Progression of GO occurs during the active phase of the disease and although several studies have sought indicators for predicting response to treatment [7–13], very few of the available data have proven useful to predict progression of GO from mild to more severe forms at the first clinical examination. To date, the most reliable method of predicting potential progression of GO relies on clinical monitoring of patients by calculating at each examination the CAS and classifying severity by NOSPECS [13, 14]. Recent work from Eckstein et al. [15] has shown that severity of GO can be predicted based on the serum levels of TRAb at 5–8 months from disease onset, but does not provide data on

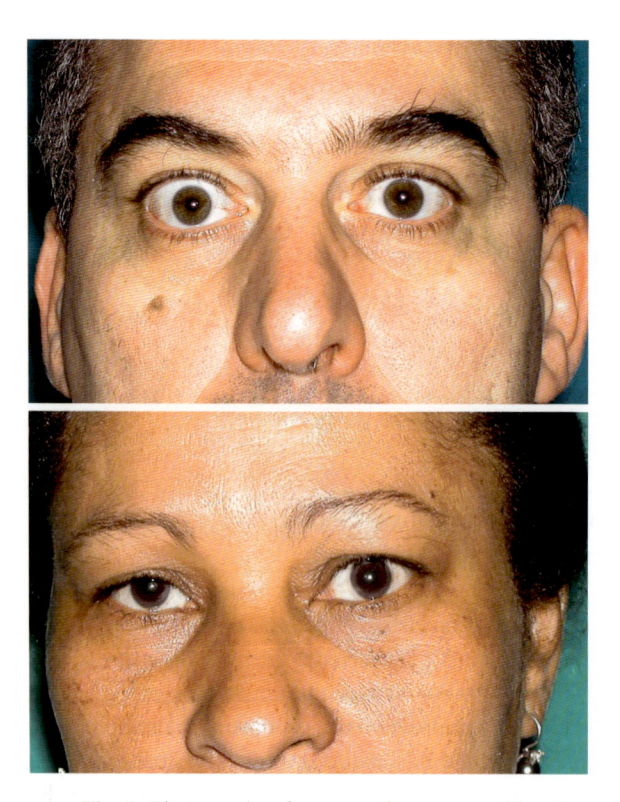

*Fig. 1.* Photographs of a man and a woman with active mild Graves' ophthalmopathy.

the number of patients with mild GO progressing to severe disease. The few data available on spontaneous progression of mild forms of GO can be drawn from two randomized controlled studies on the efficacy of radiotherapy, by looking at the follow-up data of the sham-irradiated controls groups [16, 17]. In both these studies progression was observed in 15–16% of patients. Progression of mild GO may also occur after radioactive iodine thyroid ablation for recurrence of hyperthyroidism in a limited number of patients who are to be considered at risk because of smoking, high serum TRAb and active disease [18]. Patients with mild GO account for approximately 40% of all patients with GO seen within the multidisciplinary centres of the EUGOGO [1].

## Is a 'Wait and See' Policy Justified in Mild Graves' Orbitopathy?

There are few studies addressing the issue of spontaneous evolution of GO. Perros et al. [19] have observed that up to 64% of patients with GO not subjected

*Table 1.* Management of mild Graves' ophthalmopathy

| To treat or not to treat? | |
|---|---|
| Reasons for treating | eye muscle involvement |
| | disease progression |
| | deterioration of patients' quality of life |
| | chances of relevant residual orbital disease |
| Reasons for not treating | adverse effects of treatment |
| | questionable efficacy on the degree of residual disease |
| | spontaneous improvement |
| | cost-effectiveness |

to therapy improved spontaneously when assessed at 3-monthly intervals. More recently, in a slightly larger series of 81 patients treated only with local protective agents, spontaneous improvement was observed in about 47% independently of the degree of severity according to NOSPECS (classes 2–4) [20]. In the latter study, patients with mild disease who improved with no or only local therapy were 46%, whereas another 51% remained unchanged and only one worsened. In sham-irradiated control patients from randomized studies on the effect of radiotherapy, a spontaneous improvement was observed in about 30% [16, 17]. Data from the EUGOGO centres show that about 44% patients with mild GO were indeed advised specific treatment, perhaps in relation to the reported decrease of quality of life [1] [see chapter by Wiersinga, pp. 201–211]. Reasonable arguments for treating mild GO may be based on: (1) the involvement of eye muscles, often unrecognized unless orbital imaging is performed, and solely associated to mild proptosis, as observed in some studies [see above, 'What is the degree of intra-orbital involvement in mild Graves' orbitopathy']; (2) the chances of progression, probably very low but not clearly predictable; (3) the patient's quality of life deterioration, and (4) the physician's concern about the degree of residual disease. On the other hand, arguments for not treating may also rely on: (1) the potential side effects of either steroids or radiotherapy; (2) the outcome of therapy and its actual impact on residual disease; (3) the possibility of spontaneous disease improvement; (4) the concern about the cost-effectiveness of treatment (table 1). While 'waiting and seeing', patients can be managed with supportive measures: these are in fact effective in most patients. For instance, patients can control symptoms of dry eyes with lubricating eye drops and can obviate marked lid retraction by taping their eyes shut at night to avoid excessive irritation and corneal damage. Patients should also be advised to eliminate the modifiable risk factors, such as smoking and an uncontrolled underlying thyroid dysfunction.

## Are Low-Dosage Oral Steroids Advisable or Is Orbital Irradiation Preferable?

Both therapies have a non-specific anti-inflammatory action as well as a limited immunosuppressive effect on orbital lymphocytes. The response to steroids is typically seen in 1–2 weeks and is characterized by improvement of soft tissue signs and ocular motility. Steroids are effective at high doses and, since their use is associated with morbidity even when administered intravenously, they are generally not indicated in mild GO [21]. A low-dosage therapeutic regimen of oral prednisone has only been used with a satisfactory effect by Bartalena et al. [18] in the prevention of occurrence or progression of GO after radioactive iodine administration. The therapeutic response to orbital irradiation is first seen at 2–3 weeks but a more gradual improvement is evident for several months [22]. Unless concomitant steroid treatment is used, short-term increased inflammation may initially appear as a side effect of the radiation, thereby masking the improvement in soft tissue involvement. The major advantage of orbital radiotherapy is the lack of complications. The question is if it is really effective in reducing the period of disease activity and the need for rehabilitative surgery, when the disease is burnt out. Two controlled studies have reported a significant effect of radiotherapy in GO, but were performed in patients with moderate-to-severe forms of the disease [16, 23]. Gorman et al. [24], by irradiating only one orbit and using the other one as an internal control, did not show any significant effect of therapy on the volumes of eye muscles measured by orbital CT scan in patients with mild GO. Although these negative results could have been due to the inclusion of patients with inactive disease, a proportion of whom had also been treated with steroids, that study has questioned the opportunity to treat mild GO with radiotherapy [25]. A recent randomized and controlled study by Prummel et al. [17] has shown that orbital radiotherapy is effective in mild GO and improvement, mainly on eye motility, was observed in 52% irradiated compared to 27% non-irradiated patients, likely due to the effect on eye muscle infiltrating lymphocytes. They suggest that changes of the function of eye muscles may be more relevant than those of volume when one wants to assess response to treatment in GO. It is of interest that in this study control patients with mild GO, who were sham-irradiated, showed improvement, no change or worsening of disease in line with what reported in the study on the natural history by Perros et al. [19]. Unfortunately, no conclusive answer could be given as to whether radiotherapy is better than a 'wait and see' approach in mild GO, since treatment did not improve the quality of life of patients and was not cost effective. In addition, radiotherapy did not prevent disease worsening, observed in about 15% of patients, and this data argues against an immunosuppressive effect of this treatment.

*Table 2.* Adverse effects of radiotherapy in Graves' ophthalmopathy

| Occurrence | Effect | Patients affected | Management |
|---|---|---|---|
| Short term | transient worsening of soft tissue inflammation and hair loss at the temples | many | possibly steroids |
| Long term | cataract induction | 5% (>60 years of age)* | avoid steroids, may also cause cataract |
| | definite radiation retinopathy | 0.9–2% hypertensive, diabetic patients | avoid treating diabetic patients |
| | secondary cancer | none (median follow-up 25 years) | avoid treating patients <35 years of age |

*From Marcocci et al. [32]: patients were also treated with steroids.

## Can We Reassure Patients About the Long-Term Safety of Orbital Irradiation?

Radiotherapy is well tolerated and has almost no short-term side effects, except for an acute exacerbation of soft tissue inflammation [26]. Potential long-term complications of irradiation have been a major concern for its use in GO, particularly in milder forms. While radiation-induced tumours have not been observed in GO patients [27, 28], several reports of severe retinopathy have been reported either induced by dosimetric and technique errors [29] or because of coexisting diabetes [30]. Increased cataract induction is also a concern since the lens is within the radiation beam [31]. Two recent retrospective studies have produced reassuring evidence on the long-term safety of radiotherapy in GO (table 2). Marcocci et al. [32] have studied 204 patients with moderate-to-severe GO and have observed a prevalence of cataract of 10% in patients irradiated with a high voltage linear accelerator, a figure comparable to the incidence of cataract in a non GO population of the same age. Possible radiation-induced retinopathy was detected in only 2 patients both with associated hypertension and one who also had diabctes. Wakelkamp et al. [33] conducted a follow-up study on 245 patients with moderate-to-severe GO treated with radiotherapy and found a prevalence of cataract of 29%, not different from the prevalence of 34% observed in GO patients treated with steroids only. Retinal changes were seen more frequently in irradiated than non-irradiated eyes (21 vs. 2%); however, these changes consisted mostly of 1–5 microaneurysms that did not interfere with visual acuity. Orbital irradiation was only associated with retinopathy in diabetic patients (relative risk 21, 95% confidence interval,

3–179). Diabetes mellitus is, therefore, a contraindication for orbital radiotherapy. Both these latter studies [32, 33] did not show radiation-induced tumours or increased mortality, although the duration of follow-up (median 11 years) may not be long enough to rule out an increased lifetime risk of cancer. From these data, it seems reasonable to reassure patients about the long-term safety of orbital radiotherapy, which can be proposed as a treatment option in patients with mild GO, with the exception of those with diabetes and hypertension or younger than 35 years of age [32].

## What Is the Rationale for Antioxidant Therapy in GO?

Oxygen free radicals (OFR) have been reported to be involved in the pathogenesis of GO. Studies that have linked the high prevalence of smokers to GO [34] have shown that smoking causes hypoxia within the organ tissues involved in the orbital changes of the disease [35]. OFR have been shown to be present in orbital tissues and to be involved in IL-1β-induced glycosaminoglycans accumulation [36]. OFR also induced expression of heat-shock protein 72 in retroocular fibroblasts of patients with GO [37] and caused their proliferation that could in part be inhibited by methimazole, allopurinol and nicotinamide [38]. Indices of OFR generation have been found to be increased in the serum of patients with GO and were normalized by corticosteroid therapy [39]. Despite this relevant experimental evidence, data on the clinical use of antioxidants in GO are limited. In a controlled non-randomized study vs. placebo, Bouzas et al. [40] were able to show a significant improvement of NOSPECS signs in patients treated with allopurinol and nicotinamide for 3 months. The improvement was satisfactory for soft tissue signs and motility but not for proptosis reduction. Interestingly, there were no reported side effects and the patients were all smokers. This poses the question whether smokers are more susceptible to benefit from antioxidants or, alternatively, whether non-smokers would have even a greater beneficial effect from these drugs. Pentoxifylline is a cytokine-modulating drug and is also regarded as an antioxidant. Its effect on 10 patients with active moderate-to-severe GO has been examined in a pilot, non-controlled study by Balazs et al. [41]. Eight patients showed soft tissue improvement, but no change in proptosis and ocular motility. More recently, a placebo-controlled, randomized study on 18 women with inactive GO showed significant proptosis reduction and improvement of quality of life in those treated with pentoxifylline compared to placebo [42]. In contrast to most pharmacological therapies aimed to control active GO, in this study pentoxifylline seems to offer an alternative to surgical treatment of inactive disease. All these preliminary results, albeit promising, need to be confirmed by properly conducted randomized, controlled clinical studies. Antioxidants might become an interesting option in the treatment of mild GO, perhaps in preventing progression to more severe forms.

## References

1 Prummel MF, Bakker A, Wiersinga WM, Baldeschi L, Mourits M, Kendall-Taylor P, Perros P, Neoh C, Dickinson AJ, Lazarus JH, Lane CM, Heufelder AE, Kahaly GJ, Pitz S, Orgiazzi J, Hullo A, Pinchera A, Marcocci C, Sartini MS, Rocchi R, Nardi M, Krassas GE, Halkias A: Multicenter study on the characteristics and treatment strategies of patients with Graves' orbitopathy: the first European Group on Graves' Orbitopathy experience. Eur J Endocrinol 2003;148: 491–495.
2 Mourits M, Prummel MF, Wiersinga WM, Koornneef L: Measuring eye movements in Graves' ophthalmopathy. Ophthalmology 1994;101:1341–1346.
3 Ohnishi T, Noguchi S, Murakami N, Tajiri J, Harao M, Kawamoto H, Hoshi H, Jinnouchi S, Futami S, Nagamachi S, Watanabe K: Extraocular muscles in Graves' ophthalmopathy: usefulness of T2 relaxation time measurements. Radiology 1994;190:857–862.
4 Ozgen A, Alp MN, Ariyurek M, Tutuncu NB, Can I, Gunalp I: Quantitative CT of the orbit in Graves' disease. Br J Radiol 1999;72:757–762.
5 Mikozami T, Salvi M, Wall JR: Eye muscle antibodies in Graves' ophthalmopathy pathogenic or secondary epiphenomenon? J Endocrinol Invest 2004;27:221–229.
6 Kvetny J, Puhakka KB, Rohl L: Magnetic resonance imaging determination of extraocular eye muscle volume in patients with thyroid-associated ophthalmopathy and proptosis. Acta Ophthalmol Scand 2006;84:419–423.
7 Kahaly G, Schuler M, Sewell AC, Bernhard G, Beyer J, Krause U: Urinary glycosaminoglycans in Graves' ophthalmopathy. Clin Endocrinol 1990;33:35–44.
8 Hiromatsu Y, Kojima K, Ishisaka N, Tanaka K, Sato M, Nonaka K, Nishimura H, Nishida H: Role of magnetic resonance imaging in thyroid-associated ophthalmopathy: its predictive value for therapeutic outcome of immunosuppressive therapy. Thyroid 1992;2:299–305.
9 Prummel MF, Suttorp-Schulten MSA, Wiersinga WM, Verbeck AM, Mourits MP, Koornneef L: A new ultrasonographic method to detect disease activity and predict response to immunosuppressive treatment in Graves' ophthalmopathy. Ophthalmology 1993;100:556–561.
10 Gerding MN, Prummel MF, Wiersinga WM: Assessment of disease activity in Graves' ophthalmopathy by orbital ultrasonography and clinical parameters. Clin Endocrinol 2000;52:641–646.
11 Colao A, Lastoria S, Ferone D, Pivonello R, Macchia PE, Vassallo P, Bonavolontà G, Muto P, Lombardi G, Fenzi GF: Orbital scintigraphy with [$^{111}$In-diethylenetriamine pentaacetic acid-D-phel]-octreotide predicts the clinical response to corticosteroid therapy in patients with Graves' ophthalmopathy. J Clin Endocrinol Metab 1998;83:3790–3794.
12 Krassas GE, Dumas A, Pontikedes N, Kaltsas T: Somatostatin receptor scintigraphy and octreotide treatment in patients with thyroid eye disease. Clin Endocrinol 1995;42:571–580.
13 Terwee CB, Prummel MF, Gerding MN, Kahaly GJ, Dekker FW, Wiersinga WM: Measuring disease activity to predict therapeutic outcome in Graves' ophthalmopathy. Clin Endocrinol 2005;62: 145–155.
14 Mourits MP, Prummel MF, Wiersinga WM, Koornneef L: Clinical activity score as a guide in the management of patients with Graves' ophthalmopathy. Clin Endocrinol 1997;47:9–14.
15 Eckstein AK, Plicht M, Hildegard L, Neuhauser M, Mann K, Lederbogen S, Heckmann C, Esser J, Morgenthaler NG: TSH-receptor autoantibodies are independent risk factors for Graves' ophthalmopathy and help to predict severity and outcome of the disease. J Clin Endocrinol Metab 2006;91:3464–3470.
16 Mourits MP, van Kempen-Hartenveld ML, Garcia MB, Koppeschaar HPF, Tick L, Terwee CB: Randomized placebo-controlled study of radiotherapy for Graves' ophthalmopathy. Lancet 2000; 355:1505–1509.

17  Prummel MF, Terwee CB, Gerding MN, Baldeschi L, Mourits MP, Blank L, Dekker FW, Wiersinga WM: A randomized controlled trial of orbital radiotherapy versus sham irradiation in patients with mild Graves' ophthalmopathy. J Clin Endocrinol Metab 2004;89:15–20.
18  Bartalena L, Marcocci C, Bogazzi F, Manetti L, Tanda ML, Dell'Unto E, Bruno-Bossio G, Nardi M, Bartolomei MP, Lepri A, Rossi G, Martino E, Pinchera A: Relation between therapy for hyperthyroidism and the course of Graves' ophthalmopathy. N Engl J Med 1998;338:73–78.
19  Perros P, Crombie AL, Kendall-Taylor P: Natural history of thyroid associated ophthalmopathy. Clin Endocrinol 1995;42:45–50.
20  Noth D, Gebauer M, Muller B, Burgi U, Diem P: Graves' ophthalmopathy: natural history and treatment outcomes. Swiss Med Wkly 2001;131:603–609.
21  Modjtahedi SP, Modjtahedi BS, Mansury AM, Selva D, Douglas RS, Goldberg RA, Leibovitch I: Pharmacological treatments for thyroid eye disease. Drugs 2006;66:1685–1700.
22  Cockerham KP, Kennerdell JS: Does radiotherapy have a role in the management of thyroid orbitopathy? View 1. Br J Ophthalmol 2002;86:102–104.
23  Prummel MF, Mourits MP, Blank L, Berghout A, Koornneef L: Randomized double-blind trial of prednisone versus radiotherapy in Graves' ophthalmopathy. Lancet 1993;342:949–954.
24  Gorman CA, Garrity JA, Fatourechi V, Bahn RS, Petersen IA, Stafford SL, Earle JD, Forbes GS, Kline RW, Bergstralh EJ, Offord KP, Rademacher DM, Stanley NM, Bartley GB: A prospective, randomized, double-blind, placebo-controlled study of orbital radiotherapy for Graves' ophthalmopathy. Ophthalmology 2001;108:1523–1534.
25  McNab A: Does radiotherapy have a role in the management of thyroid orbitopathy? Comment. Br J Ophthalmol 2002;86:106–107.
26  Bartalena L, Marcocci C, Tanda ML, Rocchi R, Mazzi B, Barbesino G, Pinchera A: Orbital radiotherapy for Graves' ophthalmopathy. Thyroid 2002;12:245–250.
27  Marquez SD, Lum BL, McDougall IR, Katkuri S, Levin PS, MacManus PS, Donaldson SS: Long-term results of irradiation for patients with Graves' ophthalmopathy. Int J Radiat Oncol Biol Phys 2001;51:766–774.
28  Schaefer U, Hesselmann S, Micke O, Schueller Bruns F, Palma C, Willich N: A long-term follow-up study after retro-orbital irradiation for Graves' ophthalmopathy. Int J Radiat Oncol Biol Phys 2002;52:192–197.
29  Kinyoun JL, Kalina RE, Brower SA, Mills RP, Johnson RH: Radiation retinopathy after orbital irradiation for Graves' ophthalmopathy. Arch Ophthalmol 1984;102:1473–1476.
30  Archer DB, Amoaku WM, Gardiner TA: Radiation retinopathy: clinical, histopathological, ultrastructural and experimental correlations. Eye 1991;5:239–251.
31  Beckendorf V, Maalouf T, George J-L, Bey P, Leclere J, Luporsi E: Place of radiotherapy in the treatment of Graves' orbitopathy. Int J Radiat Oncol Biol Phys 1999;43:805–815.
32  Marcocci C, Bartalena L, Rocchi R, Marinò M, Menconi F, Morabito E, Mazzi B, Mazzeo S, Sartini MS, Nardi M, Cartei F, Cionini L, Pinchera A: Long-term safety of orbital radiotherapy for Graves' ophthalmopathy. J Clin Endocrinol Metab 2003;88:3561–3566.
33  Wakelkamp IM, Tan H, Saeed P, Schlingemann RO, Verbraak FD, Blank L, Prummel MF, Wiersinga WM: Orbital irradiation for Graves' ophthalmopathy: Is it safe? A long-term follow-up study. Ophthalmology 2004;111:1557–1562.
34  Hagg E, Asplund K: Is endocrine ophthalmopathy related to smoking? Br Med J 1987;295:634–635.
35  Shine B, Fells P, Edwards OM, Weetman AP: Association between Graves' ophthalmopathy and smoking. Lancet 1990;335:1261–1263.
36  Lu R, Wang P, Wartofsky L, Sutton BD, Zweier JL, Bahn RS, Garrity J, Burman KD: Oxygen free radicals in interleukin-1β-induced glycosaminoglycan production by retro-ocular fibroblasts from normal subjects and Graves' ophthalmopathy patients. Thyroid 1999;9:297–303.
37  Heufelder AE, Wenzel BE, Bahn RS: Methimazole and propylthiouracil inhibit the oxygen free radical-induced expression of a 72 kilodalton heat shock protein in Graves' retroocular fibroblasts. J Clin Endocrinol Metab 1992;73:307–313.
38  Burch HB, Lahiri S, Bahn RS, Barnes S: Superoxide radical production stimulates retroocular fibroblast proliferation in Graves' ophthalmopathy. Exp Eye Res 1997;65:311–316.
39  Bednarek J, Wysocki H, Sowinski J: Peripheral parameters of oxidative stress in patients with infiltrative Graves' ophthalmopathy treated with corticosteroids. Immunol Lett 2004;93:227–232.

40 Bouzas EA, Karadimas P, Mastorakos G, Koutras DA: Antioxidant agents in the treatment of Graves' ophthalmopathy. Am J Ophthalmol 2000;129:618–622.
41 Balasz C, Kiss E, Vamos A, Molnar I, Farid NR: Beneficial effect of pentoxifylline on thyroid associated ophthalmopathy (TAO): a pilot study. J Clin Endocrinol Metab 1997;82:1999–2002.
42 Finamor FE, Martins JRM, Nakanami D, Paiva ER, Manso PG, Furlanetto RP: Pentoxifylline (PTX) – An alternative treatment in Graves' ophthalmopathy (inactive phase): assessment by a disease specific quality of life questionnaire and by exophthalmometry in a prospective randomized trial. Eur J Ophthalmol 2004;14:277–283.

Dr. Mario Salvi
Endocrine Unit, Department of Medical Sciences
Fondazione Ospedale Maggiore Policlinico IRCCS, University of Milan
IT–20122 Milan (Italy)
Tel. +39 02 5032 0609, Fax +39 02 5032 0605, E-Mail mariomich@lombardiacom.it

Wiersinga WM, Kahaly GJ (eds): Graves' Orbitopathy: A Multidisciplinary Approach.
Basel, Karger, 2007, pp 120–152

# Management of Moderately Severe Graves' Orbitopathy

*George J. Kahaly*

Department of Medicine I, Gutenberg University Hospital, Mainz, Germany

## Is Immunosuppression Indicated in Moderately Severe Graves' Orbitopathy?

The aim of immune modulation and/or suppression in active and moderately severe Graves' orbitopathy (GO) is to avoid surgery altogether, or to decrease the activity of the inflammation in order to improve surgical outcomes. It must be kept in mind that immunosuppressive treatment does not rule out the possibility or the need of subsequent surgery if the GO remains severe and/or active. Thus, the first step before starting specific orbital therapy is to establish whether GO is clinically severe and active [1].

The concept of disease activity in GO might explain why as many as one-third of the patients do not respond to immunosuppressive treatment, because only patients in the active stage of disease are expected to respond. Indeed, regardless of the modality applied, a beneficial response is observed in only two-thirds of the patients. What are the reasons for this consistently low response rate? First, it may be that we need stronger immunosuppressive regimens to increase the response rate. A second possible explanation for a low response rate is the selection of patients. Most physicians will use medical treatment in patients when there is moderate-to-severe GO. In other words, patients are selected on the basis of disease severity. It can be appreciated that rather severe GO can also be present in patients with inactive disease who are not likely to respond to immunosuppression. If these inactive patients with severe, though fibrotic, disease are included in studies, this will decrease the response rate considerably. It thus appears that we should select our patients not only on the basis of disease severity, but also on the basis of disease activity. Recently, in multivariate analyses, it was found that both soft tissue involvement and inflammation, as well as eye muscle reflectivity in orbital ultrasound and octreotide uptake ratio as signs of disease activity were significant predictors of a response to conservative therapy [2–4]. Again soft tissue involvement, duration of GO, and urinary glycosaminoglycan excretion were significant predictors of no change upon radiotherapy. Thus disease '(in)activity' should determine which kind of treatment should be used.

### What Are the Results of Randomized Trials with Steroids?

*Oral Glucocorticoids*

Glucocorticoids are the most common immunosuppressants used in the treatment of active and severe GO and have been used with good success since the 1950s. Numerous randomized trials have demonstrated the efficacy of steroid therapy in GO (table 1). Steroids probably serve in multiple capacities by suppressing immune function and decreasing inflammation, such as interference with the function of T and B lymphocytes; through reduction in the recruitment of monocytes, and macrophages; by inhibition of the function of immunocompetent cells [5]; by inhibition of the release of inflammatory mediators (cytokines, prostaglandins), and by decreasing glycosaminoglycan synthesis and secretion through activated orbital fibroblasts. Any patient with acute severe orbital inflammation and congestion should be considered for steroid treatment. Such patients present with significant chemosis and periorbital edema, and a course of systemic steroids in these patients will often result in a dramatic improvement in acute symptoms and health related quality of life within a matter of days [6–11]. Glucocorticoids have a proven beneficial effect on soft tissue swelling, visual acuity, and ocular motility whereas the effect on proptosis is rather limited. During the active phase of extraocular myositis early suppression of orbital inflammation by steroids may limit damage to eye muscles and decrease the risk of protracted diplopia caused by post-inflammatory intramuscular fibrosis. Steroids are also the first-line treatment for patients with severe GO, particularly where there is a threat to vision. They are most effective when given early in the course of the disease. After an initial dose of 1 mg/kg BW/day of oral prednisolone, the dose can be reduced stepwise over the ensuing few weeks depending on the response, which needs to be monitored frequently by ophthalmic assessment. The rate at which steroid dosage can be tapered will depend on the clinical response, but decreasing the daily dosage by 5–10 mg/week is usually a safe guideline. Unfortunately, some patients will develop a recurrence of symptoms during or upon completion of the steroid taper and will require long-term treatment (fig. 1). Cigarette smoking decreases the efficacy of steroid treatment [12]. In a prospective study involving patients

*Table 1.* Oral steroid monotherapy (randomized trials)

| | n | Starting dose, mg/day | Cumulative dose, g | Treatment period, weeks | Response rate | Side effects (major/moderate) |
|---|---|---|---|---|---|---|
| Bartalena et al. [30], 1983 | 12 | 70–80 | ≈4–6 | 20–24 | 10 (83%) | 3 (25%) depression: n = 1 diabetes mellitus: n = 1 | increase of intraocular pressure: n = 1 (cushingoid features in most cases) |
| Kahaly et al. [35], 1986 | 20 | 50–100 | ≈2–4 | 10 | 9 (45%) | minor side effects |
| Prummel et al. [39], 1989 | 18 | 60 | ≈4 | 12 | 11 (61%) | 17 (94%) *4 (22%) major:* sialadenitis: n = 1 nasal cellulitis: n = 1 otitis externa: n = 1 | diabetes mellitus: n = 1 depression: n = 1 *10 (56%) moderate:* hypertension: n = 1, hirsutism: n = 3, behavioural changes: n = 5, weight gain >2 kg: n = 5, cushingoid facies: n = 8, angiodermatitis: n = 1 |
| Prummel et al. [11], 1993 | 28 | 60 | ≈4 | 12 | 14 (50%) | 25 (89%) *major:* depression: n = 1 herpes zoster: n = 1 | moderate: hypertension: n = 2 hirsutism: n = 2 behavioural changes: n = 3 | severe pyrosis: n = 5 weight gain >2 kg: n = 12 cushingoid face: n = 14 |

| | | | | | |
|---|---|---|---|---|---|
| Kahaly et al. [41], 1996 | 19 | 100 | ≈6 | 20 | 12 (63%) | 16 (84%) *number of events*: 19 *major*: n = 3 diabetes mellitus: n = 1 hypertension: n = 1 | behavioural changes: n = 1 *moderate*: n = 16 weight gain: n = 3 hirsutism: n = 2 cushingoid face: n = 2 | myalgias: n = 2 nausea/pyrosis: n = 2 sleeplessness: n = 2 tiredness: n = 1 dysmenorrhoea: n = 1 headache: n = 1 |
| Kung et al. [46], 1996 | 10 | 1 mg/kg/day | ≈4 | 12 | 6 (60%) 3* complete 3* partial | 3 (30%) 1 pulmonary infection: n = 2 hypertension: n = 1 | | |
| Baschieri et al. [43], 1997 | 27 | 80 | ≈6 | 20 | 18 (67%) | 3 (11%) *number of events*: n = 36 haemorrhagic gastritis: n = 2 manic-depressive psychosis: n = 1 hypertension: n = 2 osteoporosis: n = 4/15 | abnormal glucose tolerance tests: n = 5 occult blood in the stool: n = 5 decreased bone mineral content: n = 3/15 headache: n = 3 cushingoid facies: n = 5 hirsutism: n = 6 | |

Table 1. (continued)

| | n | Starting dose, mg/day | Cumulative dose, g | Treatment period, weeks | Response rate | Side effects (major/moderate) | |
|---|---|---|---|---|---|---|---|
| Macchia et al. [14], 2001 | 26 | 60–80 | ≈4 | 16–24 | significant decrease in: GO Index and proptosis | total side effects not mentioned *number of events: n = 41* hypertension: n = 7 muscular pain: n = 6 weight gain: n = 6 cushingoid habitus: n = 5 | fluid retention: n = 4 hyperglycaemia: n = 4 petechiae and ecchymoses: n = 3 acne: n = 3 irritability: n = 2 polymenorrhoea: n = 1 | 15% drop out |
| Kauppinen- et al. [15], 2002 | 15 | 60 | ≈3 | 16 | 6 (40%) | no serious side effects, mostly weight gain | |
| Kahaly et al. [13], 2005 | 35 | 100 | ≈4 | 12 | 18 (51%) | 18 (51%) number of events: 29 major: n = 2 weight gain >3 kg: n = 9 | gastrointestinal: n = 6 sleeplessness: n = 5 myalgias: n = 3 hypertension: n = 2 | hirsutism: n = 2 depression: n = 1 palpitations: n = 1 |
| Total | 210 | | | | 104 of 184 (56%) | 85 of 164 (52%) | |

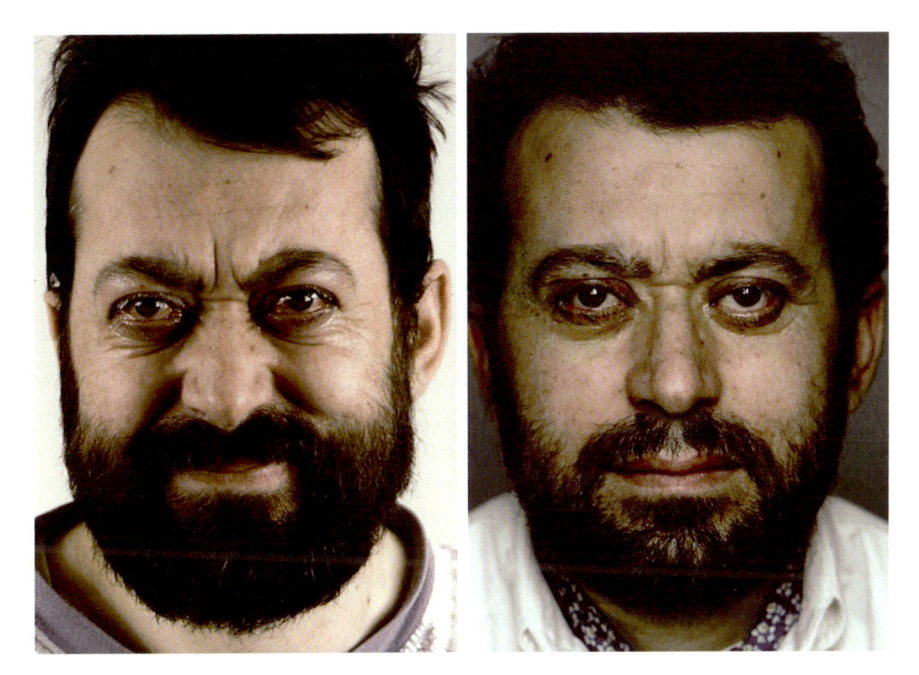

*Fig. 1.* Patient with moderately severe and active GO during oral steroid therapy and after successful immunosuppressive treatment.

with active GO, 61 of 65 non-smokers (93.8%) but 58 of 85 smokers (68.2%) only responded to high doses of oral prednisone, $p < 0.001$.

Whenever systemic steroids are used, patients should be warned about the potential for adrenocortical insufficiency associated with steroid treatment. In the months following the withdrawal of high-dose steroids, patients will require supplemental steroids in the event of trauma, surgery or infection. Given the numerous side effects of systemic steroid use (e.g. cushingoid features, diabetes, hypertension, osteoporosis), it is preferable to limit the use of steroids to a few months. Agents that protect against osteoporosis and gastric irritation should be considered. Vitamin D and calcium carbonate may be helpful in protecting bones; agents that decrease stomach acid production may be useful in protecting the gastric lining. According to recent guidelines, bisphosphonates (e.g. 70 mg alendronate once a week) should be given when starting treatment with pharmacological doses of glucocorticoids. Prophylactic potassium supplements may also be given, and additional monitoring of blood pressure, blood glucose and body weight should be made. Finally, if extended treatment is required, non-steroidal immunosuppressants or orbital irradiation should be considered as adjuvant treatments that may allow a decrease in the dosage of steroids.

*Intravenous Glucocorticoids*

The use of intravenous methylprednisolone acetate 1.0 g daily for 3 days followed by a rapid taper with prednisone has been advocated as an alternative treatment approach which may be particularly useful in patients with congestive GO [1]. One advantage of this regimen is the rapidity of the response in responsive patients. Meanwhile, various randomized trials (table 2) have demonstrated clear advantages of the intravenous pulse treatment over the oral administration in terms of effectiveness and possible side effects. In these studies, the cumulative dose of intravenous steroids ranged widely from 4.5 to 24 g. Intravenous steroids are most effective in reducing inflammatory soft tissue signs (fig. 2) and symptoms as well as eye ball motility disturbances. There is also compelling evidence that high-dose intravenous steroids abrogate circulating dendritic cells and have inhibitory effects on plasma cells [1].

In a controlled trial comparing intravenous and oral steroids [13], 70 consecutive subjects with severe and active GO were randomly assigned to receive 500 mg of methylprednisolone intravenously once weekly for 6 weeks and then 250 mg weekly for 6 weeks (total 4.5 g); or 100 mg of prednisolone orally daily for 1 week, after which the dose was reduced by 10 mg daily at weekly intervals and stopped after 12 weeks (total 4 g). The patients underwent complete ophthalmic examinations (by an examiner unaware of treatment), assessment of quality of life using the Short Form-36 questionnaire, and ultrasonography of the orbits at baseline and at 12 weeks. A response to treatment was defined as three or more of the following changes at 12 weeks: a >2 mm decrease in proptosis, a >2 mm decrease in lid width, a >3 mm decrease in ocular pressure, a >3 mm decrease in the sum of the width of the rectus muscles, and disappearance of diplopia in primary gaze or decrease in the diplopia grading, finally an increase in visual acuity. The baseline demographic characteristics were similar in each group and all patients completed the study. Among the patients who received intravenous methylprednisolone, 27 (77%) responded to treatment, as compared with 18 (51%) who received oral prednisolone. Among the patients in the intravenous group, 21 (60%) had a >2 mm decrease in proptosis, 22 (63%) had a >2 mm decrease in lid width, and 27 (77%) had a 3-point decrease in clinical activity score. Quality of life improved in patients of the intravenous group. During the 6-month follow-up period after treatment, optic neuropathy developed in 4 patients in the oral steroid group, and more patients in this group underwent orbital decompression or other ophthalmic operations. There were fewer manifestations of Cushing's syndrome and fewer adverse events in the intravenous group. In summary, a 3-month course of intravenous methylprednisolone was more effective than oral prednisolone in ameliorating ophthalmic symptoms and signs in patients with active and severe GO.

*Table 2.* Intravenous steroid monotherapy (randomized trials)

| | n | Treatment protocol | Cumulative dose, g | Treatment period, weeks | Response rate | Side effects (major/moderate) |
|---|---|---|---|---|---|---|
| Macchia et al. [14], 2001 | 25 | 1 g/week | 6 | 6 | significant decrease in: GO Index and proptosis | no relevant side effects *minor side effects* (resolved within a few hours after the end of treatment): gastric burn: n = 15 flush: n = 18 slight increase of body weight: n = 2 |
| Kauppinen-Mäkelin et al. [15], 2002 | 18 | 500 mg i.v. methylprednisolone, repeated after 48 h; then oral prednisolone (starting dose 40 mg/day) → again 2 times 500 mg i.v. (48 h interval), then again oral prednisone | 12 | 14 | 18 (89%) | no serious side effects, mostly weight gain |
| Kahaly et al. [13], 2005 | 35 | 500 mg, then 250 mg (6 weeks each) | 4.5 | 12 | 27 (77%) | 6 (17%) *number of events:* n = 8 *major:* n = 0 weight gain >3 kg: n = 1 gastrointestinal: n = 1 sleeplessness: n = 2 palpitations: n = 4 |

Table 2. (continued)

| | n | Treatment protocol | Cumulative dose, g | Treatment period, weeks | Response rate | Side effects (major/moderate) |
|---|---|---|---|---|---|---|
| Ng et al. [33], 2005 | 7 | 500 mg i.v. methylprednisolone for 3 consecutive days, followed by 0.7 mg/kg/day oral prednisolone | not mentioned | 4 | *after 52 weeks*: 2 (29%) improvement (soft tissue swelling and ocular motility | total of side effects not mentioned moon-face/weight gain/transient leucocytosis/ hyperlipidaemia: n = 3 hot flushes, gastro-intestinal upset, hypertension, insomnia, eye or nose infections: n = 2 acne: n = 1 Ramsey-Hunt syndrome: n = 1 |
| Total | 85 | | | | 45 of 53 (85%) | 6 of 35 (17%) |

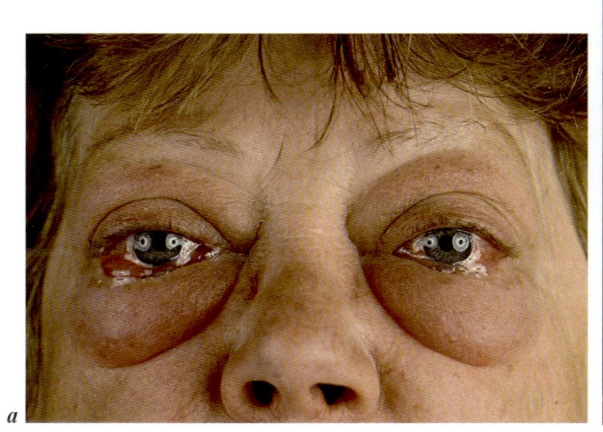

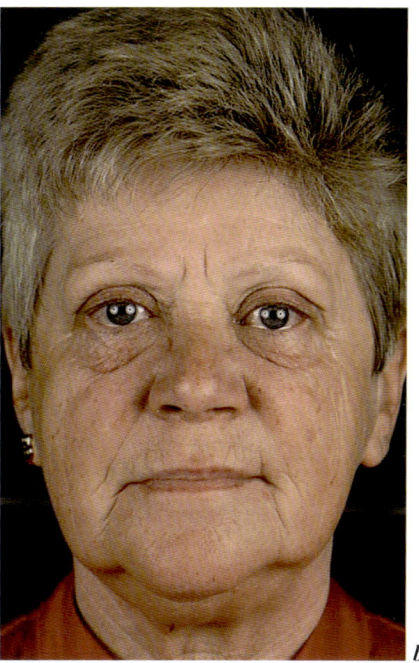

*Fig. 2.* Patient with moderately severe and active GO prior to (*a*) and after (*b*) intravenous steroid therapy.

A comparable study performed in Naples, Italy, showed similar findings although detailed demographic data, inclusion criteria, and transparent analysis of the results are lacking [14]. 25 GO patients were treated with two weekly intravenous injections of 1 g methylprednisolone for 6 weeks (total dose 12 g), and were compared to a group of 26 patients treated with oral prednisone at a dose of 60–80 mg/day progressively reduced every 2 weeks for a total duration of 4–6 months. All patients showed a significant improvement in signs and symptoms of orbital inflammation and a slight improvement in proptosis and diplopia. Relevant side effects were reported from patients receiving oral but not intravenous steroid therapy. In a further randomized trial comparing the administration of intravenous methylprednisolone pulse therapy for 3 consecutive days (3 × 1 g) followed by oral prednisolone (n = 18) for 3 months vs. oral prednisolone (n = 15) only, no significant differences in the grade of diplopia, proptosis or soft tissue activity scores were noted between both groups [15]. However, the combined therapy group required additional forms of therapy at 3 months less frequently than the oral form. In conclusion, the weekly administration of intravenous steroids is remarkably well tolerated and has become increasingly more common practice in the management of active and severe GO.

### Retrobulbar Injection of Steroids

The retrobulbar injection of steroids has been occasionally used in an attempt to treat locally the inflammation of GO while minimizing systemic side effects. In a randomized trial involving 50 patients with severe and active GO, subjects were either treated with triamcinolone or served as control [16]. The treatment group received four doses of 20 mg of triamcinolone acetate 40 mg/ml in a peribulbar injection to the inferolateral orbital quadrant. In contrast to control, there was an increase in the area of binocular vision without diplopia and a reduction in the sizes of the extraocular muscles evaluated by CT scans in the treatment group. No ocular adverse events were registered. However, this treatment has not been proven to be as effective as systemic therapy and carries the added risk of injury to the globe.

### Severe Adverse Effects of Intravenous Steroids

Acute and severe liver damage has been reported in sporadic cases during steroid pulse therapy, resulting in fatal acute liver failure in 4 patients with GO [17–19]. In those cases of liver failure following intravenous steroids, cumulative doses of intravenous methylprednisolone were 10–24 g. Thus, intravenous steroids may exert a direct toxic effect on hepatocytes and there seems to be a dose dependence of the extent and outcome of severe liver damage [20]. Pretreatment liver steatosis or diabetes are not related to liver damage, but pre-existent viral hepatitis is. Total morbidity and mortality of high doses of intravenous methylprednisolone are estimated to be 0.9 and 0.4%, respectively. In contrast, cases of hepatitis and liver failure have not been reported in patients treated with high doses of oral steroids, which may be related to the gradual withdrawal of the oral dose. Thus, the abrupt withdrawal of intravenous steroids may cause a re-exacerbation of an underlying liver autoimmune process following a prolonged immunosuppression, which may result in liver damage. Although a direct relation between intravenous steroids and severe liver damage is yet to be proven, these individual reports prompt a strict selection and a careful monitoring of patients to be subjected to intravenous therapy. Accordingly, restrictive measures have been recommended, e.g. limiting the cumulative dose of intravenous methylprednisolone to 6–8 g, assessment of liver morphology, virus markers, and auto antibodies prior to intravenous treatment and exclusion of patients at risk. Finally, monitoring liver function and morphology before, during and after intravenous treatment is warranted.

## What Are the Results of Randomized Trials Using Orbital Radiotherapy?

The rationale for the use of radiotherapy (Rx) resides in the well-established radiosensitivity of lymphocytes that infiltrate the orbit and are considered important effectors in this disorder [21, 22]. In a double-blind trial of prednisone versus Rx in patients with untreated moderately severe GO in whom euthyroidism was maintained throughout the study [11], patients were randomized to a 3-month course of oral prednisone + sham Rx or to retrobulbar Rx (20 Gy) and placebo capsules. A successful outcome was observed in 50% of the prednisone-treated and 46% of the Rx patients. Therapeutic outcome was determined by the change in the highest NO SPECS class. Successful treatment was largely caused by improvement in eye muscle motility and soft tissue swelling, associated with a decrease in eye muscle enlargement on CT scan. There were no clinically important changes in proptosis or visual acuity. The degree of improvement was not different between the two treatment groups, but prednisone patients improved more rapidly. Thus, in this study, orbital Rx and prednisone were equally effective as initial treatment in moderately severe GO although prednisone was slightly more effective on soft tissue changes and Rx was slightly more effective on eye muscle motility (table 3).

Mourits et al. [23] performed a double-blind randomized trial comparing Rx (20 Gy over 2 weeks) versus sham Rx. Enrolled were euthyroid patients with GO in the eye classes 2–4 without previous treatment. Exclusion criteria were diabetes mellitus and optic neuropathy. Definition of outcome was as follows: a decrease in NO SPECS class or grade was regarded as success, an increase in class as a failure whereas no decrease or increase was quoted as no change. According to this, success was observed in 63% after Rx vs. 31% for sham Rx, no change in 30 vs. 52% and failure was noted in 7 vs. 17%. Significant improvements for elevation of the globe, subjective eye score and clinical activity score were registered after Rx vs. significant decreases of subjective eye and activity scores in the sham group, only. With respect to the range of elevation of the globe and eye score, there were significant differences between the 2 groups. In patients with GO class 4, 82% (Rx) vs. 27% (sham) responded, but in class 2 or 3, no clear differences were noted (39 vs. 36%). Mourits et al. [23] concluded that orbital Rx improved eye motility in GO and that this treatment is effective in GO patients with motility impairment, only. A further Dutch randomized trial [24] also noted a higher response in 44 irradiated than in 44 sham-irradiated patients (52 vs. 27% at 12 months after treatment, relative risk 1.9, 95% CI 1.1–3.4; p = 0.017). Rx was effective in improving eye muscle motility and decreasing the severity of diplopia. Subsequent treatment of GO was less frequently required in the irradiated than in the sham-Rx patients

**Table 3.** Orbital radiotherapy alone (randomized trials)

| | n | Technique | Fraction dose, Gy/day | Total dose, Gy | Treatment period, weeks | Response rate | Side effects (major/moderate) |
|---|---|---|---|---|---|---|---|
| Prummel et al. [11], 1993 | 28 | 5 meV linear accelerator | 2 | 20 | 2 | 13 (46%) | 5 (18%) severe pyrosis: n = 2 weight gain >2 kg: n = 3 hair loss: n = 4 others: n = 14 (tiredness, menstrual irregularities, myalgias, headache, paresthesias, nausea, cramping of legs, vertigo, constipation) |
| Marcocci et al. [31], 1991 | 13 | 4 meV linear accelerator | 2 | 20 | 2 | 5 (38%) | some patients: mild irritative changes |
| Kahaly et al. [27], 2000 | 18 | telecobalt 60 | 1 Gy/week | 20 | 20 | 12 (67%) | 0% |
| | 22 | | 1 | 10 | 2 | 13 (59%) | 4 (18%) irradiation-induced conjunctivitis |
| | 22 | | 2 | 20 | 2 | 12 (55%) | 8 (36%) irradiation-induced conjunctivitis |
| Mourits et al. [23], 2000 | 30 | 6 MV photonbeam | 2 | 20 | 2 | 18 (60%) | 5 (17%) transient redness of the irradiated skin/transient local hair loss |
| Gorman et al. [25], 2001 | 42 | external beam accelerator | 2 | 20 | 2 | no significant difference between the treated and untreated orbit | total of side effects not mentioned |
| Prummel et al. [24], 2004 | 44 | 5 meV linear accelerator | 2 | 20 | 2 | 23 (52%) | not mentioned |
| Total | 219 | | | | | 96 (44%) | 22 of 120 (18%) |

(66 vs. 84%, p = 0.049). However, Rx was unable to prevent progression to more severe GO, which occurred in 6 irradiated and 7 sham-irradiated patients. Also, the improvement upon Rx was not associated with an increase in quality of life or a reduction in treatment costs.

Taken together, the Dutch trials provide good evidence of the efficacy – albeit modest – of retrobulbar Rx of GO patients. It is therefore difficult to reconcile these findings with the negative study from the Mayo Clinic. In the study of Gorman et al. [25], one randomly selected orbit was treated with 20 Gy of external beam Rx; sham Rx was given to the other side. Six months later, the therapies were reversed. Every 3 months for 1 year, the volume of extraocular muscle and fat, proptosis, range of extraocular muscle motion, area of diplopia fields, and lid fissure width were measured. No clinically or statistically significant difference between the treated and untreated orbit was observed in any of the main outcome measure at 6 months. At 12 months, muscle volume and proptosis improved slightly more in the orbit that was treated first. In view of the superior technical assessment of eye changes in the Mayo study, the conclusion that Rx had no benefit in their series of patients is undisputed. However, a selection bias is probable because the study recruited patients from all over the United States. Secondly, 19 (45%) of the 42 patients had been treated previously with steroids before randomization, who a priori are less likely to respond. Thirdly, not all patients were euthyroid throughout the study, as thyroid hormone levels had to be adjusted in an unknown number of patients.

*Low Irradiation Dose and Protracted Protocol*

Clinical and experimental data strongly suggest that low-dose Rx is sufficient to achieve an antiphlogistic effect on acute and chronic inflammatory processes [21]. Low-dose Rx can be repeated in cases of recurrence, and with a second series of 20 Gy, the dose of tumor therapy is almost attained. Since it is important to reduce the radiation burden for the patient, it seems attractive to reduce the total dose, especially if similar effectiveness could be proved. A retrospective evaluation of high- (20 Gy) and low-dose (10 Gy) Rx in 125 patients with GO showed no significant differences with respect to objective ophthalmic signs after a median follow-up of 5 years [26]. Recently, in patients with moderately severe and active GO efficacy and tolerability of three Rx protocols were compared in a random fashion [27]. Sixty-two euthyroid patients with untreated GO and no signs of optic neuropathy were enrolled. Orbital Rx (telecobalt 60) was administered either in 20 divided fractions of 1 Gy weekly over 20 weeks, or in 10 fractions of 1 Gy daily over 2 weeks, or in 10 fractions of 2 Gy/day/2 weeks. Therapeutic outcome was determined by the change in the highest NO SPECS class. A successful outcome was observed in 67% (1 Gy/week), 59% (1 Gy/day), and 59% (2 Gy/day) of the patients, respectively.

Objective signs regressed most in the 1 Gy/week group: visual acuity and eye muscle motility improved in this group only. Area of rectus muscles (MR imaging) decreased in all groups, significantly more in the 1 Gy/week group. Rx-induced conjunctivitis was observed in none of the 1 Gy/week group, but in 18 and 36% of the 1 and 2 Gy/day subjects, respectively. Thus, in patients with moderately severe GO, the protracted 1 Gy/week protocol was more effective and better tolerated than the short arm regimens, and subjective/objective ophthalmic signs decreased most in the groups 1 Gy/week and 1 Gy/day. Experimental evidence that the clinically observed anti-inflammatory effects of low-dose protracted Rx are due to the functional alteration of cells involved in the inflammatory response has been shown [21, 22]. A dose-dependent modulation of the nitric oxide pathway was observed with significant inhibition by the low Rx doses used in anti-inflammatory irradiation but with super-stimulation by the high Rx doses used in cancer therapy. Nitric oxide plays a central role in inflammation: it contributes to edema formation in acute inflammation, increases the vascular permeability associated with acute immune complex inflammation, and is involved in inflammatory pain. The effects of low-dose Rx have also been studied on models of inflammatory arthritis with therapeutic benefit found from a fractionated dose schedule of $4 \times 1$ Gy over 4 days, which gives a significant reduction in bone resorption and cartilage glycosaminoglycan loss. Thus, the suppressive interference of low and protracted doses of Rx with the nitric oxide pathway may be one of the radiobiological mechanisms that underlies the clinically documented efficacy of anti-inflammatory Rx. Rx-induced reductions in nitric oxide production might result in the reduction of inflammatory edema as well as in pain relief.

*Safety of Orbital Radiotherapy*

Orbital Rx for GO is a safe treatment modality, except possibly for diabetic patients. In a follow-up study in a cohort of 245 GO patients who had been treated with 20 Gy/2 weeks, 5 patients developed definite retinopathy (>5 retinal lesions). Of these, 3 had diabetes mellitus, and 1 had hypertension [28]. Diabetes was associated with both possible (p = 0.029) and definite (p = 0.005) retinopathy, with a relative risk of 21 (95% CI 3–179). In another follow-up study (n = 204, median observation 11 years), mild, asymptomatic retinopathy was observed in 14% of irradiated GO patients with diabetes and hypertension but in 3% only with hypertension alone [29]. At our institution in a long-term follow-up (17 years) study involving 125 GO patients, similar data regarding the higher risk for retinopathy in those having diabetes were noted with an applied total dose of 20 Gy [26]. Thus, diabetes mellitus, especially if associated with severe hypertension, may represent a relative contraindication for orbital Rx, as it may cause retinopathy. Also, and although no secondary tumors were detected in both studies, due to the long latency of Rx-induced tumors, Rx should preferably be restricted to subjects older than 35 years.

**Do You Favor Combination Therapy?**

Orbital Rx can be used in association with steroids to exploit the more rapid action of glucocorticoids and the more persistent effect of Rx. The combination of both classic therapies seems to be slightly more effective than when either one is given alone. However, the response to this combination is not complete and the patients may still suffer from the side effects of steroids. Although Rx and steroids do not necessary represent alternative therapeutic measures, they have been frequently used in sequence and seldom in association. At variance, at the University of Pisa during the last 20 years, orbital Rx and systemic steroids have been mostly employed in combination, in view of the possibility that the respective beneficial effects might be potentiated. With this respect, a series of controlled studies evaluating this combined treatment has been published by the Italian group. In the first report, 36 patients were treated with cobalt Rx and systemic steroids. Ten daily doses of 200 rad each were given in 2 weeks, with a cumulative dose of 2,000 rad or 20 Gy to each eye calculated on the midline. Steroids were started with 80 mg methylprednisolone daily for 3 weeks. The dose was gradually tapered by 5 mg weekly until a daily dosage of 20 mg was reached, and then the dose was subsequently reduced by 2.5–5 mg every 2–3 weeks. Treatment was discontinued after 6 months. Response to therapy was excellent in 12 (33%), good in 14 (39%), slight in 9 (25%), and in one (3%) no response was noted. Treatment with systemic methylprednisolone alone was also effective, but responses were less satisfactory; 4 of the 12 subjects of this group (33%) had good responses, 6 (50%) had slight, and 2 (17%) no response. Mean GO index decreased significantly more in the combined vs. monotherapy group. In a further trial, 44 patients with active GO were given cobalt Rx (total dose 20 Gy) and retrobulbar methylprednisolone acetate (14 bilateral injections at 20- to 30-day intervals). Excellent or good responses were observed in 11 (25%), 24 (55%) showed slight responses, and no change was found in 9 patients (20%). No major side effects were observed. The effects of retrobulbar steroid therapy and those obtained by combined therapy with systemic steroids and Rx were compared in 2 groups of 30 patients each, randomly assigned to either treatment. The results obtained in the group receiving systemic steroids were more satisfactory both clinically (excellent and good responses being observed in 60 vs. 30% of cases) and in terms of changes of the GO index [30, 31] (table 4).

Recently, in Pisa, the effect of orbital Rx with a linear accelerator (total dose 20 Gy) was evaluated either with intravenous or oral steroids [32].

Table 4. Combined standard treatment: steroids and orbital radiotherapy (randomized trials)

| | n | Dosage | Cumulative dose | Treatment period | Response rate | Side effects (major/moderate) |
|---|---|---|---|---|---|---|
| Bartalena et al. [30], 1983 | 36 | 2 Gy/day (4 meV linear accelerator) + oral prednisone starting with 70–80 mg/day; withdrawal after 5–6 months | 20 Gy ≈about 4 g | 2 weeks 20–28 weeks | 35 (97%) 26 (72%) excellent/ good; 9 (25%) slight | 3 (9%) depression: n = 1 diabetes mellitus: n = 1 increase of intraocular pressure: n = 1 (cushingoid features in most cases) → side effects of cobalt radiotherapy were not demonstrable (no signs of cataract were found after a mean follow-up period of 26 months) |
| Marcocci et al. [31], 1991 | 30 | 2 Gy/day (cobalt) + oral prednisone starting with 70–80 mg/day; withdrawal after 5–6 months | 20 Gy ≈about 4 g | 2 weeks 20–28 weeks | 18 (60%) (excellent or good) | total number of side effects not mentioned transient features of Cushing's syndrome in most cases increase of intraocular tension: n = 1, initial signs of cataract 6 months after radiotherapy (did not worsen over the following 12 months): n = 1 |
| | 30 | 2 Gy/day (cobalt) + 14 periocular injections of 40 mg (20- to 30-day intervals) | 20 Gy 0.6 g | 2 weeks 9 months | 24 (80%) 13 (30%) excellent or good | no major side effects, only a few cases of subconjunctival haemorrhages with no sequelae; no increase of intraocular pressure |
| Marcocci et al. [31], 1991 | 13 | 2 Gy/day (4 meV linear accelerator) + oral prednisone starting with 100 mg/day; withdrawal after 5–6 months | 20 Gy ≈about 6 g | 2 weeks | 9 (69%) | total number of side effects not mentioned – transient cushingoid features – 23% glycosuria – local irritative changes |

| Marcocci et al. [32], 2001 | 41 | 2 Gy/day (4 meV linear accelerator) + i.v. methylprednisolone: 15 mg/kg for 4 cycles, then 7.5 mg/kg for 4 cycles | 20 Gy 9–12 g | 14 weeks | 36 (88%) | 23 (56%) glucose intolerance: n = 9 gastritis: n = 4 urinary tract infections: n = 8 hypertension: n = 1 depression: n = 1 | cushingoid features: n = 5 hepatitis: n = 1 increase of body density: n = 1 a few hot flashes on the day after treatment |
|---|---|---|---|---|---|---|---|
| | 41 | 2 Gy/day (4 meV linear accelerator) + oral prednisone starting with 100 mg/day; withdrawal after 5 months | 20 Gy ≈about 6 g | 22 weeks | 26 (63%) | 35 (85 %) glucose intolerance: n = 8 gastritis: n = 4 urinary tract infections: n = 8 | hypertension: n = 2 depression: n = 2 cushingoid features: n = 35 hepatitis: n = 1 |
| Ng et al. [33], 2005 | 8 | 2 Gy/day (photon beams) + 500 mg i.v. methylprednisolone for 3 consecutive days, followed by 0.7 mg/kg/day oral prednisolone | 20 Gy not mentioned | 2 weeks 3 months | *after 52 weeks*: 7 (88%) improvement (soft tissue swelling and ocular motility) 5 (63%) normal eye motion | total number of side effects not mentioned moon-face/weight gain/transient leucocytosis/ hyperlipidaemia: n = 8 hot flushes, gastro-intestinal upset, hypertension, insomnia, eye or nose infections: n = 2 acne: n = 1 Ramsey-Hunt syndrome: n = 1 *associated with radiotherapy*: peri-orbital swelling and redness of the eyes: n = 3 hair loss: n = 3 | |
| Total | 199 | | | | 148 of 191 (77%) | 61 of 118 (52%) | |

82 consecutive patients with active and severe GO were randomly treated with either oral prednisone (starting dose 100 mg/day; withdrawal after 5 months) or intravenous methylprednisolone (15 mg/kg for 4 cycles and then 7.5 mg/kg for 4 cycles; each cycle consisted of 2 infusions on alternate days at 2-week intervals). A significant reduction of proptosis, lid width, and diplopia grades occurred, with no differences in both groups. The clinical activity score decreased significantly more in the intravenous group. By self-assessment evaluation, 85% intravenous and 73% oral steroid patients reported an improvement of ocular conditions, and responders in the intravenous group (88%) were more than in the oral group (63%). Side effects occurred in 56% intravenous and 85% oral steroid patients; in particular, cushingoid features developed in 5 of the intravenous and 35 of the oral steroid subjects. However, one intravenous steroid patient had severe hepatitis of undetermined origin at the end of steroid treatment, followed by spontaneous recovery. Finally, similar data demonstrating the superiority of a combined Rx-steroid therapy have been reported from China [33].

From the above data it is quite evident that the combination of Rx and oral steroids is more effective than oral steroids alone. Whether this is also true for the combination of Rx and intravenous steroids as compared to intravenous steroids alone, is not clear. In view of the greater efficacy of intravenous over oral steroids, the additional benefit of Rx may not exist when steroids are given intravenously. Addition of 20 Gy to intravenous pulses of methylprednisolone had no extra benefit in a nonrandomized study in Japan [34].

## What Are the Results of Randomized Trials Using Nonsteroid Immunosuppressants?

*Cyclosporine*

After the completion of a course of steroids, relapses of the activity of GO frequently occur. In order to avoid these recurrences and/or to keep the steroid doses low, furthermore because of the autoimmune pathogenesis of the disease, nonsteroid immunosuppressants came into use for GO in the 1970s. The drug best studied is cyclosporine which affects both humoral and cell-mediated immune reactions. It inhibits both cytotoxic T cell activation, production of cytokines and antigen presentation by monocytes and macrophages, as well as induces activation of T suppressor cells. Foremost, this agent is specific for lymphocytes and acts at an early stage of their activation. The drug binds at the lymphocyte surface on a protein (cyclophilin) and then migrates to the cell nucleus, where it has an inhibitory action on transcription of the RNA responsible for lymphokine production including that of IL-2. At our institution, a randomized trial was carried out in 40 patients with moderately severe GO [35–38]. Group 1 received prednisone in decreasing dosage, group 2 received prednisone at a comparable dosage plus cyclosporine (5 mg/kg/BW/day). Steroids were discontinued after 10 weeks in both groups. In group 2, cyclosporine was continued over 12 months. All signs of GO improved significantly in both groups whereas the improvement was significantly greater in group 2 according to a predefined score. After steroids were discontinued, inflammatory signs recurred in 9/20 patients in group 1 and in 1/20 of group 2. During the observation period of 12 months, relapses occurred in 8 in group 1 and in only 1 in group 2. Muscle thickness decreased in 9 patients in group 2, 6 months after beginning therapy. At this time, the results were not influenced in any of the 20 subjects in group 1. Both the TSH-receptor, the microsomal and the ocular muscle autoantibodies significantly decreased during cyclosporine therapy. In the cyclosporine group, *Klebsiella* pneumonia occurred 4 months after starting the immunosuppressive treatment and led to the single dropout in this trial. Prummel et al. [39] also compared the efficacy of prednisone with that of cyclosporine in 36 GO patients. During the 12-week period, 11/18 (61%) of the prednisone-treated and 4/18 (22%) of the cyclosporine-treated subjects responded. Response was manifested by decreases in eye muscle enlargement and proptosis and improvement of visual acuity, total and subjective eye scores. After 12 weeks, patients who did not respond were treated for another 12 weeks with a combination of cyclosporine and a low dose of prednisone. Among the 9 patients who initially received prednisone, the addition of cyclosporine resulted in improvement in 5 (56%), and among the 13 patients who received cyclosporine initially, 8 (62%) improved after the addition of prednisone. Combination therapy was better than prednisone treatment alone. These two studies indicated a lower efficacy of cyclosporine than prednisone as a single-agent treatment and found evidence that a combination of cyclosporine and prednisone may be more effective than either treatment alone. Thus, the use of cyclosporine might be indicated in association with steroids in patients who are resistant to steroids alone and in whom the persistent disease activity warrants continuing medical intervention. This combined treatment may be regarded as a second line alternative, especially in patients with diabetes mellitus in whom high doses of steroids and Rx should be used with caution. Side effects of cyclosporine are significant and hypertension, hepatic and nephrotoxicity may occur. Therefore, cautious dosage of this drug ($<5$ mg/kg/day) and measurement of the blood trough levels are recommended.

*Intravenous Immunoglobulin*

Intravenous administration of immunoglobulin (Ig) resulted in decreased antibody titres and clinical improvement in many autoimmune diseases [40].

Therefore, a randomized trial was done in which 19 patients with active and severe GO were treated with oral prednisolone (starting dose 100 mg/day) and 21 received 1 g Ig/kg/BW for two consecutive days every 3 weeks. The Ig course was repeated 6 times. A successful outcome was observed in 13 (62%) Ig and in 12 (63%) steroid treated patients [41]. Overall, there were no marked differences in degree of clinical improvement between the two groups. Among the patients treated with Ig, there was a marked decrease of the TSH-receptor, microsomal, and thyroglobulin autoantibodies as well as of the CD4/CD8 ratio. The significant decrease of thyroid autoantibodies in the Ig group may be viewed as a direct and local immunosuppressive effect of the drug on the intrathyroid lymphocytes. Adverse events were more frequent and severe during prednisolone than during Ig therapy. Antonelli and co-workers [42, 43] also compared the effectiveness of steroids with high-dose intravenous Ig in active GO. Response rates were 65% (n = 34) and 62% (n = 27) in patients receiving either Ig or prednisone, respectively. Soft tissue involvement improved or disappeared in 90 and 92.5% of the Ig and steroid-treated subjects, respectively. Also, the degree of diplopia decreased or diplopia disappeared in 75 and 80% in the Ig and steroid groups. Finally, proptosis decreased in 65 and 62% of the Ig and steroid patients. Orbital CT confirmed a significant reduction of eye muscle thickness in the Ig group. In both studies, intravenous Ig was safe and no major adverse events were noted. Thus, prednisolone and Ig appeared to be equally effective in treatment of severe and active GO. Nevertheless, high costs, the need for intravenous administration, and its small potential risk for transmitting infectious agents limit the routine application of Ig making them unable to replace the standard treatment with glucocorticoids (table 5).

*Azathioprine and Ciamexone*

Azathioprine competitively inhibits the incorporation of adenosine into deoxyribonucleic acid. The preparation possesses a low therapeutic index, and the dose required to inhibit T cell proliferation is almost as high as that which induces myelosuppression. Perros et al. [44] recruited 20 patients with moderately severe GO. Ten patients received azathioprine and 10 randomly matched patients served as controls. During the treatment period of one year and subsequently during a following observation year, no changes were detected in proptosis readings, visual acuity or measurement of palpebral aperture.

Ciamexone has immunomodulatory properties and inhibits antibody production in experimental models of autoimmune diseases. 51 patients with active GO were randomly allocated to two groups. Over a period of 6 months 26 patients received ciamexone 300 mg daily and 25 patients placebo [45]. All subjects additionally took prednisone in the first 4 weeks. Detailed examination did not reveal any preferential action of ciamexone on individual ophthalmic

*Table 5.* Non-steroidal immunomodulatory drugs (randomized trials)

| | Used drug | n | Dosage | Treatment period | Response rate | Adverse events (major/moderate) | |
|---|---|---|---|---|---|---|---|
| Kahaly et al. [35], 1986 | cyclosporine[1] + oral prednisone[2] | 19 | [1]5 mg/kg BW/day [2]60 mg/day | [1]1 year [2]10 weeks | 14 (74%) | 5 (26%) moderate increase of the liver enzymes: n = 4 hypertension: n = 4 pneumonia: n = 1 | swelling of the gums: n = 9 hirsutism: n=10 paresthesia: n = 12 |
| Prummel et al. [39], 1989 | cyclosporine | 18 | 7.5 mg/kg BW/day | 12 weeks | 4 (22%) | 10 (56%) 2 (11%) *major* (drop out because of diverticulitis: n = 1, irreversible rise in plasma creatinine: n = 1) | *8 (44%) moderate* (hypertension: n = 1, hirsutism: n = 3, behavioural changes: n = 5, weight gain >2kg: n = 5, congestive heart failure: n = 1) *3 (17%) minor* |
| | cyclosporine[3] + oral prednisone[4] | 22 | [3]7.5 mg/kg BW/day [4]60 mg/day | 12 weeks | 13 (59%) | 10 (45 %) *major: n=2* (drop out because of accumulation of multiple moderate side effects: n = 1, depression: n = 1) | *18 (82%) moderate* (hypertension: n = 4, hirsutism: n = 3, behavioural changes: n = 2, weight gain >2kg: n = 7, cushingoid facies: n = 2) |
| Total cyclosporine | | 59 | | | 31 (53%) | 25 (42%) | |

**Table 5.** (continued)

| | Used drug | n | Dosage | Treatment period | Response rate | Adverse events (major/moderate) |
|---|---|---|---|---|---|---|
| Kahaly et al. [45], 1990 | ciamexone | 26 | 300 mg/day | 6 months | no significant difference between treatment group and placebo | moderate increase in hepatic enzymes in patients who concomitantly took diclofenac: n = 2 |
| Perros et al. [44], 1990 | azathioprine | 10 | 150 mg/day | 12 months | no significant difference between treatment group and placebo | 0% |
| Antonelli et al. [42], 1992 | intravenous Immunglobulins | 7 | 400 mg/kg/day on 5 consecutive days (repeated 3 times every 21 days), then the same dose given for a single day for 9 additional cycles every 21 days | 10 months | 7 (100%) 3 (43%) excellent, 2 (29%) good, 2 (29%) fair | 1 (14%) headache |
| | intravenous immunglobulins + radiotherapy | 7 | 400 mg/kg/day on 5 consecutive days (repeated 3 times every 21 days), then the same dose | 10 months | 7 (100%) 3 (43%) excellent, 2 (29%) good, 2 (29%) fair | 1 (14%) headache |

| | | | | | |
|---|---|---|---|---|---|
| Kahaly et al. [41], 1996 | intravenous immun-globulins | 21 | given for a single day for 9 additional cycles every 21 days<br>+<br>2 Gy/day over (cumulative dose = 20 Gy)<br>1 g/kg body weight for 2 consecutive days every 3 weeks (repeated 6 times) | 2 weeks<br><br>18 weeks | 13 (62%) | 2 (9.5%)<br>headache: n = 1<br>fever: n = 1 |
| Baschieri et al. [43], 1997 | | 34 | 400 mg/kg/day on 5 consecutive days and repeated 3 times every 21 days, then the same dose given for a single day for 9 cycles every 21 days | 9 months | 26 (76%) | 8 (25%)<br>headache: n = 5<br>fever: n = 3 |
| Total Intravenous immunoglobulins | | 69 | | | 53 (77%) | 12 (17%) |
| Total non-steroidal immunomodulatory drugs | | 164 | | | 84 (51%) | 37 (23%) |

parameters. Orbital CT showed no significant alterations of the ocular muscle thickness.

In summary, due to the appreciable adverse effects of the agents mentioned, non-steroidal immunosuppressants should be viewed as supplementary to steroids only in active and severe GO. They should not be administered on their own. The rationale for their use is the complementary action with glucocorticoids in the acute phase of the disease and the possibility of reducing the dose of steroids (steroid-sparing effect).

## What Are the Results of Randomized Trials Using Somatostatin Analogs?

Somatostatin (SS) analogs interact with the SS receptors located on the surface of different cell types in the orbit and might inhibit the local release of IgF-1 or cytokines, which may be relevant in triggering and/or maintaining the ongoing reactions in the orbital tissue of patients with GO. In the first comparative open study [46], 18 patients with active and severe GO randomly received either Octreotide® 200 µg q8h subcutaneously (n = 8) or prednisone 1 mg/kg/day in decreasing doses (n = 10). Both Octreotide and prednisone therapy significantly decreased the palpebral aperture and activity score after 3 months, but those treated with prednisone had a lower activity score after treatment when compared to Octreotide. Only prednisone, but not Octreotide, was able to reduce intraocular pressure and muscle size as documented by MRI. Both groups showed significant elevation of urinary glycosaminoglycan excretion before therapy which was reduced after treatment. In summary, Octreotide was not as effective as prednisone in the treatment of severe GO (table 6).

Recently, four double-blind randomized studies were published. In the first trial conducted by Dickinson et al. [47], 50 euthyroid patients with active GO (median age 50 years, 39 females, NOSPECS 2–5, median duration of GO 0.9 years) received either 30 mg of the SS analog Octreotide LAR® intramuscularly or placebo every 4 weeks for 16 weeks. Both groups then received 30 mg Octreotide LAR for week 16–32 and were followed-up without treatment for a further 24 weeks. Objective assessments included all individual parameters of GO, CAS, and derived scores for soft tissue inflammation and ophthalmopathy index. During weeks 0–16 there was a significant reduction of CAS, soft tissue inflammation and subjective diplopia in the Octreotide-treated patients but the CAS and soft tissue inflammation were also reduced with placebo. During weeks 16–32 there was no significant change in the GO index in either group. Overall results (weeks 0–32) showed a slight reduction in the CAS and soft tissue inflammation in both groups, only. Thus, in this trial no significant

Table 6. Somatostatin analogs (randomized trials)

| | n | Dosage | Treatment period | Response rate | Side effects |
|---|---|---|---|---|---|
| Kung et al. [46], 1996 | 8 | Octreotide 50 μg q8h s.c. for 1 week, 100 μg for the 2nd, and subsequently 200 μg q8h | 3 months | 5 (63%) 1* complete, 4* partial | 0% (apart from abdominal colic experienced by all patients in the first week) |
| Dickinson et al. [47], 2004 | 27 | Octreotide-LAR 30 mg i.m. monthly | 4 months placebo, then 4 months octreotide-LAR treatment | *unchanged symptoms and signs in both groups* | 20 (74%) gastrointestinal, *others*: cholecystitis, increased biliary sludge |
| | 23 | Octreotide-LAR 30 mg i.m. monthly | 8 months | *unchanged symptoms and signs in both groups* | 15 (65%) gastrointestinal, *others*: cholecystitis, increased biliary sludge |
| Wemeau et al. [48], 2005 | 25 | Octreotide-LAR 30 mg i.m. monthly | 4 months | 7 (28%) | 1 (4%) gallstones *minor*: gastrointestinal (diarrhoea, abdominal pain, nausea, constipation) |
| Chang et al. [49], 2006 | 30 | Lantreotide 30 mg (slow-release formulation) i.m. every 2 weeks | 3 months | slight improvement of diplopia in upward gaze | 1 (3%) abdominal |

Table 6. (continued)

| | n | Dosage | Treatment period | Response rate | Side effects |
|---|---|---|---|---|---|
| Stan et al. [50], 2006 | 14 | Octreotide-LAR 20 mg i.m. monthly | 4 months | compared with placebo slight improvement of lid fissure width and CAS | 5 (36%) diarrhoea or abdominal cramping n = 4 mild-to-moderate abdominal pain: n = 1 |
| Total | 97 | | | 12 (12%) | 41 (42%) |

therapeutic effect of Octreotide LAR was seen. In the second multicenter trial conducted in France [48], a SS analogue (16 weeks of long-acting release formulation of Octreotide-LAR) was administered in 26 of 51 patients with active and moderate GO. The CAS was slightly reduced for patients treated with Octreotide-LAR, nevertheless no significant differences were noted vs. placebo (n = 25). Also, no treatment effect was observed for the primary end point (preventing deterioration of the disease). Orbital MRI revealed no significant changes of the eye muscle volume. This was associated with non-significant differences in class 3 grades, opening of the upper lid, the difference in ocular pressure in primary position and in upgaze, as well as in the involvement of extraocular muscles. Although Octreotide-LAR slightly and significantly reduced proptosis, the inference and overall conclusion of this study is that the drug was not suitable to mitigate activity of moderate GO. A third trial from Taiwan [49] randomly including the largest number (n = 60) of patients with active and moderately severe GO showed that 20 mg of Lanreotide® given intramuscularly every 2 weeks had absolutely no effect on the CAS and clinical course of the disease. Finally, the last study [50] involving a lower number of subjects with GO (n = 29) showed that those (n = 14) receiving Sandostatin LAR® 20 mg intramuscularly only had a slight and clinically irrelevant decrease of CAS and lid fissure, thus further questioning the role and efficacy of the SS analogs in moderately severe GO. One candidate explanation for this very low therapeutically answer might be that both Octreotide and Lanreotide have a high affinity for the SS receptor two only, a low affinity for the receptors three and five, and an almost absent affinity for the receptors one and four. This is unfortunate in view of the expression of all five subtypes of the SS receptors in orbital fibroblasts and lymphocytes of GO patients. Finally, the high costs of this treatment must also be taken into account.

### What Should You Do if Steroids Fail?

The success rate of systemic steroid treatment averages 50–75% and heavily relies on activity and duration of GO as well as on steroid dosage. For those patients not responding to steroids, alternative schemes may be offered (fig. 3). Presence of diplopia and/or impaired motility of the eye muscles are a clear indication for performing Rx alone or in combination with either intravenous steroid pulses if severe orbital inflammation is present or with a low dose of steroids (starting dose of 0.20–0.25 mg/kg BW/day) for moderate cases. The oral prednisolone dose should be tapered weekly and the steroid therapy may be stopped after termination of Rx. Severe reduction of visual acuity and/or development of optic neuropathy makes a decompression surgery mandatory. On the other hand,

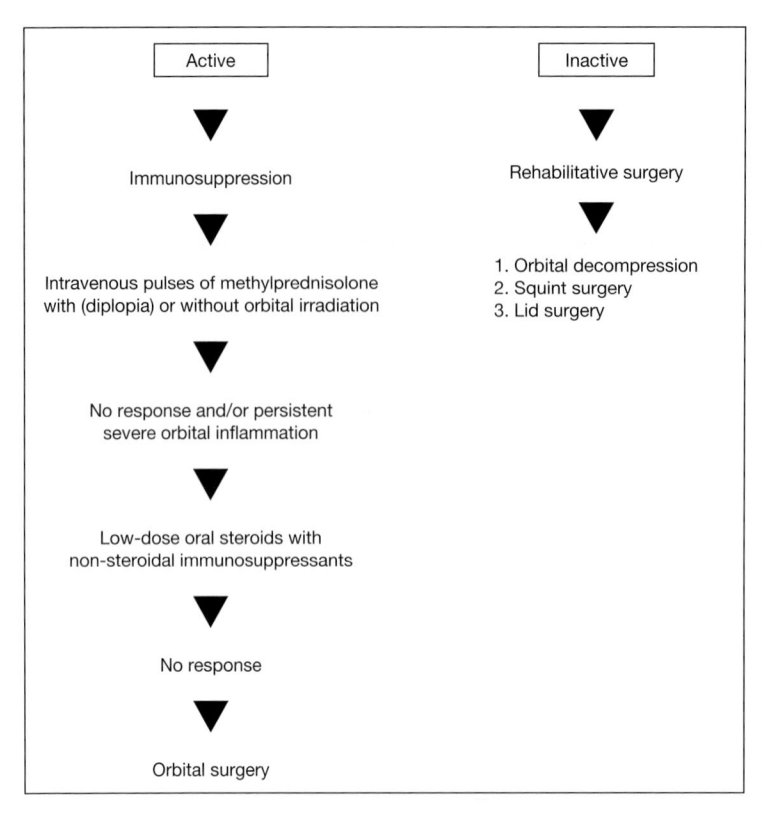

```
        Active                          Inactive
          ▼                                ▼
   Immunosuppression              Rehabilitative surgery
          ▼                                ▼
Intravenous pulses of methylprednisolone   1. Orbital decompression
with (diplopia) or without orbital irradiation   2. Squint surgery
                                           3. Lid surgery
          ▼
  No response and/or persistent
   severe orbital inflammation
          ▼
   Low-dose oral steroids with
  non-steroidal immunosuppressants
          ▼
       No response
          ▼
      Orbital surgery
```

*Fig. 3.* Recommended management of moderately severe GO.

further severe inflammation of the orbital tissue and absent signs of neuropathy may be resolved through the combined administration of non-steroid immunosuppressants and moderate doses of prednisolone (0.30–0.40 mg/kg/BW/day), as well as an intensive local therapy (eye drops and ointments).

### What Are the Actual Evidence-Based Therapeutic Recommendations for Patients with Moderately Severe Graves' Orbitopathy?

Numerous randomized well-performed controlled trials and meta-analyses have proven the beneficial effect of both intravenous methylprednisolone therapy as well as of high dose oral prednisolone in patients with active and moderately severe GO (tables 1, 2). Therefore systemic glucocorticoids are evidence-based strongly recommended (recommendation A) in this stage of the disease and are actually regarded as the first-line treatment worldwide. With respect to orbital Rx, the cited trials (table 3) have also proven the beneficial effect of Rx regarding a clinically relevant amelioration of motility disturbances of the eye muscles. Thus, this treatment is evidence-based recommended (recommendation B) in subjects with active GO and impaired motility only. The combination of the standard treatments steroids and Rx in the early stage of active GO with impaired motility is strongly evidence-based recommended (recommendation A) and, as cited before (table 4), has proven to be superior to either monotherapy. In contrast, the studies involving SS analogs did not show a relevant clinical improvement in those receiving these drugs (table 6). Therefore, SS analogs are evidence-based not recommended (recommendation D) in severe GO. Finally, in subjects with active and moderately severe GO, either not answering to prednisone or presenting a relapse after a course of intravenous steroids, a few controlled studies have proven that additional administration of non-steroid immunosuppressants, e.g. cyclosporine, is more effective that monotherapy with prednisolone alone (table 5). Thus, this combined therapy can fairly be recommended (recommendation C) since it may both decrease the activity and inflammation of the orbital connective tissue as well as reduce the rate of relapses of GO.

## Acknowledgments

The most valuable help of Anna Katharina Ponto, Medical Fellow of the Thyroid Research Laboratory, Department of Medicine I, Gutenberg University Hospital, in extensively reviewing the corresponding literature and subsequently excellently preparing the tables is greatly appreciated.

## References

1 Stemberger K, Kahaly GJ, Pitz S: Update on thyroid eye disease. Compr Ophthalmol Update 2006;7:287–298.
2 Terwee CB, Prummel MF, Gerding MN, Kahaly GJ, Dekker FW, Wiersinga WM: Measuring disease activity to predict therapeutic outcome in Graves' ophthalmopathy. Clin Endocrinol 2005;62: 145–155.
3 Kahaly GJ: Imaging in thyroid-associated orbitopathy. Eur J Endocrinol 2001;145:107–118.
4 Kahaly GJ: Recent developments in Graves' ophthalmopathy imaging. J Endocrinol Invest 2004;27: 254–258.
5 Kahaly GJ, Bang H, Berg W, Dittmar M: Alpha-fodrin as a putative autoantigen in Graves' ophthalmopathy. Clin Exp Immunol 2005;140:166–172.
6 Abalkhail S, Doi SAR, Al-Shoumer KAS: The use of corticosteroids versus other treatments for Graves' ophthalmopathy: a quantitative evaluation. Med Sci Monitor 2003;9:CR477–CR483.
7 Bartalena L, Marcocci C, Bogazzi F, Panicucci M, Lepri A, Pinchera A: Use of corticosteroids to prevent progression of Graves' ophthalmopathy after radioiodine therapy for hyperthyroidism. N Engl J Med 1989;321:1349–1352.

8    Kahaly GJ, Petrak F, Hardt J, Pitz S, Egle UT: Psychosocial morbidity of Graves' orbitopathy. Clin Endocrinol 2005;63:395–402.
9    Tehrani M, Krummenauer F, Mann WJ, Pitz S, Dick HB, Kahaly GJ: Disease-specific assessment of quality of life after decompression surgery for Graves' ophthalmopathy. Eur J Ophthalmol 2004;14:193–199.
10   Marcocci C, Bartalena L, Panicucci M, Marconcini C, Cartei F, Cavallacci G, Laddaga M, Campobasso G, Baschieri L, Pinchera A: Orbital cobalt irradiation combined with retrobulbar or systemic corticosteroids for Graves' ophthalmopathy: a comparative study. Clin Endocrinol 1987;27:33–42.
11   Prummel MF, Mourits MP, Blank L, Berghout A, Koornneef L, Wiersinga WM: Randomized double-blind trial of prednisone versus radiotherapy in Graves' ophthalmopathy. Lancet 1993;342: 949–954.
12   Bartalena L, Marcocci C, Tanda ML, Manetti L, Dell'Unto E, Bartolomei MP, Nardi M, Martino E, Pinchera A: Cigarette smoking and treatment outcomes in Graves' ophthalmopathy. Ann Intern Med 1998;129:632–635.
13   Kahaly GJ, Pitz S, Hommel G, Dittmar M: Randomized, single blind trial of intravenous versus oral steroid monotherapy in Graves' orbitopathy. J Clin Endocrinol Metab 2005;90:5234–5240.
14   Macchia PE, Bagattini M, Lupoli G, Vitale M, Vitale G, Fenzi G: High-dose intravenous corticosteroid therapy for Graves' ophthalmopathy. J Endocrinol Invest 2001;24:152–158.
15   Kauppinen-Mäkelin R, Karma A, Leinonen E, Löyttyniemi E, Salonen O, Sane T, Setälä K, Viikari J, Heufelder A, Välimäki M: High dose intravenous methylprednisolone pulse therapy versus oral prednisone for thyroid-associated ophthalmopathy. Acta Ophthalm Scan 2002;80: 316–321.
16   Ebner R, Devoto MH, Weil D, Bordaberry M, Mir C, Martinez H, Bonelli L, Niepomniszcze H: Treatment of thyroid associated ophthalmopathy with periocular injections of triamcinolone. Br J Ophthalmol 2004;88:1380–1386.
17   Weissel M, Hauff W: Fatal liver failure after high-dose glucocorticoid pulse therapy in a patient with severe thyroid eye disease. Thyroid 2000;10:521.
18   Marino M, Morabito E, Brunetto MR, Bartalena L, Pinchera A, Marcocci C: Acute and severe liver damage associated with intravenous glucocorticoid pulse therapy in patients with Graves' ophthalmopathy. Thyroid 2004;14:403–406.
19   Salvi M, Vannuchi G, Sbrozzi P, Bottari del Castello A, Carnevali A, Fargion S, Beck-Peccoz P: Onset of autoimmune hepatitis during intravenous steroid therapy for thyroid-associated ophthalmopathy in a patient with Hashimoto's thyroiditis: case report. Thyroid 2004;14:631–634.
20   Le Moli R, Baldeschi L, Saeed P, Regensburg N, Mourits MP, Wiersinga WM: Determinants of liver damage associated with intravenous methylprednisolone pulse therapy in Graves' ophthalmopathy. Thyroid 2007;17:357–360.
21   Kahaly GJ, Rösler HP, Kutzner J, Pitz S, Müller-Forell W, Beyer J, Mann WJ: Radiotherapy for thyroid-associated orbitopathy. Exp Clin Endocrinol Diab 1999;107:201–207.
22   Kahaly GJ, Gorman CA, Kal HB, Mourits MP, Pinchera A, Tan S, Prummel MF: Radiotherapy for Graves' ophthalmopathy; in Prummel MF (ed): Recent Developments in Graves' Ophthalmopathy. Boston, Kluwer Academic Publishers, 2000, pp 115–131.
23   Mourits MP, van Kempen-Harteveld ML, Garcia MB, Koppeschaar HP, Tick L, Terwee CB: Radiotherapy for Graves' orbitopathy: randomised placebo-controlled study. Lancet 2000;355: 1505–1509.
24   Prummel MF, Terwee CB, Gerding MN, Baldeschi L, Mourits MP, Blank L, Dekker FW, Wiersinga WM: A randomized controlled trial of orbital radiotherapy versus sham irradiation in patients with mild Graves' ophthalmopathy. J Clin Endocrinol Metab 2004;89:15–20.
25   Gorman CA, Garrity JA, Fatourechi V, Bahn RS, Petersen IA, Stafford SL, Earle JD, Forbes GS, Kline RW, Bergstralh EJ, Offord KP, Rademacher DM, Stanley NM, Bartley GB: A prospective, randomized, double-blind, placebo-controlled study of orbital radiotherapy for Graves' ophthalmopathy. Ophthalmology 2001;108:1523–1534.
26   Kahaly GJ, Rösler HP, Pitz S, Krummenauer F, Hommel G: Radiotherapy for Graves' ophthalmopathy. J Clin Endocrinol Metab 2001;86:2327–2328.
27   Kahaly GJ, Rösler HP, Pitz S, Hommel G: Low- versus high-dose radiotherapy for Graves' ophthalmopathy: a randomized, single blind trial. J Clin Endocrinol Metab 2000;85:102–108.

28  Wakelkamp IMMJ, Tan H, Saeed P, Schlingenmann RO, Verbraak FD, Blank LECM, Prummel MF, Wiersinga WM: Orbital irradiation for Graves' ophthalmopathy: is it safe? A long-term follow-up study. Ophthalmology 2004;111:1557–1562.
29  Marcocci C, Bartalena L, Rocchi R, Marino M, Menconi F, Morabito E, Mazzi B, Mazzeo S, Sartini MS, Nardi M, Cartei F, Cionini L, Pinchera A: Long-term safety of orbital radiotherapy for Graves' ophthalmopathy. J Clin Endocrinol Metab 2003;88:3561–3566.
30  Bartalena L, Marcocci C, Chiovato L, Laddaga M, Lepri G, Andreani D, Cavallacci G, Baschieri L, Pinchera A: Orbital cobalt irradiation combined with systemic corticosteroids for Graves' ophthalmopathy: comparison with systemic corticosteroids alone. J Clin Endocrinol Metab 1983;56: 1139–1144.
31  Marcocci C, Bartalena L, Bogazzi F, Bruno-Bossio G, Lepri A, Pinchera A: Orbital radiotherapy combined with high dose systemic glucocorticoids for Graves' ophthalmopathy is more effective than radiotherapy alone: results of a prospective randomized study. J Endocrinol Invest 1991;14: 853–860.
32  Marcocci C, Bartalena L, Tanda ML, Manetti L, Dell'Unto E, Rocchi R, Barbesino G, Mazzi B, Bartolomei MP, Lepri P, Cartei F, Nardi M, Pinchera A: Comparison of the effectiveness and tolerability of intravenous or oral glucocorticoids associated with orbital radiotherapy in the management of severe Graves' ophthalmopathy: results of a prospective, single-blind, randomized study. J Clin Endocrinol Metab 2001;86:3562–3567.
33  Ng CM, Yuen HKL, Choi KL, Chan MK, Yuen KT, Ng YW, Tiu SC: Combined orbital irradiation and systemic steroids compared with systemic steroids alone in the management of moderate-to-severe Graves' ophthalmopathy: a preliminary study. Hong Kong Med J 2005;11:322–330.
34  Ohtsuka K, Sato A, Kawaguchi S, Hashimoto M, Suzuki Y: Effect of steroid pulse therapy with and without orbital radiotherapy on Graves' ophthalmopathy. Am J Ophthalmol 2003;135: 285–290.
35  Kahaly GJ, Schrezenmeir J, Krause U, Schweikert B, Meuer S, Muller W, Dennebaum R, Beyer J: Ciclosporin and prednisone vs. prednisone in treatment of Graves' ophthalmopathy: a controlled, randomized and prospective study. Eur J Clin Invest 1986;16:415–422.
36  Kahaly GJ, Schrezenmeir J, Schweikert B, Müller W, Krause U, Beyer J: Remission-maintaining effect of cyclosporine in endocrine ophthalmopathy. Transplant Proc 1986;18:844–846.
37  Kahaly GJ, Yuan JP, Krause U, Hülbusch K, Beyer J: Ciclosporin and thyroid-stimulating immunoglobulins in endocrine orbitopathy. Res Exp Med 1989;189:355–362.
38  Kahaly GJ, Moncayo R, Bemetz U, Krause U, Beyer J, Pfeifer EF: Eye muscle antibodies in endocrine exophthalmos. Horm Metab Res 1989;12:137–141.
39  Prummel MF, Mourits MP, Berghout A, Krenning EP, van der Gaag R, Koornneef L, Wiersinga WM: Prednisone and cyclosporine in the treatment of severe Graves' ophthalmopathy. N Engl J Med 1989;321:1353–1359.
40  Kazatschkine MD, Kaveri SV: Advances in immunology: immunomodulation of autoimmune and inflammatory diseases with intravenous immune globulin. N Engl J Med 2001;345:747–755.
41  Kahaly GJ, Pitz S, Muller-Forell W, Hommel G: Randomized trial of intravenous immunoglobulins versus prednisolone in Graves' ophthalmopathy. Clin Exp Immunol 1996;106:197–202.
42  Antonelli A, Saracino A, Alberti B, Canapicchi R, Cartei F, Lepri A, Laddaga M, Baschieri L: High-dose intravenous immunoglobulin treatment in Graves' ophthalmopathy. Acta Endocrinol 1992;126:13–23.
43  Baschieri L, Antonelli A, Nardi S, Alberti B, Lepri A, Canapicchi R, Fallahi P: Intravenous immunoglobulin versus corticosteroid in treatment of Graves' ophthalmopathy. Thyroid 1997;7: 579–585.
44  Perros P, Weightman DR, Crombie AL, Kendall-Taylor P: Azathioprine in the treatment of thyroid-associated ophthalmopathy. Acta Endocrinol 1990;122:8–12.
45  Kahaly GJ, Lieb W, Müller-Forell W, Mainberger M, Beyer J, Vollmer J, Staiger C: Ciamexone in endocrine orbitopathy. Acta Endocrinol 1990;122:13–21.
46  Kung AW, Michon J, Tai KS, Chan FL: The effect of somatostatin versus corticosteroid in the treatment of Graves' ophthalmopathy. Thyroid 1996;6:381–384.
47  Dickinson AJ, Vaidya B, Miller M, Coulthard A, Perros P, Baister E, Andrews CD, Hesse L, Heverhagen JT, Heufelder AE, Kendall-Taylor P: Double-blind, placebo-controlled trial of

octreotide long-acting repeatable (LAR) in thyroid-associated ophthalmopathy. J Clin Endocrinol Metab 2004;89:5910–5915.
48   Wemeau JL, Caron P, Beckers A, Rohmer V, Orgiazzi J, Borson-Chazot F, Nocaudie M, Perimenis P, Bisot-Locard S, Bourdeix I, Dejager S: Octreotide (long-acting release formulation) treatment in patients with Graves' orbitopathy: clinical results of a four-month, randomized, placebo-controlled, double-blind study. J Clin Endocrinol Metab 2005;90:841–848.
49   Chang TC, Liao SL: Slow-release Lanreotide in Graves' opthalmopathy: a double-blind randomized, placebo-controlled clinical trial. J Endocrinol Invest 2006;29:413–422.
50   Stan MN, Garrity JA, Bradley EA, Woog JJ, Bahn MM, Brennan M, Bryant SC, Achenbach SJ, Bahn RS: Randomized, double-blind, placebo-controlled trial of long-acting release octreotide for treatment of Graves' ophthalmopathy. J Clin Endocrinol Metab 2006;91:4817–4824.

Prof. George J. Kahaly
Department of Medicine I, Gutenberg University Hospital
Langenbeckstrasse 1
DE–55131 Mainz (Germany)
Tel. +49 6131 17 3768, Fax +49 6131 17 3460, E-Mail gkahaly@mail.uni-mainz.de

# Management of Very Severe Graves' Orbitopathy (Dysthyroid Optic Neuropathy)

C.M. Lane[a], A. Boschi[b]

[a]Cardiff Eye Unit, University Hospital of Wales, Heath Park, Cardiff, UK;
[b]Department of Ophthalmology, St. Luc University Hospital, Brussels, Belgium

### How Do You Define Dysthyroid Optic Neuropathy?

Dysthyroid optic neuropathy (DON) is impairment of optic nerve function affecting approximately 3–5% of patients with Graves' orbitopathy (GO) [1]. The pathophysiological mechanism of DON is probably multifactorial, but mainly related to an increase in volume of connective tissues, particularly the extraocular muscles close to the orbital apex [2], known as apical crowding [3] (fig. 1). The enlarged muscles appear to cause optic neuropathy by direct compression on the optic nerve or its blood supply [4]. Another factor is the increase in retrobulbar pressure, consistent with a tight orbital septum and a relatively low degree of exophthalmos in patients with optic neuropathy [5]. Rarely, DON relates to optic nerve stretch, which is demonstrated radiologically as a straight rigid optic nerve which typically tents the posterior globe so that the round contour is changed to give a 'V' contour (fig. 2).

### Are There Specific Risk Factors for Dysthyroid Optic Neuropathy?

A definite systemic risk factor is diabetes, in which the incidence of DON reaches 33.3% [6]. Smoking, a well-known risk factor for vasculopathy, is also associated with severe GO, as are older patients [7].

As a local or orbital risk factor for DON, restriction of eye movements, mainly in elevation ($<30°$), is a striking abnormality ($>71\%$ of DON) [8]. The degree of enlargement of extraocular muscles has also been reported to be highly correlated with the risk of DON [2].

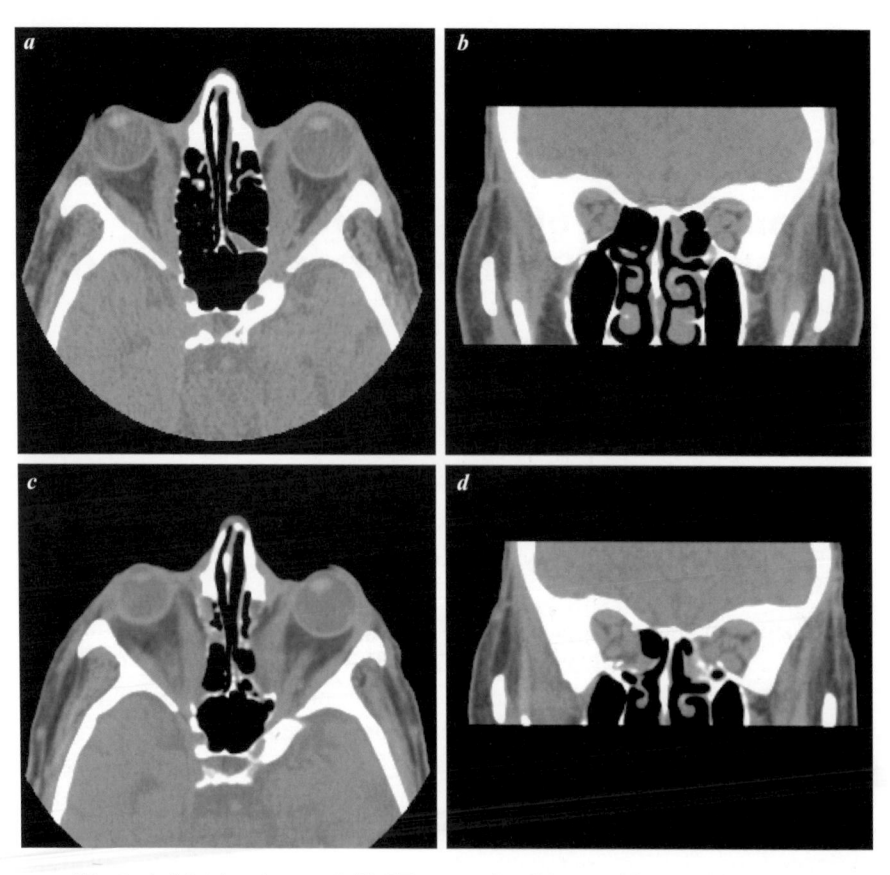

*Fig. 1.* Axial (*a*) and coronal (*b*) CT scans of an 86-year-old man with DON showing apical compression of the optic nerve with apical crowding. Axial (*c*) and coronal (*d*) CT scans of the same patient, 2 days following bilateral medial wall and medial floor orbital decompression.

## Which Symptoms Should Alert Me?

Visual dimming is often so insidious that the patient will be unaware of it until late in the clinical course. Such patients may complain of 'foggy' or 'blurred' vision which persists after blinking (so is not caused by tear film disruption), and after closing one eye (so is not caused by diplopia). Some patients can read 20/20 and have no visual complaints [9]. Light sensitivity (in the absence of corneal lesions) or dimming of colours should also alert the clinician to the possibility of DON. Orbital ache and gaze-evoked pain are not specific, but should alert the clinician in the presence of restriction of elevation (≤30°) [8].

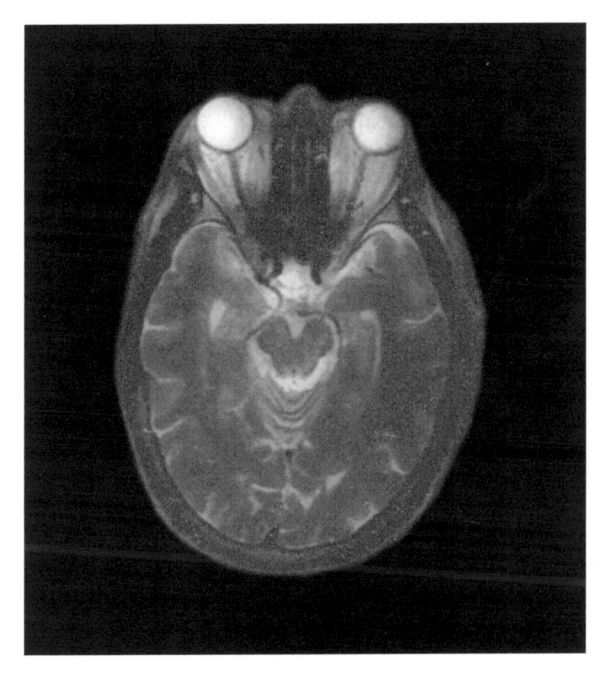

*Fig. 2.* Axial T$_2$-weighted MRI scan showing optic nerve stretch with tenting of the posterior globe in severe thyroid eye disease.

Appearance of inconstant (gaze-evoked) diplopia or constant diplopia in the primary position or reading should also warn the clinician, because diplopia has been reported in almost 50% of DON patients [2, 8].

### What Are the Ophthalmological Signs of Dysthyroid Optic Neuropathy?

Normal visual acuity does not preclude an optic neuropathy. But, in presence of a dyschromatopsia, and particularly of a relative afferent pupillary defect (RAPD), optic nerve dysfunction should always be ruled out. Many reports indicate that visual loss is similar in both eyes in about 40% of DON patients [8]; in this condition a RAPD will not be detectable [9]. Presence of active inflammatory signs and symptoms (CAS ≥ 3) has been observed in the majority of DON patients, but is not absolutely required for the diagnosis of DON [8]. The optic disc may be swollen in 30% [9] to 56% [8], rarely pale or may appear perfectly normal associated with or without retinal venous congestion (table 1).

*Table 1.* Ophthalmological examination for early detection of DON

| Test | Method | % of definite DON with this abnormality in the EUGOGO DON Study (8) | Alternative or additional tests |
| --- | --- | --- | --- |
| Visual acuity ≤0.67 | Snellen | 80 | LogMar |
| Reduced colour vision | Ishihara | 77 | red desaturation Hardy Rand Ritter |
| Automated perimetry abnormal | Humphrey 24.2 or Octopus | 71 | |
| Ocular motility defect | elevation < 30% | 71 | |
| Optic disc swelling | visualisation | 56 | fluorescein angiogram optical coherence tomography (OCT) |
| Relative afferent pupillary defect (RAPD) | N/A | 45 | testing with neutral density filters |

## Are Additional Investigations Helpful?

Automated perimetry is a necessary investigation for the evaluation of optic nerve function; the most frequent defects being a central scotoma, an arcuate or altitudinal defect, or uniform depression [8]. Pattern reversal visual-evoked potential is a complementary study which can identify early optic nerve dysfunction [10]. CT scan or magnetic resonance imaging (MRI) is essential to detect apical crowding and intracranial fat prolapse, which are highly correlated with DON [3, 8] (fig. 1). When at the orbital apex, the perineural fat effacement is greater than 50%, the diagnostic sensitivity and specificity is high (80 and 70.6%, respectively), making it a good diagnostic indicator [11]. However, as noted previously, there are occasional patients who demonstrate clinical evidence of DON without CT evidence of enlarged extraocular muscles or apical crowding of the optic nerve [8, 11].

## How Fast Can Dysthyroid Optic Neuropathy Develop? Is Urgent Treatment Necessary?

Severe GO can develop within hours of a stressful event, such as major surgery. Similar degrees of severity of disease may also be present in patients with a longer history of impairment of colour vision or visual acuity over a period of months. This is particularly likely in the tight orbit [11] where exophthalmos has not been recognised or eyelid edema has been incorrectly attributed to allergy. In any individual with active disease, the clinician has to assume that disease severity has not yet peaked and could progress rapidly; peak severity of GO follows peak activity. Acceleration of the inflammatory cascades in GO leading to compressive or inflammatory optic neuropathy or corneal exposure necessitates urgent treatment with immunosuppression and/or surgical decompression of the orbit.

Urgent treatment is not necessary if signs of optic nerve impairment are equivocal and the disease activity, as judged by the CAS [12] score, is low. Spontaneous recovery of DON in patients who have refused treatment reminds all clinicians that we are managing a condition with a finite natural history.

## What Is the Evidence Base for the Treatment of Dysthyroid Optic Neuropathy?

Currently, the evidence base for treatment of DON is unfortunately inadequate. The first reason for this is that diagnostic criteria have yet to be established and the distinction between probable and definite DON is not always clear [8]. Secondly, the numbers of patients presenting to individual units is small. This means that randomised controlled treatment trials have not been performed. There is one exception, which is a small but useful trial [13]. Fifteen patients presenting with very active GO and DON were randomised into treatment with high-dose IV steroid or surgical decompression of the orbit. Four of the nine steroid-treated and 5 of the 6 surgical patients had to be switched to the other treatment arm because of a deterioration or failure to improve visual acuity; subsequently they improved. The results favoured initial treatment with high-dose IV steroids rather than initial surgical decompression. Anecdotal evidence [14] suggests that addition of ciclosporin to pulsed intravenous steroid is needed in order to avoid surgery. Orbital radiotherapy is frequently used as an adjunctive treatment but it should be avoided in diabetics and those under 35 years of age [15]. Use of orbital decompression surgery or an alternative immunosuppressant does reduce the total steroid dose and the incidence of steroid-induced side effects including orbital Cushing's syndrome [16].

## What Is the Role of Surgery in Dysthyroid Optic Neuropathy?

Most cases of DON are due to apical optic nerve compression by enlarged extra-ocular muscles. Surgical expansion of the orbital apex by orbital decompression

*Table 2.* Advantages and disadvantages of orbital decompression surgery for DON

*Advantages*
(1) Immediate reduction in apical compression of the optic nerve
(2) Reduction in need for long-term steroid treatment
(3) Reduction in corneal exposure, if present
(4) Reduction in orbital venous pressure, reducing intraocular pressure and congestion of conjunctiva and caruncle

*Disadvantages*
(1) Surgical procedure necessitates general anaesthetic
(2) Risk of orbital haemorrhage, visual loss, diplopia, infraorbital hypoaesthesia, sinusitis (late or early) and CSF leak

is an effective method of immediate reduction of pressure on the optic nerve (fig. 1). Usually removal of the ethmoids is sufficient, but in rare cases removal of the anterior-lateral wall of the sphenoid sinus is necessary [17]. Surgery does have a long-term beneficial effect [18]. The advantages and disadvantages of surgery are listed in table 2.

## How Many Patients Become Blind due to Dysthyroid Optic Neuropathy?

Blindness has been reported in 5 of 305 cases with DON despite surgery, steroids and radiotherapy [18]. Earlier recognition of GO, an appreciation of the importance of stable thyroid function and more effective immunosuppression and surgery apparently have reduced the incidence of blindness due to DON. Late diagnosis can still result in blindness, particularly if visual loss is incorrectly attributed to another cause, such as cataract. Corneal ulceration due to exophthalmos can also cause blindness even if there is no neuropathy.

### References

1  Wiersinga WM, Bartalena L: Epidemiology and prevention of Graves' ophthalmopathy. Thyroid 2002;12:855–860.
2  Feldon S, Muramatsu MS, Weiner JM: Clinical classification of Graves' ophthalmopathy Indication of risk factors for optic neuropathy. Arch Ophthalmol 1984;102:1469–1472.
3  Birchall D, Goodall KL, Noble JL, Jackson A: Graves ophthalmopathy: intracranial fat prolapse on CT images as an indicator of optic nerve compression. Radiology 1996;200:123–127.
4  Dosso A, Safran AB, Sunaric G, Burger A: Anterior ischemic optic neuropathy in Graves' disease. J Neuroophtalmol 1994;14:170–174.

5   Koornneef L, Schmidt ED, Van der Gaag R: The orbit: structure, autoantigens, and pathology; in Wall J, How J (eds): Graves' Ophthalmopathy. Oxford, Blackwell Scientific Publications, 1990, vol 26, pp 1–21.
6   Kalman R, Mourits MP: Diabetes mellitus: a risk factor in patients with Graves' ophthalmopathy. Br J Ophthalmol 1999;83:463–465.
7   Prummel MF, Wiersinga WM: Smoking and risk of Graves' disease. JAMA 1993;269:479–482.
8   McKeag D, Lane CM, Lazarus JH, Baldeschi L, Borboridis K, Dickinson JA, Hullo A, Kahaly G, Krassas G, Marcocci C, Marino M, Mourits M, Nardi M, Neoh C, Orgiazzi J, Perros P, Pinchera A, Pitz S, Sartini MS, Wiersinga WM: Clinical features of dysthyroid optic neuropathy: a European Group on Graves' Orbitopathy (EUGOGO) survey. Br J Ophthalmol 2007;91:455–458.
9   Trobe JD: Optic nerve involvement in dysthyroidism. Ophthalmology 1981;88:388–392.
10  Tsaloumas MD, Good PA, Burdon MA, Misson GP: Flash and pattern visual evoked potentials in the diagnosis and monitoring of dysthyroid optic neuropathy. Eye 1994;8:638–645.
11  Neigel JM, Rootman J, Belkin RI, Nugent RA, Drance SM, Beattie CW, Spinelli JA: Dysthyroid optic neuropathy: the crowded orbital apex syndrome. Ophthalmology 1988;95:1515–1521.
12  Mourits MP, Koornneef L, Wiersinga WM, Prummel MP, Berghout A, van der Gaag R: Clinical criteria for the assessment of disease activity in Graves' ophthalmopathy: a novel approach. Br J Ophthalmol 1989;73:639–644.
13  Wakelkamp IM, Baldeschi L, Saeed P, Schlingemann RO, Verbraak FO, Blank LE, Prummel MF, Wiersinga WM: Surgical or medical decompression as a first-line treatment of optic neuropathy in Graves' ophthalmopathy? A randomized controlled trial. Clin Endocrinol 2006;65:132.
14  Meyer PA: Avoiding surgery for thyroid eye disease. Eye 2006;10:1171–1177.
15  Wakelkamp IM, Tan H, Saeed P, Schlingemann RO, Verbrakk FD, Blank LE, Prummel MF, Wiersinga WM: Orbital irradiation for Graves' ophthalmopathy: is it safe? A long-term follow-up study. Ophthalmology 2004;111:1557–1562.
16  Boschi A, Detry M, Duprez T, Rolland F, Plas B, De Plaen J, Eloy P: Malignant bilateral exophthalmos and secondary glaucoma in iatrogenic Cushing's syndrome. Ophthalmic Surg Lasers 1997;28:318–320.
17  Gormley PD, Bowyer J, Jones NS, Downes RN: The sphenoid sinus in optic nerve decompression. Eye 1997;11:723–726.
18  Warren JD, Spector JG, Burde R: Long term follow-up and recent observations on 305 cases of orbital decompression for dysthyroid optic neuropathy. Laryngoscope 1989;99:35–40.

Prof. Antonella Boschi
Department of Ophthalmology, St. Luc University Hospital
Avenue Hippocrate, 10
BE–1200 Brussels (Belgium)
Tel. +32 2764 1950, Ext. 1985, Fax +32 2764 29 88, E-Mail boschi@ofta.ucl.ac.be

# Rehabilitative Surgery

*L. Baldeschi*

Orbital Centre, Department of Ophthalmology, Academic Medical Center, University of Amsterdam, Amsterdam, The Netherlands

## Why Is This Chapter Called Rehabilitative Surgery and Not Cosmetic Surgery?

Graves' orbitopathy (GO) is a debilitating disease which adversely interferes with the quality of life of affected patients [1]. It is characterised by different degrees of disfigurement and alteration of vision, both of which contribute to loss of self-confidence, psycho-social stability and ability to function.

In GO, surgery, which may be necessary to protect visual function in the active phase of the disease or to correct the stable typical disfigurement and symptoms in the static post-inflammatory phase, should always be considered rehabilitative as it is aimed to restore the individual integrity disrupted by the disease and ultimately the lost ability to function.

Commonly, however, surgery performed primarily to treat potentially sight-threatening conditions such as optic neuropathy or exposure keratopathy is referred to as *functional*, while procedures primarily aimed at correcting disfigurement and symptoms are referred to as *rehabilitative*. For didactic purposes, we like to maintain this distinction between functional and rehabilitative surgery although it is necessary to admit that besides the above-listed semantic considerations, a clear-cut distinction between the two does not exist as surgery aimed primarily at restoring function also has positive effects on disfigurement and vice versa.

The definition *cosmetic surgery*, which does not stress the impact of the orbital disease in affected patients, appears inadequate and should be avoided. Surgery is in fact aimed at restoring a patient's appearance as close as possible to that preceding the onset of GO, and not at changing his or her somatic tracts making them more beautiful. *Cosmetic/aesthetic rehabilitation* has often been used and can be considered an acceptable compromise when defining surgery mainly aimed at correcting disfigurement due to GO.

## What Are the Steps and Timing of Rehabilitative Surgery?

During the post-inflammatory phase of GO, after a 6- to 8-month period of stable endocrinological and ophthalmic clinical picture, surgical rehabilitation can be performed if required. Depending on the severity of the disease surgical rehabilitation can be more or less extensive, the full treatment consisting of decompression surgery, squint surgery, eyelid lengthening, blepharoplasty and eyebrow plasty.

The first rehabilitative step mainly consists of orbital bony decompression and early intervention soon after stabilisation had been advocated [2]. Fibrosis due to long-lasting orbital disease or as a possible consequence of retrobulbar irradiation administrated in the early phase of GO has been questioned to be a possible cause of poor distensibility and plasticity of the soft orbital tissues resulting in scarce effectiveness of orbital expansion surgery [3–6]. Recent studies, however, have demonstrated that long-lasting GO or pre-operative radiotherapy do not adversely interfere with the results of orbital bony decompression; thus, when the stabilisation of Graves' disease and orbitopathy has occurred, rehabilitative surgery can be started at any time and no adverse effects from common preceding treatments such as retrobulbar irradiation are to be expected [7, 8].

Decompression surgery causes a reduction of exophthalmos as well as reduction of upper and lower eyelid displacement [7]. It may positively influence extra-ocular muscle restriction, but displacement of the soft orbital tissues caused by decompression procedures may also cause strabismus. Eventual squint surgery should therefore follow orbital decompressions but considering that vertical tropias may influence eyelid position, squint surgery should precede eventual correction of eyelid position. Finally, when necessary the finishing touch can be given by blepharoplasty and eyebrow plasty.

In short, surgical rehabilitation needs to respect the given order since the preceding step may influence the step that follows. When all the steps are necessary the entire rehabilitation may require between 1.5 and 2 years. In particular cases, exceptions are possible and the rehabilitation can be favourably sped-up by carrying out more than one procedure at the same time.

## How Should Patients Be Selected for Rehabilitative Surgery

Patients should be selected on the basis of their motivation to undertake a long-lasting, potentially risky, and somewhat exhausting trail. Multiple interventions may also be necessary in the case that full treatment, starting with orbital decompression, is not required. Patients should be fully aware of the risks and benefits of each possible procedure and should accept the possibility of partial results or temporary worsening of their inability to function in the course of rehabilitation. Information provided by the physicians, although precise, may be inadequate to the patients and potential candidates for surgery can better build up realistic expectancies by contact with patient associations. The psychological impact of GO on the affected patient is consistent but should not itself be a reason to undertake a surgical treatment with potential distressing effects in the same respect. It is up to the physician to understand when the patient has matured the necessary acquisition of consciousness for being admitted to surgical rehabilitation, and the ophthalmologic controls necessary to assess disease stability should also be finalised according to this.

Besides the patient's determination to accept major surgeries, the possibility to aim at attaining only partial results should always be weighed in the light of patients' characteristics such as age, general health conditions, profession, education and psyco-social environment. Often conservative surgery is of maximal benefit to the patient in spite of modest final results that may be unattractive to the surgeon.

## References

1  Terwee CB, Dekker FW, Prummel MF, Wiersinga WM: Graves' ophthalmopathy through the eyes of the patient: a state of the art on health-related quality of life assessment. Orbit 2001;20:281–290.
2  Härting F, Koornneef L, Peeters HJF, Gillisen JPA: Fourteen years of orbital decompression in Graves' disease: a review of technique, results and complications. Orbit 1986;5:123–129.
3  Wilson WB, Manke WF: Orbital decompression in Graves' disease: the predictability of reduction of proptosis. Arch Opthalmol 1991;109:343–345.
4  Goldberg RA, Weinberg DA, Shorr N, Wirta D: Maximal three-wall orbital decompression through a coronal approach. Ophthalmic Surg Lasers 1997;28:832–843.
5  Kazim M, Trokel S, Moore S: Treatment of acute Graves' orbitopathy. Ophthalmology 1991;98: 1443–1448.
6  Clauser L, Galie M, Sarti E, Dallera V: Rationale of treatment in Graves' ophthalmopathy. Plast Reconstr Surg 2001;108:1880–1894.
7  Baldeschi L, Wakelkamp IMMJ, Lindeboom R, Prummel MF, Wiersinga WM: Early versus late orbital decompression in Graves' orbitopathy: a retrospective study in 125 patients. Ophthalmology 2006;113:874–878.
8  Baldeschi L, MacAndie K, Koetsier E, Blank L, Wiersinga WM: The influence of previous orbital irradiation on the outcome of rehabilitative decompression surgery in Graves' orbitopathy. Am J Ophthalmol, in press.

Dr. Lelio Baldeschi
Room D2–436, Orbital Center, Department of Ophthalmology
Academic Medical Center, University of Amsterdam
Meibergdreef 9
NL–1105 AZ Amsterdam (The Netherlands)
Tel. +31 20 566 3580, Fax +31 20 566 9053, E-Mail l.baldeschi@amc.uva.nl

# Orbital Decompression

*L. Baldeschi*

Orbital Centre, Department of Ophthalmology, Academic Medical Center, University of Amsterdam, Amsterdam, The Netherlands

## What Is Orbital Decompression?

The autoimmune process at the basis of Graves' orbitopathy (GO) induces swelling of the soft tissues contained within the boundary of the bony orbit, this causes impairment of venous out flux towards the cavernous sinus and reverse of the flux in direction of facial circulation.

This positive feedback circle leads to increase of the intraorbital pressure which is first responsible for the progression of GO and later for its typical signs and symptoms [1]. Any surgical procedure aimed at decreasing the raised intraorbital pressure and its effects by means of enlargement of the bony orbit and/or removal of the orbital fat is defined as orbital decompression.

## What Are the Aims of Orbital Decompression?

For almost one century decompression surgery had been used to treat GO. First it was used only to address sight-threatening conditions such as optic neuropathy refractory to medical therapy, or exposure keratopathy unresponsive to local measures and/or minor eyelid surgeries. More recently, the indications of orbital decompression were extended to the treatment of disfiguring exophthalmos and symptoms. Eyeball subluxation which may be a possible cause of acute optic neuropathy and exposure keratopathy [2], postural visual obscuration in patients with congestive inactive GO [3] and choroidal folds due to eyeball indentation by enlarged extraocular muscles represent other, more recently recognised functional indications for decompression surgery.

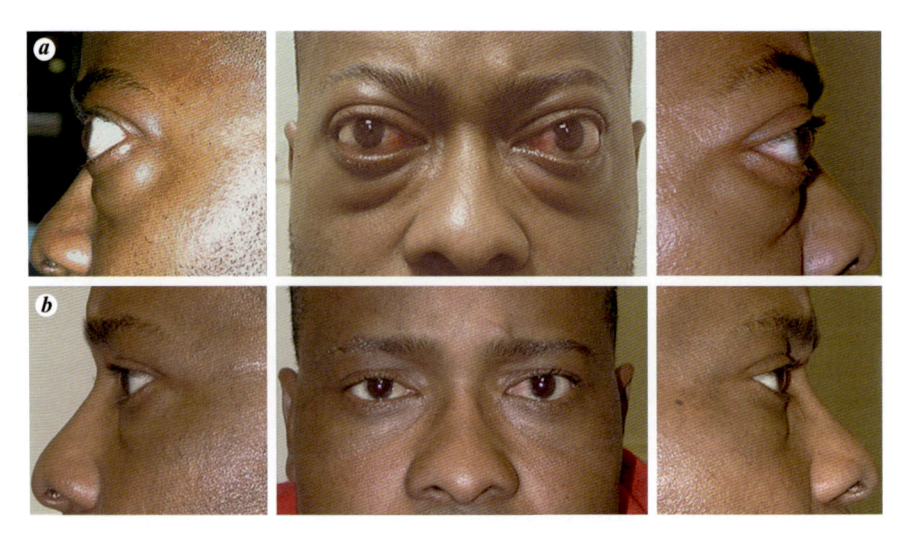

*Fig. 1.* A patient with severe GO and optic neuropathy unresponsive to glucocorticoids and orbital irradiation. *a* At admittance for orbital decompression. *b* 6 months after extensive three-wall orbital decompression performed through a combined transinferior conjunctival fornix and coronal approach. Visual function was restored and disfigurement treated.

## Functional Aims

According to a large retrospective study decompression surgery can offer a rapid solution to dysthyroid optic neuropathy with an acceptable list of adverse effects (fig. 1) [4]. A more recent randomised controlled clinical trial comparing surgical to medical decompression as a first-line treatment of dysthyroid optic neuropathy led to the conclusion that immediate decompression surgery did not result in a better outcome in terms of increase in visual acuity and therefore intravenous followed by oral glucocorticoids appeared to be the first-choice therapy [5]. In line with these latter results, it was also the trend of clinicians of three European professional organisations potentially involved in the treatment of patients with GO, who answered a questionnaire sent by the European Group on Graves' Orbitopathy (EUGOGO) [6, 7].

In GO exophthalmos, increased palpebral fissure width, blink rate alterations, lid lag, lagophthalmos, deficit of elevation and poor Bell's phenomenon can all be potentially connected with drying of the ocular surface. In the course of active GO, ocular surface damage correlated significantly with a reduced tear secretion due to autoimmune lacrimal gland impairment, but not with increased ocular surface or impaired upgaze [8]. Other studies had shown that in patients with short duration of GO tear secretion was not abnormal and exophthalmos, lid lag and lagophthalmos did not correlate with ocular surface damage, while the damage to the ocular surface depended principally on widened palpebral fissure which is the cause of increased ocular surface evaporation resulting in an elevated tear film osmolarity similar to that of sicca kerato-conjunctivitis [9]. The influence of decompression rehabilitative surgery on increased eyelid aperture has recently been reported. A decrease in eyelid aperture based equally on decreased upper and lower lid displacement was found in about 50% of the patients presenting with preoperative increased eyelid aperture and decompressed by means of a 3-wall coronal approach which leaves the upper and lower lid retractors undisturbed [10].

The effect of decompression surgery on severe corneal alteration had never been studied specifically and although most of the studies on orbital decompression report a reduction in symptoms associated with exposure keratopathy, a case of severe corneal ulcer refractory to decompression surgery has also been published [11].

Eyeball subluxation is a rare (0.1%), recurrent complication of GO that deserves urgent referral to a specialist centre as it represents a potential cause of visual loss [2, 12]. In light of the current literature, eyeball subluxation seems to occur in the type I, 'lipogenic' variant of GO as described by Nureny and never in the type II 'myopathic' variant. Globe subluxation in fact requires extensibility of the extraocular muscles [2, 13]. For this, it is conceivable that a definitive treatment of this sight-threatening condition can benefit either from bony and/or orbital fat decompression, but studies addressing this issue are missing.

Among patients with inactive congestive orbitopathy there appear some with borderline optic nerve perfusion: a blood flow that is just able to maintain neural function. Such patients would seem to be liable to visual obscuration whenever there is a fall in systemic blood pressure due to postural changes, diabetics appearing particularly susceptible to this phenomenon. The vascular embarrassment of the optic nerve depending on elevated intraorbital pressure is very effectively relieved by orbital decompression and leads to an immediate cessation of postural visual obscuration [3].

Organised choroidal fold consecutive to eyeball indentation by enlarged extraocular muscles had been thought to be refractory to orbital decompression [14] until recently when a positive response of this complication to bony decompression surgery has been reported [15].

*Rehabilitative Symptomatic Aims*

In GO, severe functional complications due to increased intraocular pressure are rare, different degrees of venous congestion, strabismus, eyelid puffiness and retraction, exophthalmos and symptoms such as retroocular pressure and/or grittiness due to chronic corneal exposure are more frequent. Decompression surgery is the mainstay method to treat stable disfiguring

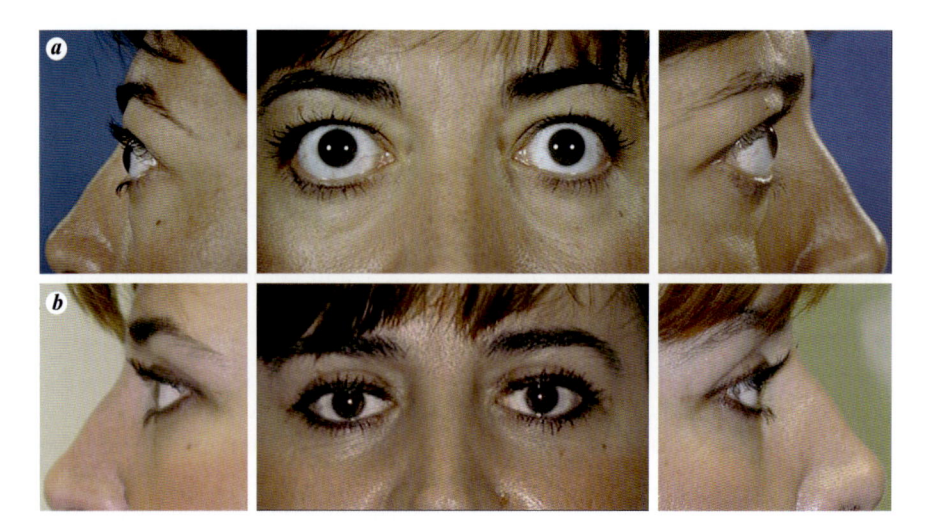

*Fig. 2.* A patient with moderately severe non-active GO. *a* The patient at admittance for orbital decompression. *b* The patient at the end of the surgical rehabilitation which included bilateral transinferior fornix inferomedial orbital decompression, upper lid lengthening by means of transconjunctival Müllerectomy, and upper lid blepharoplasty.

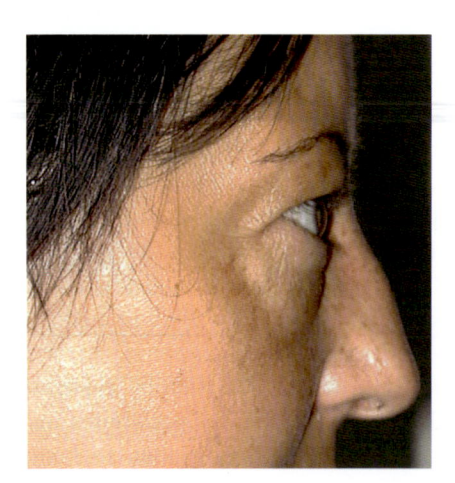

*Fig. 3.* A patient affected with GO, and presenting a flat forehead, and a scarce anterior projection of the zygomatic eminence. The patient appears disfigured by exophthalmos although her exophthalmometric value is only 18 mm.

alterations and/or symptoms that can typify the inactive post-inflammatory phase of the disease (fig. 2). Decompression surgery is not necessarily required only when exophthalmos exceeds the normal reference range. Patients with a flat forehead, scaree brow bossing, and scarce anterior projection of the zygomatic eminence or patients with deep-set eyes before GO may result or feel disfigured at normal exophthalmometric values (fig. 3). Evaluation of pre-GO

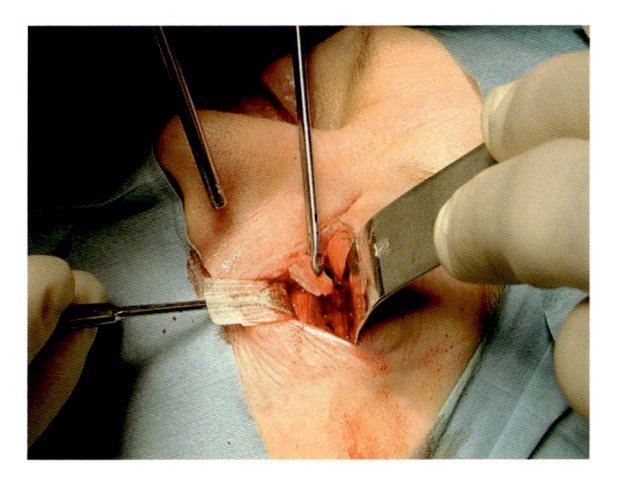

*Fig. 4.* Bone removal in course of transinferior fornix inferomedial orbital decompression.

face photographs may help the surgeon to restore a patient's appearance as close as possible to how it was before the onset of orbital disease.

### Which Surgical Technique Should Be Preferred?

The raised intraorbital pressure and its consequences can be surgically addressed by expansion of the bony orbital boundary and/or by means of fat removal. For about one century, the two possibilities developed through parallel routes; only recently did it become clear that they should no longer be considered alternatives but complementary approaches concurring in tailoring the most adequate treatment to the specific patient's needs (figs. 4, 5) [16–18]. Through the years many have been the proposed techniques and many their variations. This has been largely due to the multifaceted nature of the disease, the different indications for decompression surgery, surgeon preferences and expertise, variations in orbital osteology, patients' expectations and attitude towards intervention. Furthermore, the constant attempt to implement the beneficial effects of this type of surgery simultaneously decreasing the aesthetic impact of surgical scars, convalescence periods and risks for iatrogenic complications in general, and consecutive strabismus in particular, has further extended the case scenario (figs. 6, 7).

Any type of fat removal or osteotomy has been hypothesized to cause a critical relief of pressure at the apex, which can be beneficial for optic nerve disfunction [19, 20]. The current trend is to directly relieve the apical pressure

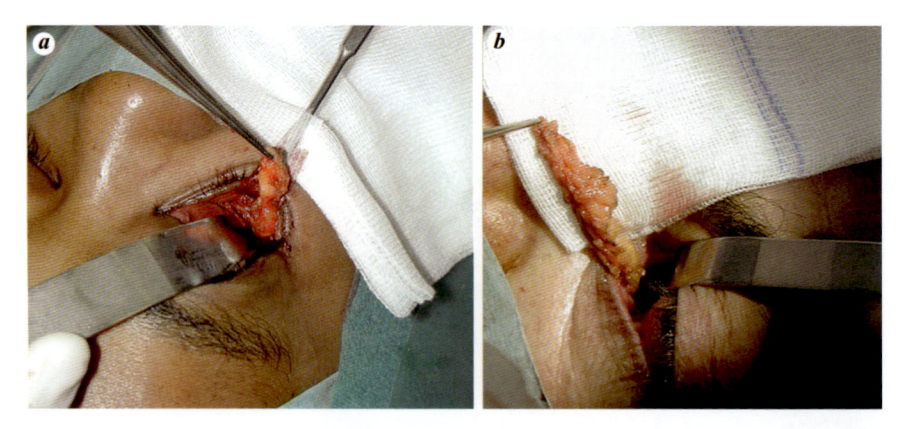

*Fig. 5.* Orbital fat removal. *a* Removal of the fat located in the inferior lateral orbital quadrant as a part of a combined transinferior conjungtival fornix inferomedial bone/inferior lateral fat decompression procedure. *b* Removal of the fat located in the inferior medial orbital quadrant during an extensive three-wall/fat decompression procedure performed through a combined transinferior conjunctival fornix and coronal approach.

as much as possible by increasing the apical volume of the bony orbit. This is obtained by removing the medial orbital wall (fig. 7b) [18]. In particularly severe cases, preventive removal of the lateral wall including its rim can prove convenient (fig. 7a). Forces exerted by retractors in an attempt to achieve apex decompression along the medial orbital wall can increase the already high retro-bulbar pressure up to critical levels for optic nerve fibres and vasculature. The preventive removal of the lateral orbital wall permits to address more smoothly the deepest orbit, reducing in fact, the risk to add an iatrogenic component to the pathologically high orbital pressure at the basis of the neuropathy. Several are the possible options to remove the medial orbital wall, and transconjunctival routes either transcaruncular or transinferior fornix, which leaves no scars, can adequately serve this scope and to date are the preferred [21, 22]. The endoscopic transnasal approach, described first and relatively recently by Kennedy et al. [23], addressing the orbital apex without any substantial increase of the intraorbital pressure can also be a valid alternative.

During the last two decades, when the number of rehabilitative orbital decompression started to rise [24], it became of primary importance to balance a given technique in terms not only of effectiveness in reducing exophthalmos, but also and mostly in terms of safety. At that time the antral-ethmoidal decompression by a transantral approach, as described by Walsh and Ogura in 1957, was the mainstay technique [25, 26]. The major disadvantage reported with transantral surgery was a subsequent motility imbalance as high as 52% [27], and therefore alternative procedures were sought in an attempt to decrease the

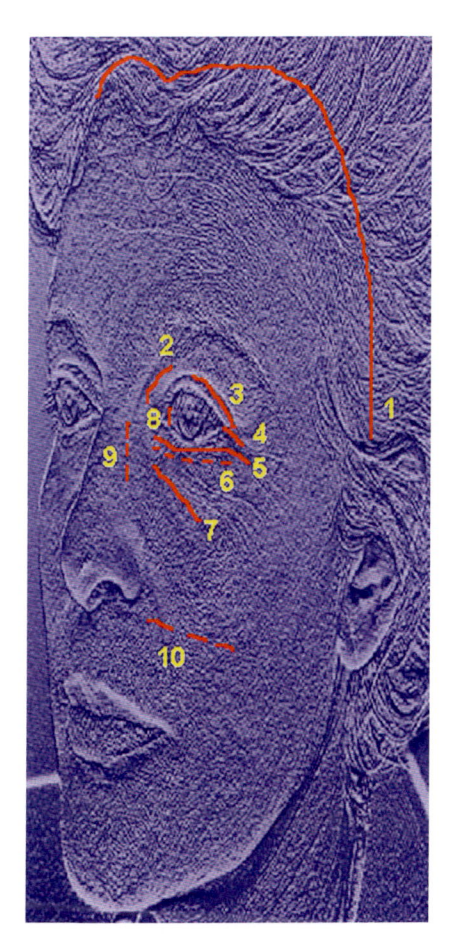

*Fig. 6.* Common surgical incisions for orbital decompression: (1) coronal; (2) 'Lynch'; (3) upper skin crease; (4) lateral canthus; (5) sub-ciliary; (6) inferior fornix; (7) direct translower lid; (8) transcaruncular; (9) transnasal; (10) transoral; (4 + 6) swinging eyelid.

risk of decompression-induced diplopia. In cases of mild exophthalmos, translid antral-ethmoidal decompression appeared to be a valid alternative, with a risk of iatrogenic diplopia in only 4.6% of patients [24]. For more severe exophthalmos, infero-medial decompression was used in combination with lateral decompression. Such procedures were also related with a low incidence of consecutive diplopia [26]. In 1989, Leone et al. [28], in an attempt to further reduce post decompression strabismus proposed balancing the decompression by removing the medial and lateral orbital walls while sparing the floor. This technique, which theoretically should have minimised the risk of iatrogenic diplopia, later appeared to be associated with a higher risk of such a complication as compared with removal of the lateral orbital wall alone, or with inferomedial and three wall techniques [29, 30].

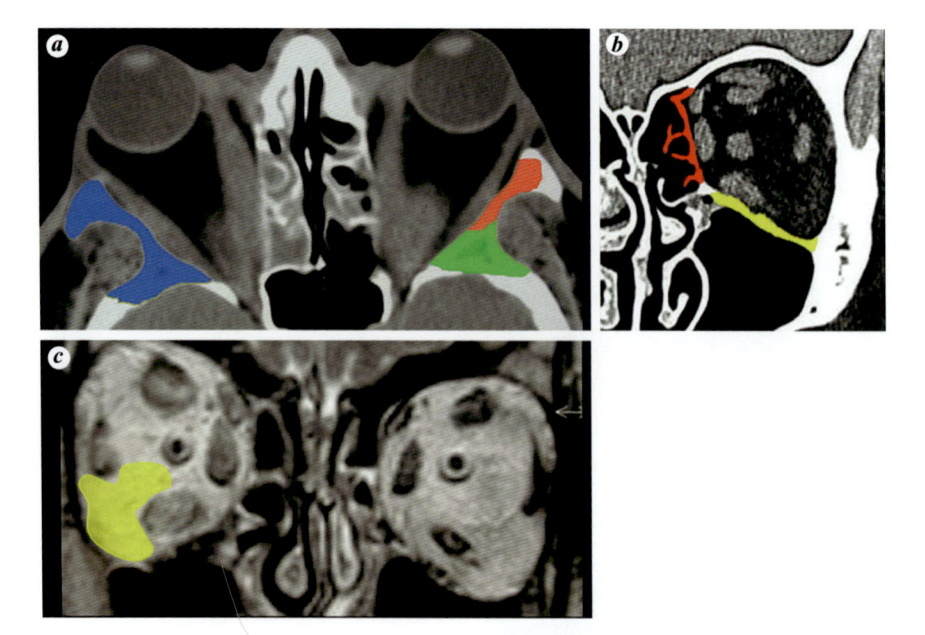

*Fig. 7.* Common zones of bone and fat removal for orbital decompression. *a* Axial projection of an orbital computer tomography scan which highlights possible lateral wall osteotomies: conservative anterior (red), deep (green), extended (red + green), total (blue). *b* Coronal projection of an orbital computer tomography scan which highlights possible osteotomies: inferior (yellow), medial (red), inferomedial (yellow + red). *c* Coronal projection of an orbital magnetic resonance scan with the typical zone of fat removal highlighted in yellow in one of the orbits.

At present the medial wall, the orbital floor and the lateral wall continue to be addressed during bony decompression surgery (fig. 7a, b), while orbital roof removal has been abandoned due to the fact that its contribution to orbital expansion was minimal and consistent with potential complications and side effects. Minimally invasive approaches and hidden incisions such as conjunctival and upper skin creases are currently preferred (fig. 6).

Depending on the severity of exophthalmos the effect of inferomedial decompression can be implemented adding lateral wall decompression and/or removal of the fat, usually of the inferior lateral orbital quadrant (fig. 5a, 7c). In view of reducing post-operative diplopia, an opposite sequence which imply firstly the removal of the lateral wall, associated or not to fat excision, and secondly, if necessary, the removal of the medial and inferior walls has been suggested [31]. This strategy represents a significant conceptual departure from the traditional approach which began with inferomedial decompression and suggests regarding to the lateral orbital wall, and in particular its deep portion, as being the region of first choice for orbital decompression in the case of rehabilitative surgery (fig. 7a). Removal of the lateral orbital wall which appears to be connected with a low risk of consecutive diplopia or severe complications, such as cerebrospinal fluid leak, perfectly fits the needs of the increasingly demanding patient population [18, 31]. It was recently reported that removal of the deep lateral wall as a part of a rehabilitative coronal-approach 3-wall decompression gives a 32% enhancement of exophthalmos reduction without increasing the risk of consecutive diplopia as compared with traditional more conservative 3-wall decompression [32]. The same study, however, confirmed the known high interindividual variability of the volume of the deep lateral wall. In light of this, the deep lateral wall is to be considered an effective although not always available zone of possible orbital volume expansion when dealing with rehabilitative decompression surgery [32]. The effect of pure lateral wall decompression on exophthalmos reduction may result as modest if not associated with medial wall removal, but in this case the risk of consecutive diplopia rises, while the result of lateral wall decompression can be implemented by intraconal fat removal without substantially increasing the risk for iatrogenic strabismus. On the contrary, removal of the lateral orbital wall and intraconal fat resulted as being beneficial in reducing pre-operative primary gaze diplopia [33].

Rehabilitative decompression surgery aimed at addressing the tiresome retro-ocular tension that may characterise the post-inflammatory stage of GO can be performed with minimally invasive techniques leading to minimal, if any, impact on extraocular motility or complications in general [34].

Orbital fat decompression was first described by Moore [35] in 1920. A mean exophthalmos reduction of 6 mm and an improvement of extraocular eye motility have been reported by Olivari on a large series of patients, but the same results were not confirmed by other authors [36–38]. During the last years the combination of bone decompression associated with fat removal (fig. 5) has been gaining popularity in view of its claimed safety and increased effectiveness as compared with bone or fat decompression alone [16–18].

Most of the techniques currently used seem to be effective in reverse restoring eye position and/or congestive symptomatology and disfigurement of the periorbital region; nevertheless, an unbiased analysis of the current literature in terms of effectiveness versus safety is extremely difficult due to the great heterogeneity of the patients included in the published studies and variations applied to surgical techniques. Furthermore, it should be noted that the evidence in the literature concerning rehabilitative decompression surgery is modest, being basically based on retrospective case series. In order to estimate the effectiveness of various surgical techniques, a prospective comparison of different treatment modalities along with different decompression surgeries, using a powerful tool such as the GO quality of life questionnaire [39], had been advocated [34].

## What Are the Possible Complications of Orbital Decompression?

Orbital fat decompression has never reached the popularity of bone decompression due to the theoretic more than real possible feared complications that seem to be connected with this approach and which encompass damages to oculomotor ciliary and lacrimal nerves, orbital vasculature, extraocular eye muscles, optic nerve and the eyeball itself [38]. Also, in the case of bone orbital decompression, in spite of theoretical expectations, severe complications are rare in clinical practice. Common complications of this surgical approach are consecutive strabismus, infraorbital hypoaesthesia and sinusitis [40], lower lid entropion [41] and eyeball dystopia [42], while leakage of cerebrospinal fluid, infections involving the central nervous system, damages to the eye and optic nerve or their vasculature, cerebral vasospasm, ischaemia and infarction are rare events [3, 43]. Reactivation of GO after rehabilitative bony orbital decompression is another rare complication very recently described in 3 of 239 patients not treated with perioperative glucocorticoids. The phenomenon consisted of the onset of typical sings and symptoms of active GO with radiologic evidence of extraocular muscle enlargement a few weeks after surgery and following a normal convalescence period. Based on its clinical characteristics, the observation was named delayed decompression-related reactivation (DDRR). Although the incidence of DDRR appeared to be in the order of 1.3% and could be controlled with systemic immunosuppression or retrobulbar irradiation, it is a complication which deserves to be known by physicians and to be mentioned to those patients undertaking rehabilitative decompression surgery [44].

## Can Complications Be Forecasted or Prevented?

Most of the possible complications cannot be forecasted and their prevention is based on recommendation which are not specific in nature, and which include careful manipulation of the orbital content, accurate dissection of the orbital fat, and avoidance of extensive use of diathermy within the orbit.

Other complications with know pathogenesis such as sinusitis can be simply prevented by taking care to create an adequate sinus aeration as a part of the surgical procedure at the time of decompression.

The occurrence of other complications, namely infraorbital hypoesthesia, eyeball dystopia leakage of cerebrospinal fluid and possible consecutive infectious involvement of the central nervous system, can be reduced by means of accurate evaluation of preoperative imaging, adequate planning of surgical intervention, and the use of prophylactic antibiotics.

Strict respect of this methodology helps detecting patients at an increased risk of possible complications. A low lamina cribrosa for instance should be regarded as a possible source of cerebrospinal fluid leak for those patients planned for medial wall decompression. Late-onset enophthalmos and hypoglobus can be prevented simply by avoiding inferomedial decompression when dealing with patients recognised at higher risk due to their anatomical substrate. The complication had in fact been described as dependent on prolapse of orbital fat into the ethmoidal infundibulum in the presence of a predisposing anatomy which includes septal deviation to the affected side and eventual abnormal middle turbinate whose inferior part, directed laterally, also crows the maxillary infundibulum [42].

Diplopia has a considerable impact on the quality of life of patients with GO, and is a feared complication that often refrains patients and physicians from undertaking decompression rehabilitative surgery. In light of the current literature, strabismus subsequent to decompression surgery has been linked to mechanical and neurological implications connected with the 'lipogenic or myopathic' types of GO [13], the surgical route, the extension and location of the osteotomy, and the respect of structures such as the maxillary ethmoidal strut or the anterior periorbit. Differing type of motor and/or sensory capacities for compensation of induced muscle imbalance may also play a role [10]. A better understanding of all of the possible factors involved in the pathogenesis of diplopia consecutive to decompression surgery may help its prevention.

## References

1  Bahn RS: Pathophysiology of Graves' ophthalmopathy: the cycle of disease. J Clin Endocrinol Metab 2003;88:1939–1946.
2  Rubin PAD, Watkins LM, Rumelt S, Sutula FC, Dallow RL: Orbital computed tomographic characteristics of globe subluxation in thyroid orbitopathy. Ophthalmology 1998;105:2061–2064.
3  Rose GE: Postural visual obscurations in patients with inactive thyroid eye disease; a variant of 'hydraulic' disease. Eye 2006;20:1178–1185.
4  Soares-Welch CV, Fatourechi V, Bartley GB, Beartty CW, Gorman CA, Bahn RS, Bergstralh EJ, Schlech CD, Garrithy BS: Optic neuropathy of Graves' disease: results of transantral orbital decompression and long-term follow-up in 215 patients. Am J Ophthalmol 2003;136:433–441.
5  Wakelkamp IMMJ, Baldeschi L, Saeed P, Mourits MP, Prummel MF, Wiersinga WM: Surgical or medical decompression as a first line treatment of optic neuropathy in Graves' ophthalmopathy? A randomized controlled trial. Clin Endocrinol (Oxf) 2005;63:323–328.

6 www.eugogo.org.
7 Perros P, Baldeschi L, Boboridis K, Dickinson AJ, Hullo A, Kahaly GJ, Kendall-Taylor P, Krassas GE, Lane CM, Lazarus JH, Marcocci C, Mourits MP, Nardi M, Orgiazzi J, Pinchera A, Pitz S, Prummel MF, Wiersinga WM: A questionnaire survey on the management of Graves' orbitopathy in Europe. Eur J Endocrinol 2006;155:207–211.
8 Eckstein AK, Finkenrath A, Heiligenhaus A, Renzing-Kohler K, Esser J, Kruger C, Quadbeck B, Steuhl KP, Gieseler RK: Dry eye syndrome in thyroid-associated ophthalmopathy: lacrimal expression of TSH receptor suggests involvement of TSHR-specific autoantibodies. Acta Ophthalmol Scand 2004;82:291–297.
9 Gilbard JP, Farris RL: Ocular surface drying and ocular tear film osmolarity in thyroid eye disease. Acta Ophthalmol (Copenh) 1983;61:108–116.
10 Baldeschi L, Wakelkamp IMMJ, Lindeboom R, Prummel MF, Wiersinga WM: Early versus late orbital decompression in Graves' orbitopathy: a retrospective study in 125 patients. Ophthalmology 2006;113:874–878.
11 Heinz C, Eckstein A, Steuhl KP, Meller D: Amniotic membrane transplantation for reconstruction of corneal ulcer in Graves' ophthalmopathy. Cornea 2004;23:524–526.
12 Wiersinga WM, Perros P, Kahaly GJ, Mourits MP, Baldeschi L, Boboridis K, Boschi A, Dickinson AJ, Hullo A, Kendall-Taylor P, Krassas GE, Lane CM, Lazarus JH, Marcocci C, Marino M, Nardi M, Neho C, Orgiazzi J, Pinchera A, Pitz S, Prummel MF, Sartini MS, Stahl M, von Arx G: Clinical assessment of patients with Graves' orbitopathy: the European group for Graves' orbitopathy recommendations to generalists, specialists and clinical researchers. Eur J Endocrinol 2006;155: 387–389.
13 Nunery WR: Ophthalmic Graves' disease: a dual theory of pathogenesis. Ophthalmol Clin North Am 1991;4:73–87.
14 Mourits MPh, Rose GE, Garrity JA, Nardi M, Matton G, Koornneef L: Surgical management of Graves' ophthalmopathy; in Prummel MF (ed): Recent Developments in Graves' Ophthalmopathy. Dordrecht, Kluwer Academic Publishers, 2000.
15 Jorge R, Scott IU, Akaishi PM, Velasco Cruz AA, Flynn HW Jr: Resolution of choroidal folds and improvement in visual acuity after orbital decompression for Graves' orbitopathy. Retina 2003;23: 563–565.
16 Goldberg RA: The evolving paradigm of orbital decompression surgery. Arch Ophthalmol 1998;116:95–96.
17 Unal M, Leri F, Konuk O, Hasanreisoglu B: Balanced orbital decompression combined with fat removal in Graves' ophthalmopathy: do we really need to remove the third wall? Ophthal Plast Reconstr Surg 2003;19:112–118.
18 McCann JD, Goldberg RA, Anderson RL, Burroughs JR, Ben Simon GJ: Medial wall decompression for optic neuropathy but lateral wall decompression with fat removal for non vision-threatening indications. Am J Ophthalmol 2006;141:916–917.
19 Dollinger J: Die Druckentlastung der Augenhöhle durch Entfernung der äusseren Orbitawand bei hochgradigem Exophthalmos (Morbus Basedowii) und konsekutiver Hauterkrankung. Dtsch Med Wochenschr 1911;37:1888–1890.
20 Kazim M, Trokel SL, Acaroglu G, Elliot A: Reversal of dysthyroid optic neuropathy following orbital fat decompression. Br J Ophthalmol 2000;84:600–605.
21 Liao SL, Chang TC, Iin LL: Transcaruncular orbital decompression: an alternate procedure for Graves' ophthalmopathy with compressive optic neuropathy. Am J Ophthalmol 2006;14:810–818.
22 McCord CD: Orbital decompression for Graves' disease: exposure through lateral canthal and inferior fornix incision. Ophthalmology 1981;88:533–541.
23 Kennedy DW, Goldstein ML, Miller NR, Zinreich SJ: Endoscopic transnasal orbital decompression. Arch Otolaryngol Head Neck Surg 1990;116:275–282.
24 Mc Cord CD: Current trends in orbital decompression. Ophthalmology 1985;92:21–33.
25 Walsch TE, Ogura JH: Transantral orbital decompression for malignant exophthalmos. Laryngoscope 1957;67:544–568.
26 Mourits MPh, Koornneef L, Wiersinga WM, et al: Orbital decompression for Graves' ophthalmopathy by inferomedial, by inferomedial plus lateral, and by coronal approach. Ophthalmology 1990;97:636–641.

27 De Santo LW: Transantral orbital decompression; in Gorman CA, Waller RR, Dyer JA (eds): The Eye and Orbit in Thyroid disease. New York, Raven Press, 1984, pp 231–251.
28 Leone CR, Piest KL, Newman RJ: Medial and lateral wall decompression for thyroid ophthalmopathy. Am J Ophthalmol 1989;108:160–166.
29 Goldberg RA, Perry JD, Hortoleza V, Tong JT: Strabismus after balanced medial plus lateral wall versus lateral wall only orbital decompression for dysthyroid orbitopathy. Ophthal Plast Reconstr Surg 2000;16:271–277.
30 Paridaens D, Hans K, van Buiten S, Mourits MPh: The incidence of diplopia following coronal and translid orbital decompression in Graves' orbitopathy. Eye 1998;12:800–805.
31 Goldberg RA: The evolving paradigm of orbital decompression surgery. Arch Ophthalmol 1998;116:95–96.
32 Baldeschi L, MacAndie K, Hintschich C, Wakelkamp IMMJ, Prummel MF, Wiersinga WM: The removal of the deep lateral wall in decompression surgery: its contribution to exophthalmos reduction and influence on consecutive diplopia. Am J Ophthalmol 2005;140:642–647.
33 Ben Simon GJ, Wang L, McCann JD, Goldberg RA: Primary-gaze diplopia in patients with thyroid-related orbitopathy undergoing deep lateral orbital decompression with intraconal fat debulking: a retrospective analysis of treatment outcome. Thyroid 2004;14:379–383.
34 Ben Simon GJ, Schwarcz RM, Mansury AM, Wang L, McCann JD, Goldberg RA: Minimally invasive orbital decompression: local anesthesia and hand-carved bone. Arch Ophthalmol 2005;123:1671–1675.
35 Moore RF: Exophthalmos and limitation of eye movements of Graves' disease. Lancet 1920;ii:701.
36 Olivari N: Transpalpebral Decompression-Operation bei endokriner Orbitopathy (Exophthalmus). Wien Med Wochenschr 1988;18:138–142.
37 Trokel S, Kazim M, Moore S: Orbital fat removal, decompression for Graves' ophthalmopathy. Ophthalmology 1993;100:674–682.
38 Adenis JP, Rober PY, Lasudry JGH, Dalloul Z: Treatment of proptosis with fat removal orbital decompression in Graves' ophthalmopathy. Eur J Ophthalmol 1998;8:246–252.
39 Terwee CB, Dekker FW, Mourits MPh, Gerdings MN, Baldeschi L, Kalmann R, Prummel MF, Wiersinga WM: Interpretation and validity of changes in scores on the Graves' ophthalmopathy quality of life questionnaire (GO-QOL) after different treatments. Clin Endocrinol 2001;54:391–398.
40 Carrasco JR, Castillo I, Bilyk JR, Pribitkin EA, Savino PJ: Incidence of infraorbital hypesthesia and sinusitis after orbital decompression for thyroid-related orbitopathy: a comparison of surgical techniques. Ophthal Plast Reconstr Surg 2005;21:188–191.
41 Goldberg RA, Christenbury JD, Shorr N: Medial entropion following orbital decompression for dysthyroid ophthalmopathy. Ophthal Plast Reconstr Surg 1988;4:81–85.
42 Rose GE, Lund VJ: Clinical features and treatment of late enophthalmos after orbital decompression: a condition suggesting cause for idiopathic 'imploding antrum' (silent sinus) syndrome. Ophthalmology 2003;110:819–826.
43 McCormick CD, Bearden WH, Hunts JH, Anderson RL: Cerebral vasospasm and ischemia after orbital decompression for graves ophthalmopathy. Ophthal Plast Reconstr Surg 2004;20:347–351.
44 Baldeschi L, Lupetti A, Vu P, Wakelkamp IMMJ, Prummel MF, Wiersinga WM: Reactivation of Graves' orbitopathy after rehabilitative orbital decompression. Ophthalmology 2007 Feb 21;[Epub ahead of print].

Dr. Lelio Baldeschi
Room D2–436, Orbital Center, Department of Ophthalmology
Academic Medical Center, University of Amsterdam
Meibergdreef 9
NL–1105 AZ Amsterdam (The Netherlands)
Tel. +31 20 566 3580, Fax +31 20 566 9053, E-Mail l.baldeschi@amc.uva.nl

# Eye Muscle Surgery

*M. Nardi*

Ophthalmology, Neuroscience Department, University of Pisa, Pisa, Italy

## What Is the Cause of Ocular Motility Impairment?

Ocular motility disorders in Graves' orbitopathy (GO) are non-concomitant, i.e. the angle of strabismus varies in different directions of gaze. Non-concomitant deviation may be paralytic or restrictive: restrictive differs from paralytic strabismus because, while the latter is due to a paralysis with insufficient contraction of an extraocular muscle, the former is due to a mechanical obstacle to ocular rotation. Usually, in GO extraocular muscle involvement is characterized by a myositis followed by fibrosis: this makes the muscle stiff and inextensible (fig. 1). Restriction limits eyeball rotation in the direction opposite to the involved muscle because it is no longer able to lengthen (this type of lash effect is called direct restriction); moreover, when the antagonist of the restricted muscle contracts, the eyeball is pulled into the orbit and there is a temporary increase in intraocular pressure [1]. In extreme cases of fibrosis the muscle may shorten, rotating the globe toward its direction of action and causing a deviation also in primary position of gaze.

The distinction between paralytic and restrictive strabismus is fundamental for treatment: in paralysis you have to reinforce the action of the involved muscle while in restriction you have to weaken the involved muscle.

## How Do You Identify the Affected Muscles?

Identification of the affected muscles may appear complex because a multitude of test has been proposed but, considering that we face a restrictive disorder, few simple tests are sufficient in order to establish a diagnosis and formulate a surgical plan. A very simple and quick diagnostic flow is presented here.

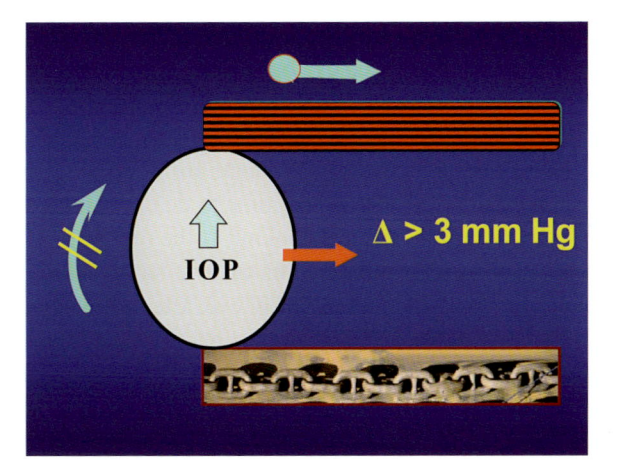

*Fig. 1.* In attempting elevation, a restriction of the inferior rectus muscle causes a deficit of elevation and, pushing the eye into the orbit, a temporary rise in intraocular pressure.

Observe the orbital region of the patient while he is looking straight ahead (primary position of gaze): this is important for a gross impression of the presence of monolateral or bilateral proptosis, the type of dislocation of the eyeball (if present), and/or the presence of a manifest strabismus (looking at the corneal reflex).

Examine ductions (ductions are monocular movements of the eye): this is done by patching the controlateral eye and asking the patient to look at a penlight that is moved along the diagnostic positions of gaze, starting from the primary position. If the eye does not reach the maximal excursion, a restrictive disorder of the opposite rectus muscle is very probable. The test may be also performed in a quantitative way with an arc perimeter following the indication of Mourits et al. [2].

Examine versions (versions are binocular movements of the eyes): this is done by asking the patient to look at a penlight that is moved along the diagnostic positions of gaze starting from the primary position. It gives different information in respect to duction testing, because it evaluates the relative position of both eyes during ocular rotations. This is fundamental for the surgical plan, because in the frequent case of multiple or bilateral restrictions you must tailor your surgery, not only in order to reduce the angle of strabismus (working on the most involved muscle) but also to make ocular movements more concomitant as possible, with the aim of obtaining a useful field of single binocular vision. So, e.g., if we are facing a symmetric restriction of the inferior rectus muscle (IRM) in both eyes (OO), the patient may have a good field of single binocular vision and may not need surgery; or if the restriction is asymmetric, operating only on one eye you must plan your surgery in order to symmetrize and not to normalize ductions in the most affected eye because in this latter case you will get a vertical hypercorrection.

Cover tests are essential for determining the presence of strabismus, its type and for an objective measurement of the angle. There are substantially 3 types of cover test: (1) The cover-uncover test which aims to detect manifest strabismus: it is performed by covering one eye and looking at the other eye in order to see if it makes a movement of refixation. In this case, a manifest strabismus is detected. The manoeuvre is repeated on the other eye, after allowing a moment of binocularity. (2) The alternate cover test which aims to detect latent strabismus (the ocular deviations that are masked by fusion). In this test, the eyes are covered alternately without giving moments of binocularity (this is in order to dissociate fusion). The test is positive for latent strabismus when there is evidence of refixation movements. (3) The prism cover test which measures the deviation in both latent and manifest strabismus: it is performed in the same way as the alternate cover test, interposing a bar prism in front of one eye and finding the prism that neutralizes the refixation movement.

Measurement of intraocular pressure in upgaze: an increase more than 3 mm Hg in upgaze may indicate the presence (also not evident in ocular motility assessment) of a restriction of the inferior rectus muscle.

Forced duction test: this test is fundamental for assessing the presence of a restriction. It may be performed under local or general anaesthesia and consist of taking the perilimbal conjunctiva with a forceps and trying to move the eye passively in the direction of action of the extraocular rectus muscles. If there is some resistance the presence of a restriction of the antagonist muscle is confirmed. This test has to be performed before surgery for confirming the presence of a restriction, and during and at the end of surgery in order to assess that the restrictions have been relieved.

## How Can You Avoid Diagnostic Errors in Complex Cases?

In order to avoid errors we must remember:
(1) In GO impairment of ocular motility is always due to restriction and never to hyperfunction or paralysis.
(2) Multiple restrictions are often present and must be detected for a correct surgical plan.
(3) Some signs may be misleading [3] and may induce a wrong diagnosis. Among these we consider:
    (a) Apparent overaction of the inferior oblique muscle (IOM): On examination, these patients show an apparent hypertropia of the adducted eye

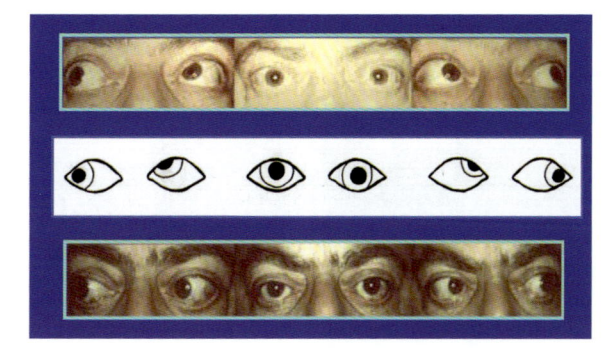

*Fig. 2.* Restriction of inferior rectus muscle gives hypotropia of the affected eye which increases in abduction: this may simulate inferior oblique overaction (pseudo overaction of the inferior oblique muscle; above). This is a bilateral case and surgery on both inferior rectus muscles solved the problem (below).

simulating inferior oblique muscle (IOM) hyperfunction, common in concomitant strabismus. The hypertropia of the adducted eye in GO is usually due to a restriction of the controlateral IRM: in this case IRM has to be weakened (fig. 2) and surgery on IOM will result in a disaster [4].
(b) Pseudoparalysis of the superior oblique muscle (SOM): The diagnosis of paralysis is usually made after performing the three-step test of Parks; this test is valid for diagnosis of a paralytic cyclovertical disorder but is unattainable in restrictive disorders. In this case the disorder is again due to a restriction of the controlateral IOM. It is often accompanied by torticollis with head tilt towards the controlateral shoulder. Again, operating on SOM may result in a disaster and surgery has to be performed on the controlateral IRM (fig. 3).
(c) Excyclotorsion on attempted upgaze: This finding may be interpreted as a paretic involvement of a SOM but once again it is due to a homolateral restriction of the IRM. It is due to hyperactivation of the IOM in attempted elevation, when the superior rectus muscle (SRM) is unable to elevate the eye: the problem is solved weakening the omolateral IRM [3].

### How Can You Evaluate the Need for Surgery?

The need for surgery is evaluated considering:
(1) The disability of the patient which is usually related to the diplopia field.
(2) The prognosis for a favourable result.
(3) Rarely the aesthetic problem.

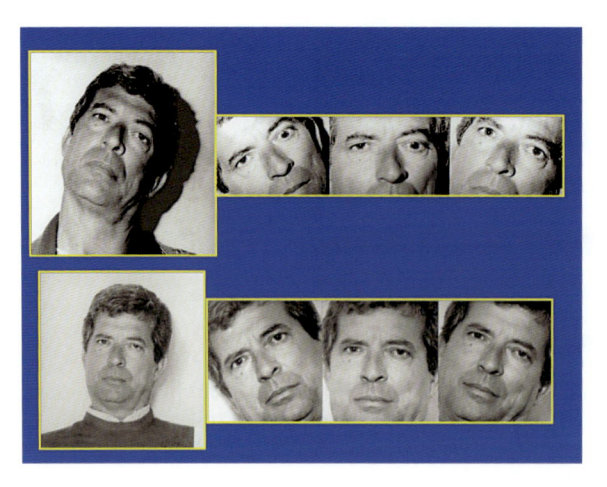

*Fig. 3.* A positive head tilt test may simulate a controlateral superior oblique palsy at the Parks' three-step test (above). In GO, a positive head tilt test is due to inferior rectus muscle restriction and is confirmed by the fact that surgery on this muscle will result in a negative head tilt test and reduction of torticollis (below).

Disability is the most important factor when considering surgery: it is usually linked to the field of diplopia more than to the angle of strabismus (this because the same angle of strabismus may or may not give diplopia in different patients due to the entity of fusional amplitudes). The extent of diplopia may be quantified by examining the field of single binocular vision (FSBV). This test is performed with an arc or bowl perimeter: the patient, with both eyes open, is asked to look at a target which is moved from the area of the field of gaze in which it appears single toward the area in which it appears double. In this manner, the limits of the area of single binocular vision can be determined and reported in a graph (fig. 4). Obviously, diplopia in the primary position of gaze and/or in downgaze is the most disabling.

Disability may also be due to an anomalous head posture (torticollis oculi, not infrequently causing pain in the back of the neck) and this may be a strong indication for surgery (fig. 3).

The prognosis progressively worsens from pure horizontal deviation, to pure vertical deviation and to mixed deviation (figs. 5, 6). Particularly problematic are those eyes with multiple heavy restriction and deficit of ductions in the opposite direction of gaze or in all directions of gaze (frozen eyes): in these eyes one must be very careful when performing surgery because, for the restriction of the homolateral antagonist, a mild degree of weakening surgery may induce a conspicuous hypercorrection.

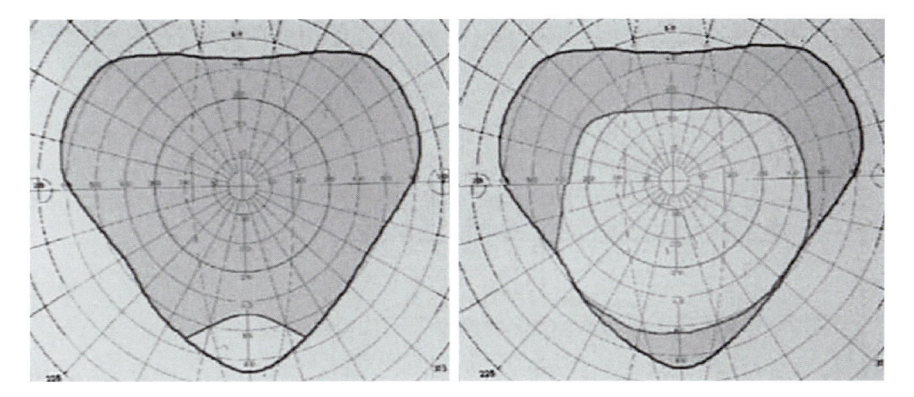

*Fig. 4.* Field of single binocular vision in a patient with left inferior rectus muscle restriction before (left) and after (right) a lengthening procedure on the left inferior rectus muscle.

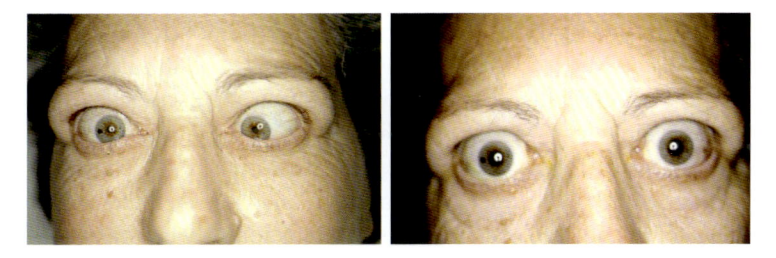

*Fig. 5.* A mixed deviation (horizontal and vertical) before (left) and after (right) surgery.

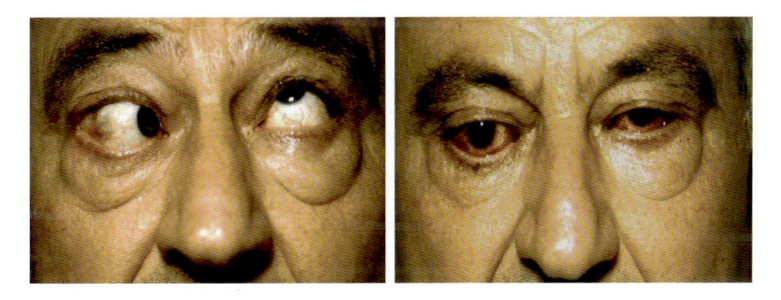

*Fig. 6.* A mixed deviation (horizontal and vertical) before (left) and after (right) surgery. This patient did not attain SBV after surgery: however, he ignored diplopia and after further surgery on the right inferior lid he was happy with the result.

The prognosis for a favourable result other than the type of deviation is related to the presence of potential single binocular vision (SBV). This may be checked neutralizing the angle with a prism and asking the patient if he is seeing double. Obviously, this test may be misleading but usually it is a good indicator of a possibly good result.

Moreover, any decision has to be made on the basis of patient's needs, and surgery must be asked for by the patient himself.

### When Is the Right Time for Surgery?

At least 6 months after normalization of thyroid function, loss of activity of GO and stabilization of ocular motility. For the stability of the results, it is important to operate when GO is inactive.

### What Can You Realistically Expect from Surgery?

Obviously, the results expected vary in relationship to the form of ocular motility disorder. More often a good result may be considered by the attainment of a useful field of SBV, comprising both primary position and downgaze [5]. It is important immediately after surgery to obtain an area of single binocular vision: this area, also if limited, will usually enlarge with time, due to development of fusional amplitudes (fusional amplitudes are plastic: when there is no area of SBV they are not utilized and will reduce; after surgery, when an area of SBV is present, they will increase with exercise in casual seeing).

### How Should You Advise the Patient?

Very often GO patients have unrealistic expectations from surgery, sometimes generated by optimistic press releases from physicians. Speaking about extraocular muscle surgery, the surgeon must specify that:
(1) It is an incompletely predictable surgery: in the best series success is about 80–85% with one surgery and rises to 92–93% with more than one procedure. Obviously, it depends not only on the appropriateness of the surgical plan but also on factors related to the patient that may not be detectable on preoperative examination.
(2) An acceptable result is to obtain a useful field of single binocular vision (so diplopia in lateral and superior gaze may probably persist).
(3) In some cases, there may be the need to operate on both eyes and more than one muscle per eye (maximum 2 rectus muscles).

(4) If adjustable sutures are planned there will be an adjustment under topical anaesthesia on the following day.
(5) The surgical plan may be modified during surgery if the surgeon detects some restrictions which were not detected during the preoperative examination.

**The Surgical Plan: What Procedures Are Recommended?**

The surgical plan is the focal point: surgery has to be planned taking in account that:
(1) It is important to aim at obtaining an area of single binocular vision with a single surgery: this area, also if limited, will usually enlarge with time, due to development of fusional amplitudes with spontaneous exercise in casual viewing; for that reason we have to operate on more than one muscle and on both eyes at one time, if needed; in adult patients you can perform surgery safely only on two rectus muscles in each eye, for the fear of anterior segment ischaemia [6]. You must plan your surgery and reoperations thinking that you must not detach more than two rectus muscles from the globe (this must be taken in account also in eventual subsequent procedures, because there is no evidence that this will avoid anterior segment ischaemia).
(2) Usually only weakening procedures (recessions, recession on adjustable sutures, lengthening procedures) are performed, due to the restrictive nature of the disorder. Pay attention, a strengthening procedure (that has invariably to be coupled to a weakening procedure on the antagonist) will usually result in a marked hypercorrection; moreover, in such a situation, having operated on two rectus muscle of the same eye, any other surgery on the remaining rectus muscles will be precluded.
(3) Misleading signs (pseudo inferior oblique overaction, pseudo superior oblique paresis, excyclotorsion during elevation, head tilt on a shoulder) are due to restriction of the inferior rectus muscles and not to involvement of an oblique muscle.
(4) In vertical deviation always aim for a slight hypocorrection. After surgery there is very often a slow updrift of the operated eye and this may result in late hypercorrection. A mild hypocorrection will afford single binocular vision in downgaze and primary gaze (with or without a temporary prism) and the area of single binocular vision will enlarge with time. I worry about a late hypercorrection if I get a full correction of the vertical deviation on the day after surgery [7].
(5) The procedures recommended are, as stated, weakening procedures: these comprise recessions, recession on adjustable sutures, lengthening procedures and conjunctival recession. In the last years much has changed in

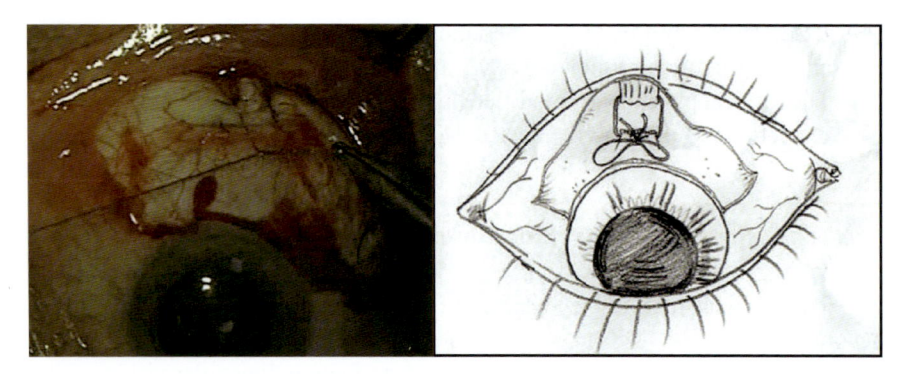

*Fig. 7.* Adjustable suture. The muscle is recessed with a loop anchored to the original insertion. A temporary knot affords intra-operative and early post-operative adjustment.

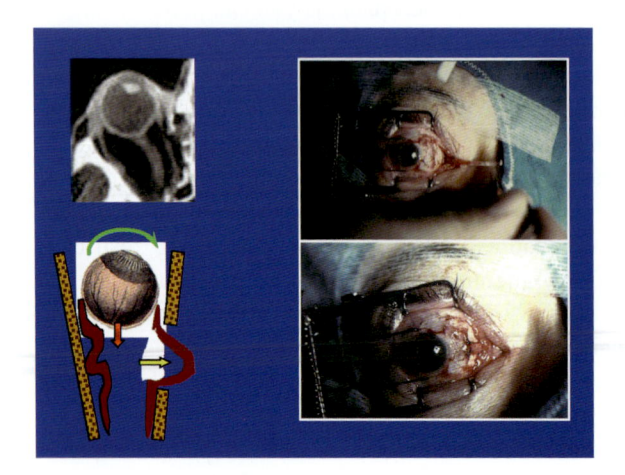

*Fig. 8.* Lengthening procedures are useful in some cases, particularly when, after decompression, the tendon is displaced, or in presence of very strong restrictions: in these circumstances it is important to maintain an arc of contact and lengthening the tendon is indicated.

strabismus surgery with the introduction of topical anaesthesia and adjustable sutures. Topical anaesthesia (eventually implemented with subtenonian injection and general sedation) allows intra-operative assessment of the results, while adjustable suturing allows fine tuning of the results on the following day (fig. 7). Lengthening procedures are useful in some cases, particularly when, after decompression, the tendon is displaced (fig. 8), or in the presence of very strong restrictions.

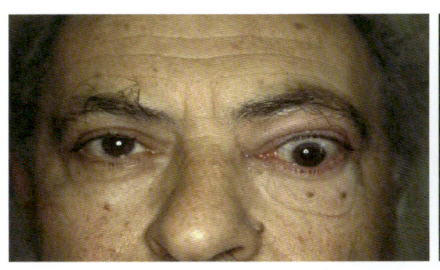

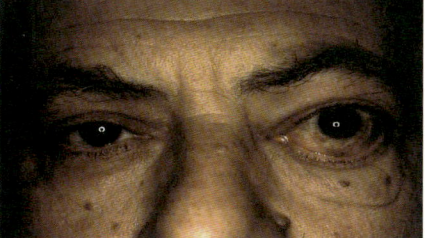

*Fig. 9.* Late vertical hypercorrection and left lower lid ptosis after weakening procedure on the left IRM.

(6) Weakening of both the inferior and medial rectus muscles may cause a divergence in downgaze (the so-called A pattern of deviation) with diplopia in the reading position. To avoid this problem, it is important to transpose the medial rectus muscle insertion upward during the weakening procedure: in this way, the adduction in downgaze will be reinforced [8].

### What Are the Possible Complications of Surgery and How Can I Avoid or Manage Them?

There are two types of surgical complications: those common to every strabismus surgery (e.g. perforation of the sclera, postoperative infections, and adherence syndrome) and those more frequent or more dangerous in GO patients. The latter include:
(1) Lost or slipped muscle: This is really a threatened complication: usually the slipped muscle will retract deeply into the orbit without the possibility of being recovered. Very often the presence of a contracture of the homolateral antagonist will cause a marked overcorrection: this is very difficult to treat surgically and for this reason every effort has to be made in order to prevent muscle slippage.
(2) Late vertical hypercorrections (fig. 9): Late vertical hypercorrection may be due to concomitant restriction of the homolateral antagonist or restriction of the controlateral inferior rectus muscle (fig. 10). The treatment is based on prism prescription in mild cases or more often in a new surgical procedure: in order to plan surgery, we again must detect the muscles involved and take in account that not more than 2 rectus muscles for each eye can be severed from the sclera.

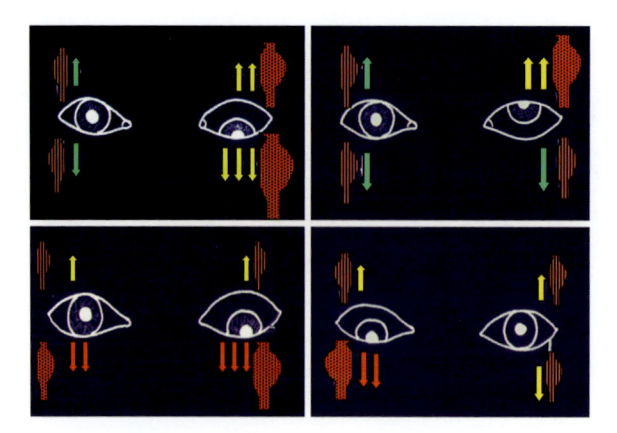

*Fig. 10.* Late vertical hypercorrection may be due to concomitant restriction of the homolateral antagonist (above: left before surgery, right after surgery) or restriction of the controlateral inferior rectus muscle (below: left before surgery, right after surgery).

(3) Change in eyelid position: Surgery on vertical rectus muscles may affect eyelid position: the commonest event is inferior lid retraction after surgery on the inferior rectus muscle and this may be prevented to a certain degree by freeing the inferior rectus muscle from other inferior lid retractors and from the Lockwood ligament. However, in marked weakening procedures on IRM, some degree of inferior lid retraction has to be taken in account. The patient has to be informed of this together with the possibility of further surgery on the inferior lid [5].

(4) Persistent diplopia: When diplopia persists after an acceptable alignment of the eyes (fig. 6), we have to recheck the patient in order to understand if this is due to:

  (a) Marked reduction of fusional amplitudes: in this case the temporary prescription of prisms may be of help, giving an area of SBV and the possibility of developing fusional amplitudes with exercise.

  (b) Cyclotorsional component: in this case it is important to remember that it is usually due to a vertical muscle and oblique muscles must be considered only as the last resort.

  (c) Absence of fusion: This is very rare (usually post-traumatic) and is characterized by the presence of superimposition of the images (when the residual angle is neutralized with prism or synoptophore) and absence of fusional amplitudes. In this case, there is nothing which can be done and if the patient cannot manage with his diplopia, occlusion of one eye must be considered.

# References

1 Nardi M, Bartolomei MP, Romani A, Barca L: Intraocular pressure changes in secondary position of gaze in normal subjects and in restrictive ocular motility disorders. Graefe's Arch Klin Exp Ophthalmol 1988;226:8–10.
2 Mourits MP, Prummel MF, Wiersinga WM, Koorneef L: Measuring eye movements in Graves' ophthalmopathy. Ophthalmology 1994;101:1341–1346.
3 Nardi M, Bartolomei MP, Pinchera A, Barca L: Misleading signs in inferior rectus restrictive disorders. It J Ophthalmol 1990;4:91–94.
4 Shimek SE: Surgical management of ocular complications of Graves' disease. Arch Ophthalmol 1972;87:655–664.
5 Mourits M, Rose GE, Garrity JA, Nardi M, Matton G, Koorneef L: Surgical management of Graves' ophthalmopathy; in Prummel MF (ed): Recent Developments in Graves' Ophthalmopathy. Boston, Kluwer Academic Publishers, 2000, pp 133–169.
6 Saunders RA, Bluestein EC, Wilson ME, Berland JE: Anterior segment ischemia after strabismus surgery. Surv Ophthalmol 1994;38:456–466.
7 Nardi M, Barca L: Hypercorrection of hypotropia in Graves' ophthalmopathy. Ophthalmology 1993;100:1–2.
8 Nardi M, Sellari S, Laddaga F, Marabotti A, Pinchera A: Extraocular muscle surgery in Graves' disease. Operative Tech Oculoplastic Orbital Reconstruct Surg 1999;2:89–94.

Prof. Marco Nardi
Institute of Ophthalmology, Neuroscience Department
University of Pisa, Via Roma, 56
IT–56100 Pisa (Italy)
Tel. +39 050 993385, Fax +39 050 992019, E-Mail marco.nardi@med.unipi.it

# Eyelid Surgery

C. Neoh[a], A. Eckstein[b]

[a]Eye Department, Claremont Wing, Royal Victoria Infirmary, Newcastle upon Tyne, UK;
[b]Department of Ophthalmology, Essen University Clinic, Essen, Germany

## What Are the Indications for Eyelid Surgery in Patients with Graves' Orbitopathy?

Eyelid lengthening with or without blepharoplasty (dermatochalasis correction) is usually the final step of surgical rehabilitation. A pleasing outcome after orbital decompression and squint surgery, if indicated, is very much dependent on correcting any remaining lid deformity satisfactorily. This is often more challenging than the preceding surgery.

The most common indication for lid surgery is upper lid retraction with poor cosmesis meriting rehabilitative intervention and functional loss particularly when incomplete lid closure is present. Lid retraction worsens the proptotic appearance. Lagophthalmos and incomplete blinking lead to instability of the tear film and secondary ocular surface disturbance.

Surgery is recommended for significant lid retraction of >1 mm and asymmetry of palpebral apertures. Another indication is lateral (temporal) flare (fig. 1) [see chapter by Dickinson, pp. 1–26].

True lid retraction has to be differentiated from pseudo lid retraction due to fibrosis of the inferior rectus muscle. The latter resolves after inferior rectus recession.

Lower lid lengthening is indicated in lower lid retraction after inferior rectus recession. Bilateral lower lid retraction with proptosis should be primarily referred for orbital decompression. The cosmetic result following lower lid lengthening in patients with disfiguring proptosis who decline orbital decompression is poor. This is due to negative orbital vector where the angle of tilt of the lower lid is unnatural and not vertical in disposition.

Lid retraction can resolve when hyperthyroidism is treated and surgery should always be delayed till after a period of euthyroidism has elapsed.

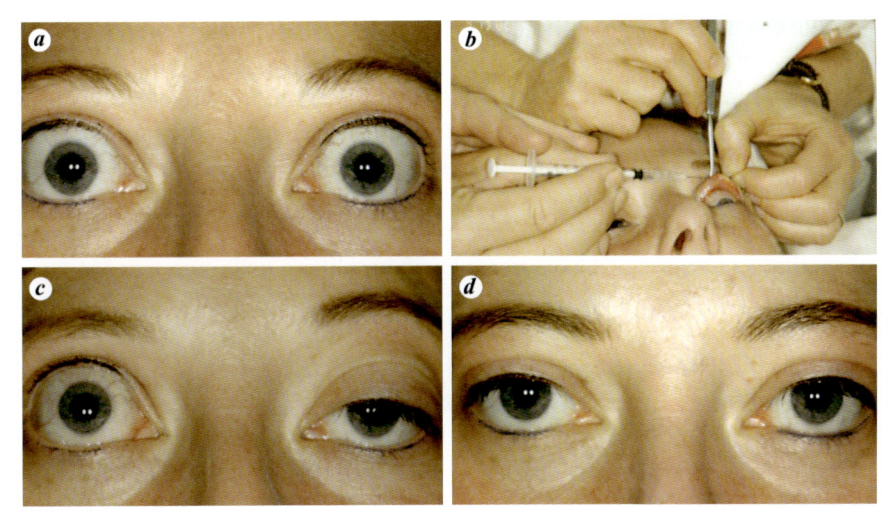

*Fig. 1. a* Patient with bilateral upper lid retraction. *b* Transconjunctival injection of 10 IU botulinum toxin in the Mueller muscle. *c* Effect 3 days after injection of left upper lid. *d* Effect after injection of both eyes.

Another indication for eyelid surgery is increased preaponeurotic and subdermal fat, resulting in bulging of the lids. This can be treated during blepharoplasty when redundant lid skin is excised.

## Is Botulinum Toxin Useful?

Botulinum toxin is produced by the bacterium *Clostridium botulinum* and acts on the motor endplate. Reversible chemodenervation lasting 4–6 weeks results in paralysis of the muscle injected. Botulinum toxin is commercially available.

The indications for botulinum toxin in Graves' orbitopathy (GO) (ophthalmopathy) are upper lid retraction, marked extraocular muscle fibrosis in the fixing eye and glabella and corrugator superciliaris overaction prior to definitive surgery (fig. 1).

Upper lid retraction can be reduced by injecting 5–15 IU of botulinum toxin subconjunctivally or transcutaneously in the levator/Mueller muscle, as shown in figure 1. Full effect is evident after 2–3 days and persists for about 4–6 weeks. The outcome is variable and the dose of botulinum toxin has to be adjusted individually. Transient double vision and ptosis can occur in 10–20% [1–5].

Further injection should therefore be avoided for about 8 weeks before surgery.

Botulinum toxin can also be used in case of marked fibrosis of extraocular muscles if fixation is affected and the patient can only attain primary position with a marked abnormal head posture. The injection of botulinum toxin is best performed under EMG control.

Deep furrowing in the glabellar area due to overaction of the corrugator superciliaris muscle can also be treated with botulinum toxin injection [6].

## Is Surgical Intervention Indicated in Corneal Ulceration Secondary to Exposure Keratopathy?

Corneal ulceration is a serious sight threatening complication of ocular surface damage due to reduced tear production, upper and lower lid retraction and impaired Bell's phenomenon due to inferior rectus fibrosis [7]. Attempted lid closure normally induces reflex elevation of the globe and lubrication of the cornea by the upper lid (Bell's phenomenon). Patients with GO and tight inferior recti may have impaired Bell's phenomenon and are therefore at risk of exposure keratopathy and corneal ulceration.

Patients with inactive disease, lagophthalmos, increased lid aperture and inferior rectus fibrosis can be surgically corrected by orbital decompression, mono- or bilateral inferior rectus recession and lid lengthening.

When lid lengthening has to be postponed due to active disease, chemodenervation-induced ptosis (30 IU botulinum toxin injection into the levator muscle) and/or a temporary lateral tarsorrhaphy can be performed.

Intensive artificial tears, serum eye drops and topical antibiotics are the mainstay. In case of delayed repair of the epithelial surface and marked corneal inflammatory reaction, the corneal surface can be shielded with amniotic membrane transplantation [8] (fig. 2). AMT can be used as an adjunctive approach to reduce inflammation and promote epithelial wound healing [9]. The amniotic membrane graft is reabsorbed without severe inflammation and stromal fibrosis with reduced transparency is avoided.

## Does Orbital Decompression Have Any Effect on Lid Retraction?

Lid retraction, when present preoperatively, does not always resolve after orbital decompression. There have been reports of reduction of lid retraction after orbital decompression by the bicoronal approach [10–12]. Orbital decompression,

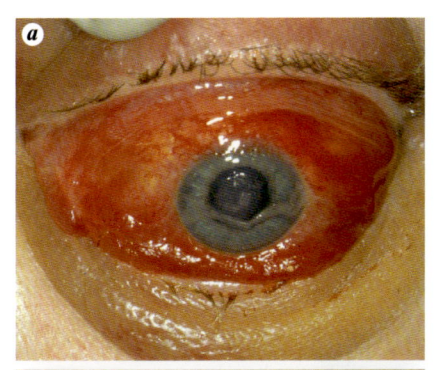

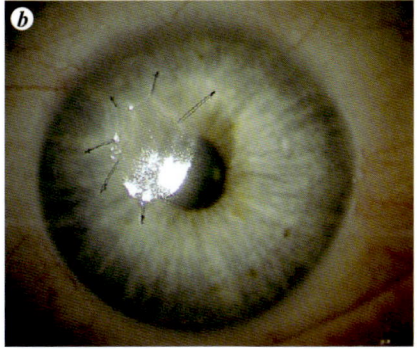

*Fig. 2. a* Corneal ulcer due to lagophthalmos in patient with marked proptosis before decompression surgery. *b* Two weeks after amniotic membrane transplant and emergency 3-wall orbital decompression, inlay membrane has become more transparent. The corneal epithelial defect is healed and ocular surface inflammation is drastically reduced.

however, can facilitate lid closure in patients with proptosis, lagophthalmos and tense orbits.

### Does Squint Surgery Influence the Lid Configuration?

The levator and superior rectus muscles share their nerve supply. When upgaze is restricted due to fibrosis of the inferior rectus, upper lid retraction may be induced on attempted upgaze. This upper lid retraction in intended upgaze resolves after inferior rectus recession (fig. 3).

Ligaments connect the Tenon capsule of the inferior rectus muscle with the lower lid retractors. The lower lid retractors originate as the capsulopalpepral head from attachments to the terminal muscle fibres of the inferior rectus muscle approximately 15 mm from the limbus. Recession of the inferior rectus results in posterior displacement of the capsulopalpepral head and can cause disfiguring lower lid retraction (fig. 3).

This can be successfully prevented by simultaneous sharp detachment of the fascia of the capsulopalpepral head [13]. Lysis of the surrounding check

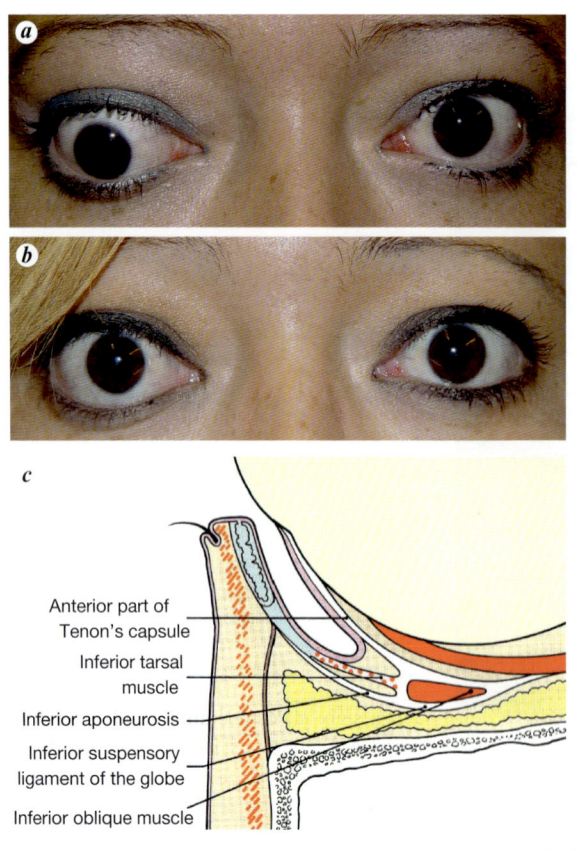

*Fig. 3. a* Patient with inferior rectus fibrosis and pseudo upper lid retraction due to coinnervation of levator and superior rectus muscle. *b* Patient after inferior rectus recession of 7 mm. Upper lid retraction has completely resolved; lower lid retraction has developed. *c* Anatomy of the lower lid. Ligaments connect the Tenon capsule of the inferior rectus muscle with inferior tarsus muscle (lower lid retractor); recession of inferior rectus without disconnection of these ligaments can cause lower lid retraction.

ligaments and fascial attachments does not have an adequate effect [14]. Meyer et al. [15] have described a primary infratarsal lower eyelid retractor lysis to prevent eyelid retraction after inferior rectus muscle recession. If disfiguring lower lid retraction appears, lower lid lengthening is necessary (see below, 'What surgical procedures are available for correction of lower lid retraction?'; fig. 5).

Large recessions or tendon elongation can cause an increase of proptosis.

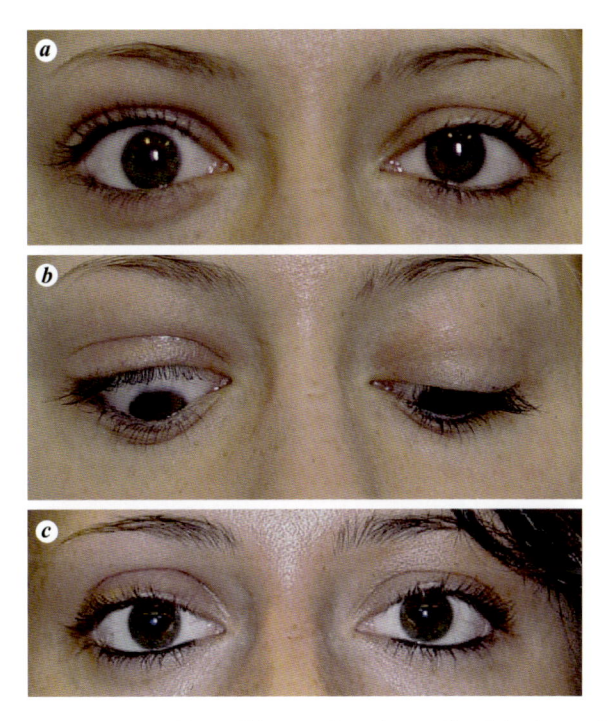

*Fig. 4. a* Upper lid retraction. *b* von Graefe's sign. *c* Postoperative result after full thickness medial and lateral blepharotomy (conjunctiva, Müller muscle and levator aponeurosis) with acceptable result and mild lid crease recession.

## What Surgical Procedures Are Available for Correction of Upper Lid Retraction?

Many different techniques have been described to lengthen the upper lid. Methods and results are reviewed in table 1. Criteria for successful correction of upper lid retraction are covering of 1–2 mm of the superior cornea, smooth lid margin contour, upper lid skin crease between 7 and 10 mm, bilateral symmetry and patient satisfaction (fig. 4). Most of the surgical procedures are described with success rates of about 70–80%.

A summary of upper lid lengthening procedures from Mourits et al. [10] is shown in table 1: Acceptable/good/success implies at least (1) upper eyelid margin from 0.5 above to ≤ 2 mm below the limbus, (2) difference less than 2 mm between eyes, (3) smooth lid margin contour, (4) lid crease within 7–10 mm of the lid margin, (5) symmetrical skin folds, and (6) patient satisfaction and no further treatment. Perfect results are included in this group.

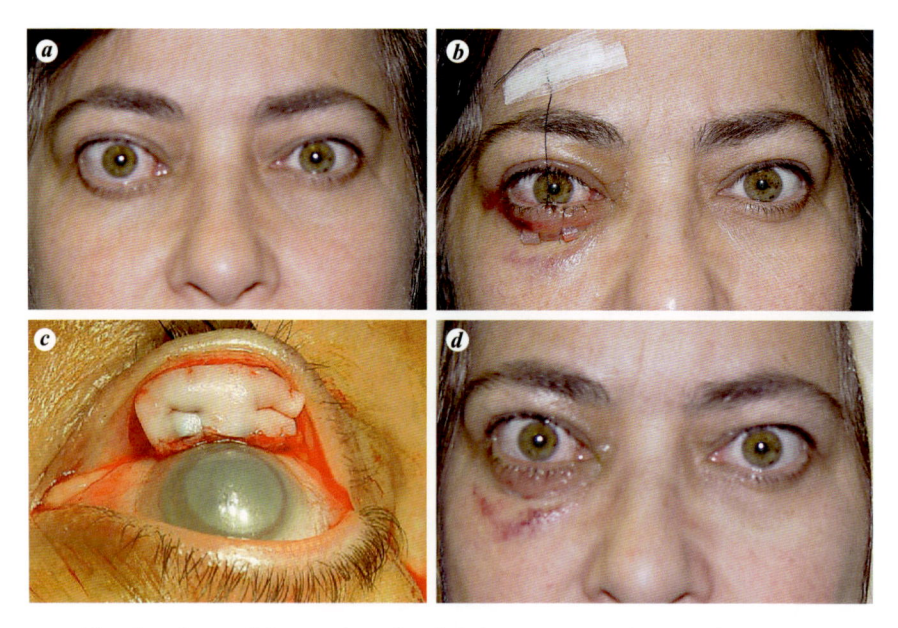

*Fig. 5. a* Lower lid retraction after inferior rectus muscle recession. *b* Transconjunctival surgical correction with 6 mm implant (Tutopatch). The spacer is first sutured to the recessed retractors and then to the tarsus. *c* Day 1 after surgery with supporting sutures. *d* Day 14 after removal of the sutures.

Varying recommendations for functional and stable outcomes have been made. Since lateral retraction (flare) is the most important aspect of upper lid retraction in patients with GO, division of the lateral horn of the aponeurosis is necessary in most cases. Sutures can be placed between the tarsal plate and the detached aponeurosis to prevent spontaneous disinsertion. When sutures are used, it is important to have conjunctival cover to protect the cornea.

Myotomies without spacers (grafts) need the cooperation of the patient but they are easy to perform for all degrees of retraction. If patient cooperation is poor, lid spacers can be used under general anaesthesia. The vertical height of the implant should be approximately twice the measured eyelid retraction [23] or measured eyelid retraction +2 mm, respectively [32].

Further investigation into whether levator lengthening accompanied by fat excision is needed. Mourits and Sasim [29] reported more failure in patients in whom fat had been excised as well, but the numbers were too small for statistical analysis. Modest fat excision is sometimes unavoidable and probably safe. However, excision of larger amounts of fat and skin should be postponed till another operation because of possible reactivation of fibrosing factors and recurrence of lid retraction.

*Table 1.* Methods and results

| Author | Type of surgery | Results |
|---|---|---|
| Puttermann et al. [16] | graded müllerotomy ± levator aponeurosis recession | success: 81% |
| Doxanas et al. [17] | sclera interposition | success: 61% |
| Harvey et al. [18] | müllerotomy, levator aponeurosis recession, lateral horn cut | good/acceptable: 76% |
| Thaller et al. [19] | Müller recession | acceptable: 73% |
| | levator aponeurosis recession | acceptable: 89% |
| | levator aponeurosis recession + sclera | acceptable: 89% |
| | Z-myotomy | acceptable: 100% |
| Hedin et al. [20] | müllerectomy + levator division | acceptable: 90% |
| Harvey et al. [21] | levator aponeurosis recession + Müller recession | good: 86% |
| Levine et al. [22] | levator aponeurosis recession + Müller recession | success: 87% |
| Mourits et al. [23] | Sclera interposition | acceptable: 77% |
| Liu et al. [24] | central aponeurosis disinsertion | acceptable: 77% |
| Uccello et al. [25] | free levator complex recession | acceptable: 73% |
| Ceisler et al. [26] | müllerectomy + levator aponeurosis transposition | acceptable: 98% |
| Tucker et al. [27] | adjustable levator recession | good: 75% |
| | nonadjustable levator recession | good: 34% |
| Woog [28] | adjustable levator recession | acceptable: 86% |
| Mourits et al. [29] | lateral levator recession, Müller recession | acceptable: 82% |
| Elner et al. [30] | lateral full thickness levator, Müller, conjunctiva recession | desired height: 88% |
| Hintschich et al. [31] | medial and lateral full thickness levator, Müller, conjunctiva recession | good ± 1 mm: 97% |

Lateral tarsorrhaphy is unsatisfactory because stretching results in blunting and rounding of the lateral canthal angle and lateral flare becomes evident again. However, a small tarsorrhaphy in combination with lid lengthening procedures can improve the result by disguising proptosis.

## Are There Complications?

Overcorrection can occur due to dissecting the aponeurosis and Müller's muscle too far medially. This leads to flattening of the medial contour. Patients should be evaluated in an upright position before skin closure especially when myotomy has been carried out.

Undercorrection, especially lateral, can occur and leave a temporal obliquity of the lid. Cutting of the lateral horn of the aponeurosis has to be done very carefully. Asymmetry can occur as consequence of over/undercorrection, lid crease recession and a thickened eyelid after graft utilisation.

Lacrimal production can be reduced by transconjunctival Müller's muscle myotomy [33].

Extrusion, shrinkage or migration of allograft material spacer can also occur [34].

## What Surgical Procedures Are Available for Correction of Lower Lid Retraction?

Recession of lower lid retractors alone is insufficient to correct more than 1 mm of lid retraction and an interposition graft or spacer is needed if there is significant lower lid retraction (fig. 5). Spacers act as scaffolding and help overcome the effects of gravity.

The lower lid retractors can be approached by anterior subciliary or posterior subtarsal transconjunctival approach. After detaching the lower lid retractors from the inferior border of the tarsus, the sheet of muscle is dissected free of the conjunctiva till the remaining lid with attached tarsus can be easily elevated to cover the inferior cornea.

The spacer is first sutured to the recessed retractors and then to the inferior border of the tarsus. The vertical size of the spacer should be three times the lid retraction in mm [23]. Apart from hard palate mucosal graft, other spacers should be covered with conjunctiva.

## Should This Be Combined with Horizontal Lid Tightening?

Lower lid horizontal laxity often accompanies lid retraction especially after orbital decompression. This can be addressed by lateral wedge excision, tarsal strip procedure and/or lateral tarsorrhaphy [35]. Anterosuperior fixation of the tarsal strip improves changes of the lateral canthus.

It is important not to overtighten the lower lid which can result in exacerbating lower lid retraction in a proptosed eye by pulling the lower lid under the globe.

Lateral tarsorrhaphy can initially appear to reduce the palpebral fissure but the effect is not permanent.

## Which Materials Are Suitable for Use as Spacers? Should the Use of Allogeneic Grafts Be Avoided?

Various materials have been used for spacers. These include auricular cartilage [36], hard palate mucosa [37], expanded polyethylene (Medpor

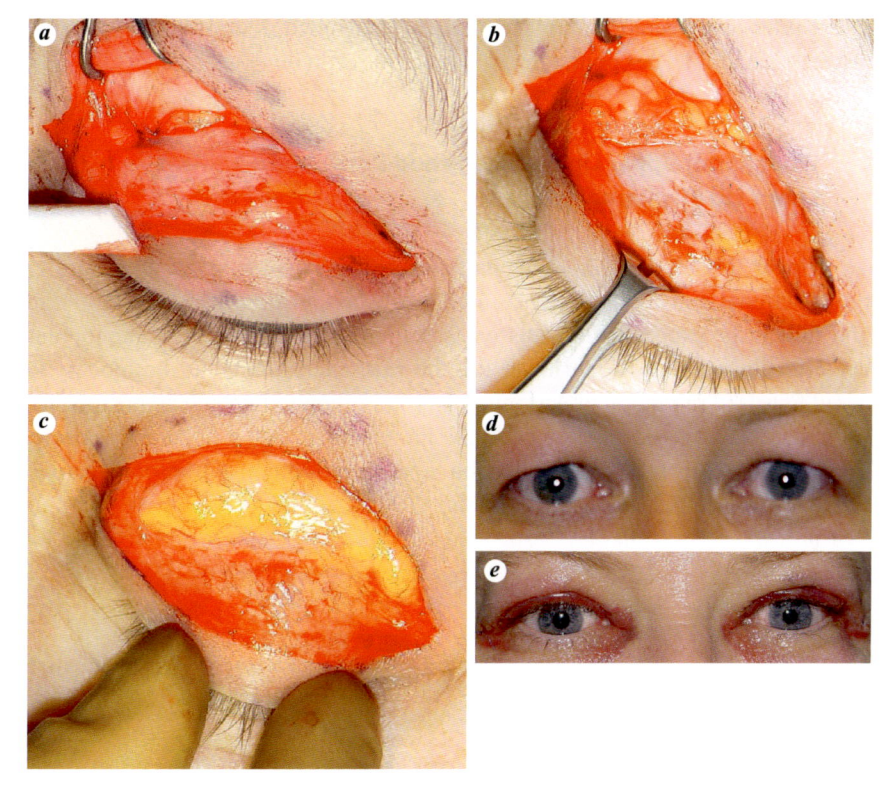

*Fig. 6. a* Preaponeurotic fat after opening of the orbital septum. *b* Persistent lacrimal gland prolapse after fat removal. *c* Post-repositioning of lacrimal gland with two sutures. *d, e* Pre-operatively and 1 day after levator recession, fat removal and blepharoplasty.

microplates [38]) and donor sclera/pericardium [32, 39]. Donor sclera has the tendency to retract and is no longer a popular choice because of the possible risk of disease transmission. Autogenous material like auricular cartilage and hard palate mucosa would not carry any risk of virus or prion transmission. Conchal cartilage is a good spacer material but should be thinned very carefully to overcome its inherent stiffness [10, 40].

### Are There Complications?

Extrusion, shrinkage or migration of allograft material spacer can occur. This is less common with autogenous grafts. Meticulous closure after secure placement of the spacer is vital to reduce extrusion [38].

Under- and overcorrection can usually be avoided. Rarely, a stiff spacer is also static and intrudes on the inferior field of vision on downgaze.

## What About Upper Lid Debulking and Upper and Lower Lid Blepharoplasty?

Upper lid debulking and blepharoplasty is the final surgical procedure in the functional and cosmetic rehabilitation of the GO patient. Redundant skin and fat can be excised using scissors and bipolar cautery, laser or monopolar cauterisation needle. In the lower lid, the skin excision should be modest to avoid lower lid retraction or ectropion. It is important to remove the preaponeurotic fat (fig. 6) and even subdermal fat together with orbicularis muscle. Prolapsing lower lid fat can also be removed through a transconjunctival approach in patients without excess skin.

### References

1 Dintelmann T, Sold J, Grehn F: Botulinum toxin injection treatment of upper lid retraction in thyroid eye disease. Ophthalmology 2005;102:247–250.
2 Shih MJ, Liao SL, Lu HY: A single transcutaneous injection with Botox for dysthyroid lid retraction. Eye 2004;18:466–469.
3 Uddin JM, Davies PD: Treatment of upper eyelid retraction associated with thyroid eye disease with subconjunctival botulinum toxin injection. Ophthalmology 2002;109:1183–1187.
4 Traisk F, Tallstedt L: Thyroid associated ophthalmopathy: botulinum toxin A in the treatment of upper eyelid retraction – a pilot study. Acta Ophthalmol Scand 2001;79:585–588.
5 Ebner R: Botulinum toxin type A in upper lid retraction of Graves' ophthalmopathy. J Clin Neuroophthalmol 1993;13:258–261.
6 Olver JM: Botulinum toxin A treatment of overactive corrugator supercilii in thyroid eye disease. Br J Ophthalmol 1998;82:528–533.
7 Eckstein AK, Finkenrath A, Heiligenhaus A, Renzing-Kohler K, Esser J, Kruger C, Quadbeck B, Steuhl KP, Gieseler RK: Dry eye syndrome in thyroid-associated ophthalmopathy: lacrimal expression of TSH receptor suggests involvement of TSHR-specific autoantibodies. Acta Ophthalmol Scand 2004;82:291–297.
8 Heinz C, Eckstein A, Steuhl KP, Meller D: Amniotic membrane transplantation for reconstruction of corneal ulcer in graves ophthalmopathy. Cornea 2004;23:524–526.
9 Solomon A, Meller D, Prabhasawat P, John T, Espana EM, Steuhl KP, Tseng SC: Amniotic membrane grafts for nontraumatic corneal perforations, descemetoceles, and deep ulcers. Ophthalmology 2002;109:694–703.
10 Mourits M, Rose GE, Garrity J, Nardi M, Matton G, Koornneef L: Surgical management of Graves' ophthalmopathy; in Prummel MF (ed): Recent Developments in Graves' Ophthalmopathy. Boston, Kluwer Academic Publishers, 2000, pp 133–170.
11 Garrity JA, Fatourechi V, Bergstralh EJ, Bartley GB, Beatty CW, DeSanto LW, Gorman CA: Results of transantral orbital decompression in 428 patients with severe Graves' ophthalmopathy. Am J Ophthalmol 1993;116:533–547.

12 Baldeschi L, Wakelkamp IM, Lindeboom R, Prummel MF, Wiersinga WM: Early versus late orbital decompression in Graves' orbitopathy: a retrospective study in 125 patients. Ophthalmology 2006;113:874–878.
13 Liao SL, Shih MJ, Lin LL: A procedure to minimize lower lid retraction during large inferior rectus recession in graves ophthalmopathy. Am J Ophthalmol 2006;141:340–345.
14 Kushner BJ: A surgical procedure to minimize lower-eyelid retraction with inferior rectus recession. Arch Ophthalmol 1992;110:1011–1014.
15 Meyer DR, Simon JW, Kansora M: Primary infratarsal lower eyelid retractor lysis to prevent eyelid retraction after inferior rectus muscle recession. Am J Ophthalmol 1996;122:331–339.
16 Putterman AM, Fett DR: Muller's muscle in the treatment of upper eyelid retraction: a 12-year study. Ophthalmic Surg 1986;17:361–367.
17 Doxanas MT, Dryden RM: The use of sclera in the treatment of dysthyroid eyelid retraction. Ophthalmology 1981;88:887–894.
18 Harvey JT, Anderson RL: The aponeurotic approach to eyelid retraction. Ophthalmology 1981;88: 513–524.
19 Thaller VT, Kaden K, Lane CM, Collin JR: Thyroid lid surgery. Eye 1987;1:609–614.
20 Hedin A: Eyelid surgery in dysthyroid ophthalmopathy. Eye 1988;2:201–206.
21 Harvey JT, Corin S, Nixon D, Veloudios A: Modified levator aponeurosis recession for upper eyelid retraction in Graves' disease. Ophthalmic Surg 1991;22:313–317.
22 Levine MR, Chu A: Surgical treatment of thyroid-related lid retraction: a new variation. Ophthalmic Surg 1991;22:90–94.
23 Mourits MP, Koornneef L: Lid lengthening by sclera interposition for eyelid retraction in Graves' ophthalmopathy. Br J Ophthalmol 1991;75:344–347.
24 Liu D: Surgical correction of upper lid retraction. Ophthalmic Surg 1993;24:323–327.
25 Ucello G, Vassallo P, Strianes D, Bonavolonta G: Free levator complex reccession in Graves's ophthalmopathy. Orbit 1994;13:119–122.
26 Ceisler EJ, Bilyk JR, Rubin PA, Burks WR, Shore JW: Results of Mullerotomy and levator aponeurosis transposition for the correction of upper eyelid retraction in Graves' disease. Ophthalmology 1995;102:483–492.
27 Tucker SM, Collin R: Repair of upper eyelid retraction: a comparison between adjustable and non-adjustable sutures. Br J Ophthalmol 1995;79:658–660.
28 Woog JJ, Hartstein ME, Hoenig J: Adjustable suture technique for levator recession. Arch Ophthalmol 1996;114:620–624.
29 Mourits MP, Sasim IV: A single technique to correct various degrees of upper lid retraction in patients with Graves' orbitopathy. Br J Ophthalmol 1999;83:81–84.
30 Elner VM, Hassan AS, Frueh BR: Graded full-thickness anterior blepharotomy for upper eyelid retraction. Trans Am Ophthalmol Soc 2003;101:67–73; discussion 73–75.
31 Hintschich C, Haritoglou C: Full thickness eyelid transsection (blepharotomy) for upper eyelid lengthening in lid retraction associated with Graves' disease. Br J Ophthalmol 2005;89: 413–416.
32 Esser J, Eckstein A: Ocular muscle and eyelid surgery in thyroid-associated orbitopathy. Exp Clin Endocrinol Diabetes 1999;107(suppl 5):S214–S221.
33 George JL, Tercero ME, Angioi-Duprez K, Maalouf T: Risk of dry eye after mullerectomy via the posterior conjunctival approach for thyroid-related upper eyelid retraction. Orbit 2002;21: 19–25.
34 Fenton S, Kemp EG: A review of the outcome of upper lid lowering for eyelid retraction and complications of spacers at a single unit over five years. Orbit 2002;21:289–294.
35 Feldman KA, Putterman AM, Farber MD: Surgical treatment of thyroid-related lower eyelid retraction: a modified approach. Ophthal Plast Reconstr Surg 1992;8:278–286.
36 Waller RR: Eyelid malpositions in Graves' ophthalmopathy. Trans Am Ophthalmol Soc 1982;80:855–930.
37 Cohen MS, Shorr N: Eyelid reconstruction with hard palate mucosa grafts. Ophthal Plast Reconstr Surg 1992;8:183–195.

38  Tan J, Olver J, Wright M, Maini R, Neoh C, Dickinson AJ: The use of porous polyethylene (Medpor) lower eyelid spacers in lid heightening and stabilisation. Br J Ophthalmol 2004;88: 1197–1200.
39  Olver JM, Rose GE, Khaw PT, Collin JR: Correction of lower eyelid retraction in thyroid eye disease: a randomised controlled trial of retractor tenotomy with adjuvant antimetabolite versus scleral graft. Br J Ophthalmol 1998;82:174–180.
40  Waller RR: Lower eyelid retraction: management. Ophthalmic Surg 1978;9:41–47.

Dr. C. Neoh
Eye Department, Claremont Wing, Royal Victoria Infirmary
Newcastle upon Tyne NE1 4LP (UK)
Tel. +44 191 282 5315, Fax +44 191 282 5315, E-Mail christopher.neoh@nuth.nhs.uk

# Quality of Life

*Wilmar M. Wiersinga*

Department of Endocrinology and Metabolism, Academic Medical Centre, University of Amsterdam, Amsterdam, The Netherlands

## What Is Quality of Life?

'From a beautiful young woman I changed into a "creep" who stared at people pop-eyed. Children backed away, adults nudged one another. Having a squint made me quit my hobbies and make mistakes at work.' This description by a patient who suffered from GO clearly illustrates the negative impact of the disease on her quality of life (QoL). The concept of QoL has developed slowly. In 1964, Lyndon B. Johnson declared in a report on national goals in the United States that '… goals cannot be measured by the size of our bank balance. They can only be measured in the quality of the lives that our people lead …'. But only in 1977, did quality of live become a key word in the Medline database. Still, there is no consensus on a single definition of the concept of QoL.

There seems to be agreement on a few points. First, QoL by definition can only be rated by the patients themselves. Second, QoL is a multi-dimensional concept, including physical, mental, and social aspects. Third, most clinicians prefer the term health-related quality of life (HRQL) since they are most interested in those aspects of QoL that are directly related to health. Consequently, HRQL can be defined as 'the physical, psychological, and social domains of health, seen as distinct areas that are influenced by a person's experiences, beliefs, expectations, and perceptions' [1].

## What Is the Usefulness of Quality of Life Measurements?

From the patient's perspective, clinical measures like proptosis or visual acuity are of little interest. They often correlate poorly with physical, emotional and social functioning in daily life. For example, in a clinical trial on prednisone

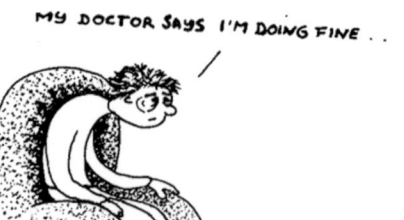

*Fig. 1.* Cartoon illustrating the need for involvement of patients in assessing therapeutic outcome.

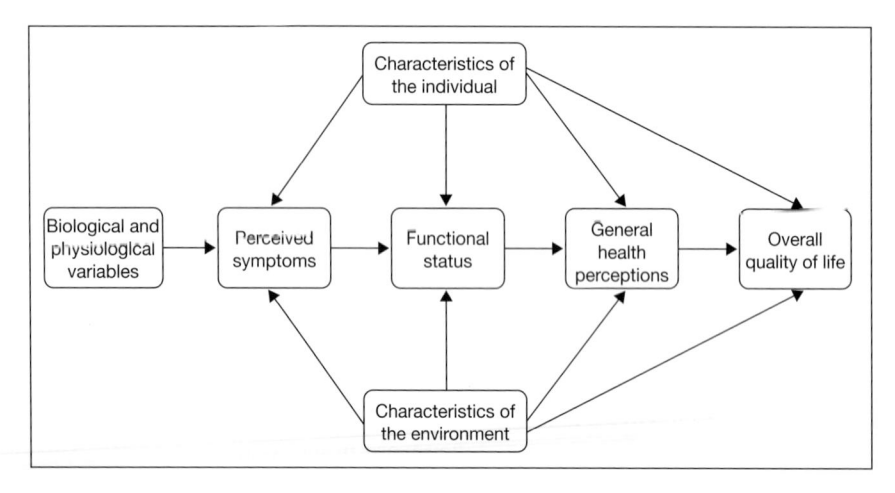

*Fig. 2.* A health-related QoL model of patients outcomes. Adapted from Wilson and Cleary [3].

versus radiotherapy, it was observed that a clinical success rate of about 50% was associated with only a modest mean benefit on the subjective eye judgement by the patient [2]. A significant reduction in proptosis of 2 mm might be labelled as a successful outcome by the physician, but will be hardly perceived as a real improvement by the patient (fig. 1).

These discrepancies between clinical measures and patient's experiences can be explained by the fact that the degree of daily functioning and general health as perceived by the patient is not only determined by the severity of signs and symptoms, but also by the characteristics of the individual and the environment such as expectations, coping ability, motivation, social support, the physician-patient relationship. These relationships are illustrated in a HRQL model of patients' outcomes (fig. 2) [3]. Clinical measures like proptosis or eye muscle motility are on the left side of the model. The perception of these clinical findings by the patients is expressed in perceived symptoms such as pain or diplopia. These symptoms can lead to functional limitations in daily activities such as driving or reading, which influences the general health perceptions and overall QoL, the latter also including other aspects of life besides health, such as financial situations, job satisfaction, etc.

Outcome levels referring to symptoms, functional status and general health perceptions can all be considered HRQL measures. The different levels of outcome are causally related but are influenced by personal factors and characteristics of the environment. The more you move to the right of the model, the larger the influence of these factors. As a consequence, the correlation with clinical measures becomes weaker. The model explains why two people with the same clinical disease status (based on physiological measures) can have a very different perception of their daily functioning and general health.

HRQL measures can be of important additional value in the description of disease severity because they highlight a different outcome level of interest. HRQL measures can also be important indicators of treatment success, and are especially useful in the evaluation of treatments that include side effects [4]. Finally, HRQL measures are often the most important outcomes of medial care, and are among the best predictors of the use of general medical and mental health sources.

## What Is Known about General Health-Related Quality of Life in Graves' Orbitopathy?

As HRQL is considered a subjective concept, the only approach to measuring HRQL is to ask the patients themselves. Several short and simple validated self-assessment questionnaires are used internationally. General HRQL questionnaires are mostly multidimensional and designed to measure the most important aspects of HRQL that apply to many different impairments, patients and populations. Examples are the Medical Outcomes Study short-form health surveys (SF-36 or MOS-24) and the Sickness Impact Profile (SIP).

In 70 consecutive patients with various degrees of severity of Graves' orbitopathy (GO) (all euthyroid at the time of investigation) low scores on the MOS-24 were found in comparison with a large reference group: mean ± SD scores (difference from reference group between brackets) were for physical functioning 58 ± 31 (−28), role functioning 72 ± 40 (−15), social functioning 78 ± 25 (−14), mental health 67 ± 18 (−10), health perceptions 46 ± 22 (−26), and bodily pain 68 ± 28 (−6) [5]. MOS-24 scores did not correlate with the duration, severity or activity of GO. This implies that the subjective health as perceived by the patient is different between subjects: the same degree of ophthalmopathy can have a different impact on the well-being of different patients. When compared with patients with other conditions, GO patients scored worse than patients with diabetes, emphysema, or heart failure, but scores were comparable to patients with inflammatory bowel disease [5].

Similar results are obtained with the SF-36 questionnaire [6–8]. Applying the Hospital Anxiety and Depression scale, it was observed that anxiety (40%) and depression (22%) were more frequent in GO patients than in the reference population (5 and 8%, respectively); anxiety and depression correlated positively with depression coping and negatively with SF-36 scales [8]. A high level of emotional distress is also reported using the Profile of Mood States: GO patients had significant mood disturbances, especially when disfiguring signs were predominant [9].

It must be concluded that general HRQL is markedly decreased in GO patients.

### Is There a GO-Specific Quality of Life Questionnaire?

Generic HRQL questionnaires (like the MOS-24, SF-36) are applicable across different diseases and different populations, allowing direct comparison among patient groups. However, these questionnaires are often too general and their questions too broadly based to detect small but clinically important changes within diseases. Disease-specific questionnaires are more focussed on those aspects of QoL particularly affected by a specific disease and may have greater detail or more items containing specific relevant aspects.

A disease-specific QoL questionnaire has been developed for GO, the so-called GO-QoL [10]. It contains 16 questions, 8 on the consequences of double vision and decreased visual acuity on visual functioning, and 8 on the psychosocial consequences of a changed appearance (table 1). The questions are answered on a three-point Likert scale: one point is given for the answer 'yes, seriously limited', two points for 'yes, a little limited', and three points for 'no, not limited at all'. The points given to questions 1–8 and 9–16 are added up to obtain two raw scores ranging from 8 to 24 points, one for visual functioning and one for appearance. The two raw scores are then transformed to two total scores by the formula: Total score = (raw score − 8) / 16 × 100.

The range of both scores is from 0 to 100, higher scores indicating better health. While limitations in bicycling are important for Dutch patients, they may be less important for patients in other countries. In that case, the item on bicycling can be excluded, leaving 7 questions for the subscale on visual functioning; the total score is then calculated as (raw score − 7) / 14 × 100.

Principal component analysis confirmed the division in the two subscales. Cronbach's alphas for the correlations of items within subscales were 0.83 for

*Table 1.* A disease-specific QoL questionnaire for GO: the GO-QoL

The following questions deal specifically with your thyroid eye disease.
Please focus on the past week while answering these questions
During the past week, to what extent were you limited in carrying out the following activities, because of your thyroid eye disease?
Tick the box that matches your answer. The boxes correspond with the answers above them.
Please tick only one box for each question.

|  | Yes, seriously limited | Yes, a little limited | No not at all limited |
|---|---|---|---|
| 1 Bicycling [never learned to ride a bike ☐] | ☐ | ☐ | ☐ |
| 2 Driving [no driver's licence ☐] | ☐ | ☐ | ☐ |
| 3 Moving around the house | ☐ | ☐ | ☐ |
| 4 Walking outdoors | ☐ | ☐ | ☐ |
| 5 Reading | ☐ | ☐ | ☐ |
| 6 Watching TV | ☐ | ☐ | ☐ |
| 7 Hobby or pastime, i.e…………… | ☐ | ☐ | ☐ |

|  | Yes, severely hindered | Yes a little hindered | No not at all hindered |
|---|---|---|---|
| 8 During the past week, did you feel hindered from something that you wanted to do because of your thyroid eye disease? | ☐ | ☐ | ☐ |

The following questions deal with your thyroid eye disease in general

|  | Yes, very much so | Yes, a little | No, not at all |
|---|---|---|---|
| 9 Do you feel that your appearance has changed because of your thyroid eye disease? | ☐ | ☐ | ☐ |
| 10 Do you feel that you are stared at in the streets because of your thyroid eye disease? | ☐ | ☐ | ☐ |
| 11 Do you feel that people react unpleasantly because of your thyroid eye disease? | ☐ | ☐ | ☐ |
| 12 Do you feel that your thyroid eye disease has an influence on your self confidence? | ☐ | ☐ | ☐ |
| 13 Do you feel socially isolated because of your thyroid eye disease? | ☐ | ☐ | ☐ |
| 14 Do you feel that your thyroid eye disease has an influence on making friends? | ☐ | ☐ | ☐ |
| 15 Do you feel that you appear less often on photos than before you had thyroid eye disease? | ☐ | ☐ | ☐ |
| 16 Do you try to mask changes in appearance caused by your thyroid eye disease? | ☐ | ☐ | ☐ |

*Table 2.* GO-QoL scores before, during and after treatment of GO [10–12]

|  | Before treatment (n = 70) | During treatment (n = 93) | After treatment (n = 163) |
|---|---|---|---|
| Visual functioning | 54.7 ± 22.8 | 65.6 ± 26.1 | 78.2 ± 23.7 |
| Appearance | 60.1 ± 24.8 | 61.0 ± 27.4 | 77.0 ± 22.4 |

visual functioning and 0.87 for appearance. Older patients and patients with more severe eye motility disturbances reported more problems with visual functioning, and females reported more with appearance, further supporting the construct validity. Like the general HRQL measurements using the MOS, the GO-QoL scores correlated only moderately with clinical measurements of severity and activity of GO. In a test-retest reliability study, substantial intra-class correlation coefficients of >0.80 were found for both subscales of the GO-QoL, indicating the subscales differentiate well between patients with different degrees of functioning [11].

The GO-QoL questionnaire thus seems to be valid (as judged from its construct validity it actually measures what it is supposed to measure) and reliable (as judged from its accuracy reflected by the small measurement error and from its reproducibility). The Go-QoL is now available in six languages (Dutch, English, French, German, Greek and Italian) and can be downloaded for free from the website (www.eugogo.com).

### What Are the Results of the GO-QoL?

Table 2 shows the GO-QoL scores obtained in cross-sectional studies of Dutch patients before, during and after treatment of GO [10–12]. Because the GO-QoL specifically measures limitations in functioning as a result of GO, healthy subjects should score 100 points (no limitations). It is clear that QoL is severely impaired in untreated patients, and not fully restored after treatment. The scores obtained in the untreated Dutch patients are in good agreement with those in Australian patients using a slightly modified GO-QoL (59.0 for visual functioning and 54.4 for appearance) [13].

### Can You Explain Response Shift in Quality of Life?

HRQL measures can be important indicators of treatment success. However, HRQL measures incorporate the effects of adaptation to the illness that happens over time. HRQL is a dynamic construct, which means that a person's ideas about poor functioning and general health can change over time as a consequence of coping strategies, seeking social support, changing expectations, etc. For example, patients with physical disabilities, e.g. spinal cord injuries, may place greater emphasis on mental abilities and selectively focus on aspects that make them appear better off than other people ('brain is more important than brawn'). These changes are inherent to the process of adjustment to the illness and are called response shift [14].

Response shift can interact with the effects of treatment, raising questions on the validity of within-subject comparison of changes in HRQL scores over time. Alternatively, response shift can be viewed as an adoptive characteristic of the individual, changing certain patient outcome levels in the HRQL model (fig. 1) while other levels remain stable. There is no consensus how to deal with response shift. One can argue that response shift is not a bias but a determinant of a reported change in HRQL. It can either be considered as part of the intervention strategy (active) or natural adaptation process (passive).

## Can GO-QoL Be Used as a Separate Outcome Measurement in GO?

Assessment of therapeutic outcome in GO patients is usually done by quantitative measurements of severity (lid aperture, proptosis, etc.) and activity (CAS). However, the primary goal of treatment is to improve functioning and general health, and consequently therapeutic outcome should also be evaluated in terms of functioning and general health perceptions (that is by HRQL). In other words, treatments should not only *work* from the physician's perspective, but they should also *help* from the patient's perspective. In 1992, the four international thyroid associations endorsed a joint statement that patient self-assessment should be included in the evaluation of treatment effects [15]. The GO-QoL was specifically designed for patient self-assessment and is recommended as a separate outcome measurement, especially in clinical trials [16].

In a prospective study patients completed the GO-QoL questionnaire before and three or six months after treatment, depending on the procedure (table 3) [17]. The direction and amount of change in GO-QoL scores on visual functioning or appearance after different treatments were in accordance with our pre-specified hypotheses about treatment effects (except for changes after eye muscle surgery, possibly related to improvement of diplopia in only 50% of patients in this series). Effect sizes in the GO-GoL subscales were higher than effect sizes of general HRQL subscales (like SF-36, SIP), supporting the longitudinal validity of the GO-QoL.

*Table 3.* GO-QoL scores for visual functioning (VF) and appearance (AP) in patients with GO before and after specific eye treatment

|  |  | Before treatment | After treatment | p value | Mean change | Effect size |
|---|---|---|---|---|---|---|
| Radiotherapy | VF | 37.0 | 45.1 | 0.05 | **8.1** | **0.39** |
|  | AP | 72.0 | 73.6 | NS | 2.0 | 0.11 |
| Decompression (sight loss) | VF | 27.1 | 47.4 | 0.01 | **20.3** | **0.90** |
|  | AP | 51.0 | 55.0 | NS | 4.0 | 0.20 |
| Decompression (exophthalmos) | VF | 64.8 | 68.0 | NS | 3.2 | 0.13 |
|  | AP | 44.7 | 55.8 | <0.001 | **11.0** | **0.45** |
| Eye muscle surgery | VF | 50.5 | 53.3 | NS | **2.8** | **0.12** |
|  | AP | 65.1 | 67.7 | NS | 2.6 | 0.13 |
| Eyelid lengthening | VF | 66.7 | 70.4 | NS | 3.7 | 0.14 |
|  | AP | 63.4 | 67.6 | 0.05 | **4.2** | **0.18** |
| Blepharoplasty | VF | 64.7 | 64.9 | NS | 0.2 | 0.01 |
|  | AP | 58.6 | 68.8 | 0.02 | **10.2** | **0.35** |

Scales on which treatment was expected to have the highest effect are shown in **bold** figures. NS = Not significant. Effect size = Mean change divided by SD of pre-treatment score.

A clinical response to treatment was associated with an increase in GO-QoL scores of approximately 10–20 points after major treatments (radiotherapy or decompression) and of 3–10 points after minor surgery (eye muscle and eye lid surgery). The minimal clinically important difference (MCID) in either GO-QoL subscale appeared to be 6–10 points (the MCID has been defined as the smallest difference in score on the domain of interest which patients perceive as benefit and which would mandate, in the absence of troublesome side effects and costs, a change in the patient's management). One could consider a mean change of at least 6 points on one or both GO-QoL subscales an important change in daily functioning for GO patients. For more invasive therapies, a change of at least 10 points is recommended as MCID.

### Is Quality of Life Fully Restored after Treatment of GO?

After a median follow-up of 10 years of 120 GO patients, 32% of patients reported that their eyes still did not appear normal, and 28% were not satisfied with the appearance of their eyes [18]. Similar findings are reported applying HRQL questionnaires in 163 GO patients at a median of 11.7 years after treatment [12]. GO-QoL scores were 23.5 points higher on visual functioning and

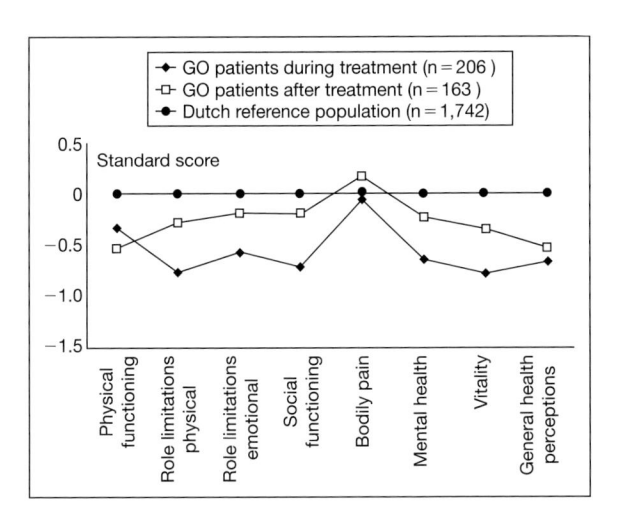

*Fig. 3.* General HRQL (expressed as SF-36 Z-scores) of GO patients after completion of treatments compared with GO patients during treatment and a Dutch reference population [12].

17 points higher on appearance than the newly diagnosed GO patients before treatment (table 2), but after treatment 12 and 13% of patients still scored below 50 points for visual functioning and appearance respectively; only 30% scored 100 points for visual functioning and 19% scored 100 points for appearance. Applying the SF-36 general HRQL questionnaire, GO patients after treatment likewise reported more limitations compared with the reference population, especially in physical functioning and general health perceptions (fig. 3).

GO has thus a marked negative effect on HRQL, even many years after treatment. The findings suggest that GO can be considered a chronic disease. An interesting comparative study on HRQL in a wide range of chronic disorders shows how HRQL data can be used to pinpoint areas that may be worthy of extra attention [19]. The suggestion has been made that research funds should be allocated to patient groups with those chronic diseases who are in greatest need as judged from their HRQL [20]. The field of GO certainly meets such criteria for more funding.

## Can I Apply the GO-QoL in My Own Practice?

It has not been studied formally if application of the GO-QoL is useful in individual patients, although this is very likely to be the case from experience with HRQL questionnaires in cancer patients. Two randomized clinical trials have demonstrated that incorporating standardized HRQL assessments in daily clinical oncology practice facilitates the discussion of HRQL issues, resulting in benefits for patients by improving their QoL and emotional functioning [21, 22]. In GO patients, psychosocial morbidity and especially emotional distress are frequently present; HRQL questionnaires could identify patients who are in need of further counselling, as recommended by several authors [8, 9, 13].

## References

1 Testa MA, Simonson DC: Assessment of quality of life outcomes. N Engl J Med 1996;334: 834–840.
2 Prummel MF, Mourits MP, Blank L, Berghout A, Koornneef L, Wiersinga WM: Randomized double-blind trial of prednisone versus radiotherapy in Graves' ophthalmopathy. Lancet 1993;342: 949–954.
3 Wilson IB, Cleary PD: Linking clinical variables with health-related quality of life. JAMA 1995;273:59–65.
4 Terwee CB, Dekker FW, Prummel MF, Wiersinga WM: Graves' ophthalmopathy through the eyes of the patient: a state of the art on health-related quality of life assessment. Orbit 2001;20: 281–290.
5 Gerding MN, Terwee CB, Dekker FW, Koornneef L, Prummel MF, Wiersinga WM: Quality of life in patients with Graves' ophthalmopathy is markedly decreased: measurements by the Medical Outcomes Study Instrument. Thyroid 1997;7:885–889.
6 Kahaly GJ, Hardt J, Petrak F, Egle UT: Psychosocial factors in subjects with Graves' ophthalmopathy. Thyroid 2002;12:237–239.
7 Elberling TV, Rasmussen AK, Fedt-Rasmussen U, Hording M, Perrild H, Waldemar G: Impaired health-related quality of life: a prospective study. Eur J Endocrinol 2004;151:549–555.
8 Kahaly GJ, Petrak T, Hardt J, Pitz S, Egle UT: Psychosocial morbidity of Graves' orbitopathy. Clin Endocrinol 2005;63:395–402.
9 Farid M, Roch-Leveq A-C, Levi L, Brody BL, Granet DB, Kikkawa DO: Psychological disturbances in Graves' ophthalmopathy. Arch Ophthalmol 2005;123:491–496.
10 Terwee CB, Gerding MN, Dekker FW, Prummel MF, Wiersinga WM: Development of disease-specific quality of life questionnaire for patients with Graves' ophthalmopathy: the GO-QoL. Br J Ophthalmol 1998;82:773–779.
11 Terwee CB, Gerding MN, Dekker FW, Prummel MF, van der Pol JP, Wiersinga WM: Test-retest reliability of the GO-QoL: a disease-specific quality of life questionnaire for patients with Graves' ophthalmopathy. J Clin Epidemol 1999;52:875–884.
12 Terwee CB, Wakelkamp I, Tas S, Dekker F, Prummel MF, Wiersinga WM: Long-term effects of Graves' ophthalmopathy on health-related quality of life. Eur J Endocrinol 2002;146:751–757.
13 Park JJ, Sullivan TJ, Mortimer RH, Wagenaar M, Perry-Keene DA: Assessing quality of life in Australian patients with Graves' ophthalmopathy. Br J Ophthalmol 2004;88:75–78.
14 Terwee CB, Dekker FW, Wiersinga WM, Prummer MF, Bossuyt PM: On assessing responsiveness of health-related quality of life instruments: guidelines for instrument evaluation. Qual Life Res 2003;12:349–362.
15 European, American, Latin-American, Japanese and Asia-Oceania Thyroid Associations: Classification of eye changes of Graves' disease. Thyroid 1992;2:235–236.
16 The European Group on Graves' Orbitopathy (EUGOGO): Clinical assessment of patients with Graves' orbitopathy: the European Group on Graves' Orbitopathy recommendations to generalists, specialists and clinical researchers. Eur J Endocrinol 2006;155:387–389.
17 Terwee CB, Dekker FW, Mourits MP, Gerding MN, Baldeschi L, Kalmann R, Prummel MF, Wiersinga WM: Interpretation and validity of changes in scores on the Graves' ophthalmopathy quality of life questionnaire (GO-QoL) after different treatments. Clin Endocrinol 2001;54: 391–398.

18  Bartley GB, Fatourechi V, Kadrmas EF, Jacobson SJ, Hstrup DM, Garrrity JA, Gorman CA: Long-term follow-up of Graves' ophthalmopathy in an incidence cohort. Opthalmology 1996;103: 958–962.
19  Sprangers MAG, de Regt EB, Andries F, van Agt HME, Bijl RV, Boer JB, Foets M, Hoeymans N, Jacobs AE, Kempen GJJM, Miedema HS, Tijhuis MAR, de Haes HCJM: Which chronic conditions are associated with better or poorer quality of life? J Clin Epidemiol 2000;53:895–907.
20  Fayers P, Bjordal K: Should quality-of-life needs influence resource allocation? Lancet 2001; 357:978.
21  Detmar SB, Muller MJ, Schornagel JH, Wever LDV, Aaronson NK: Health-related quality-of-life assessments and patient-physician communication. A randomized controlled trial. JAMA 2002; 288:3027–3034.
22  Velikova G, Booth L, Smith AB, Brown PM, Lynch P, Brown JM, Selby PJ: Measuring quality of life in routine oncology practice improves communication and patient well-being: a randomized contolled trial. J Clin Oncol 2004;22:714–724.


Prof. Wilmar M. Wiersinga
Department of Endocrinology and Metabolism, Academic Medical Centre
Room F5–171, University of Amsterdam
Meibergdreef 9
NL–1105 AZ Amsterdam (The Netherlands)
Tel. +31 20 566 6071, Fax +31 20 691 7682, E-Mail w.m.wiersinga@amc.uva.nl

## Atypical Manifestations

G. von Arx

basedow.ch, Interdisziplinäres Zentrum für Endokrine Orbitopathie, Olten, Switzerland

### What Are the Atypical Manifestations of Graves' Orbitopathy?

The clinical features of Graves' orbitopathy (GO) with eyelid retraction (Dalrymple's sign), lid-lag (von Graefe's sign), lagophthalmos, exophthalmos, motility disorders and dysthyroid optic neuropathy (DON) are all well known. The underlying disease is autoimmune thyroid disease and it is often associated with pretibial myxedema and acropachy. The combination of bilateral exophthalmos, lid retraction, stare and enlarged thyroid are virtually pathognomonic for GO. Some ocular signs are relatively specific and these include proptosis and lid-lag or stare, proptosis plus restrictive extraocular myopathy, or the presence of isolated enlarged vessels over the insertions of the medial or lateral rectus muscles. Conjunctival or periorbital edema is also quite common in GO. These typical manifestations of GO have already been described in previous chapters. This chapter reviews the most common atypical manifestations of GO: unilateral or asymmetric exophthalmos, euthyroid GO and globe subluxation as an extreme variant of exophthalmos.

### How Do You Explain Unilateral Graves' Orbitopathy (We Don't have Graves' Hyperthyroidism in Just One Thyroid Lobe, Have We?)

Hyperthyroidism of Graves' disease is known to involve the entire thyroid gland, unlike GO which clinically may either be unilateral or bilateral. To our knowledge only one case of 'single-lobe' autoimmune hyperthyroidism is known in the literature. Dimai et al. reported a 31-year-old Caucasian female patient who presented with clinical and laboratory evidence of hyperthyroidism and unilateral goitre [1]. High-resolution ultrasonography of the thyroid gland revealed a morphology indicative of an autoimmune thyroid disease strictly limited only to the right lobe. $^{123}$I-scintigraphy showed a homogenous, several-fold increased uptake of the radionuclide in the right lobe of the thyroid gland, whereas the uptake in the left lobe did not differ from the uptake in normal controls. Cytology of the fine-needle aspirate of the right lobe revealed a remarkable inflammatory background mainly by presence of lymphocytes, a finding which was not seen in the cytology of the left lobe. Furthermore, both serum antibodies to TSH receptors and thyroid peroxidase were significantly increased. Consequently, hyperthyroidism of Graves' disease with involvement of only one lobe of the thyroid gland was diagnosed.

GO is the most common cause of both unilateral and bilateral proptosis in adults [2–8, 22, 23]. The literature about real unilateral GO is relatively scarce and heterogeneous. However, to date there are no conclusive data and explanations for unilateral GO. Sattler [9] and others have noted more prominent orbital findings on the ipsilateral side of prominent thyroid enlargement in cases of asymmetric thyroid gland swelling, but this thyroid abnormality has rarely been observed and described in patients with unilateral GO ever since. Drescher and Benedict [2] have made the most accurate statement in evaluating unilateral or asymmetric GO when they stated: 'The data presented... are not intended to be comparable..., since dissimilar criteria were used.... in the selection of cases'. The mean prominence in their series of 200 normal eyes was 17.3 mm Hertel readings. The mean of measurements for the 'base eye' in all cases in their series, excluding cases of exophthalmic goitre and those of exophthalmos of unknown origin was 17.2 mm. This compares closely with the normal figure. The mean of measurements for the 'base eye' for the group with exophthalmic goitre, however, was 19.1 mm, thus a difference of 1.9 mm. This variation was statistically significant and exceeded 5-fold the standard deviation of the mean. Thus, they found that in cases of unilateral exophthalmic goiter the supposedly uninvolved eye that lies within the 'normal' range of prominence is more prominent by an average of almost 2 mm than the eye in cases of exophthalmos of any other cause. Accordingly, since exophthalmos obviously involves both orbits, it is believed preferable to use the term 'asymmetric exophthalmos' when discussing cases of exophthalmic goitre in which clinically ocular involvement appears to be unilateral (figs. 1–3). Hence, almost all patients with GO, even asymptomatic cases, show some degree of clinical signs with extraocular muscle involvement demonstrable by an abnormal ultrasound pattern or raised intraocular pressure in upgaze [10–17]. In our own series of 105 patients with Graves' disease, 76 (72.3%) patients had only minor clinical signs of thyroid eye disease (NOSPECS class 2), but 100 (95.2%) had a sound evidence of GO ultrasonographically with enlarged extraocular muscles and altered ultrasound pattern of the enlarged extraocular muscles correlating with GO. Six patients (5.7%) had unilateral disease of whom 1 patient (0.9%) with monomuscular active GO (enlarged inferior rectus muscle

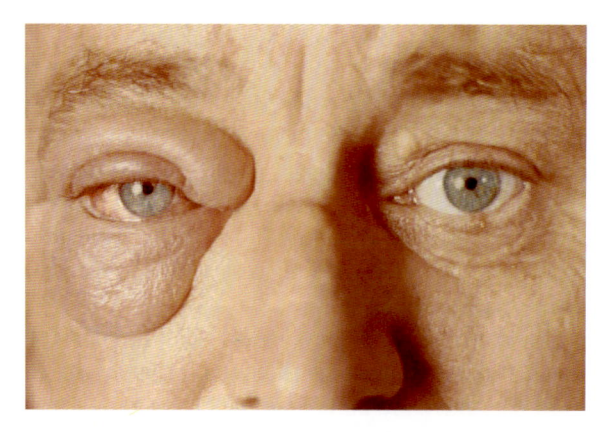

*Fig. 1.* Unilateral GO in an elderly male diabetic patient who was a heavy smoker and presented dysthyroid optic neuropathy restricted to the right eye.

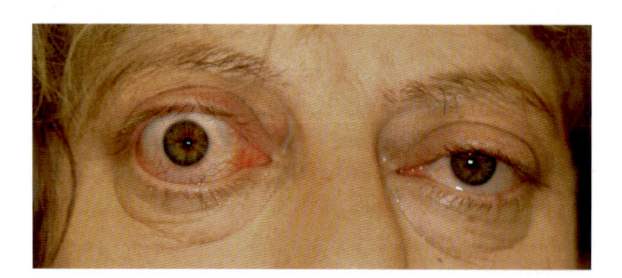

*Fig. 2.* Asymmetric active GO.

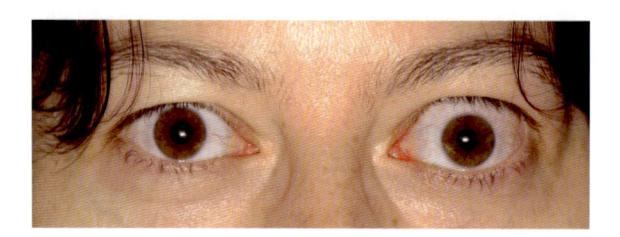

*Fig. 3.* Asymmetric inactive GO.

with low reflectivity) and another patient with inactive fibrotic changes of his right inferior and medial rectus muscle (enlarged muscles with high reflectivity) were shown. All others had involvement of at least two or more extraocular muscles. Two patients were borderline in relation to thickness and reflectivity of their extraocular muscles but developed clinical signs of bilateral GO 3 and 7 months

Table 1. Characteristics of unilateral versus bilateral eye disease in 90 patients with untreated GO

|  | Unilateral eye disease (group A, n = 13) | Bilateral eye disease (group B, n = 77) | p value (A vs. B) |
|---|---|---|---|
| Sex | 9 F, 4 M | 57 F, 20 M | n.s. |
| Age at study entrance, years | 49.7 ± 16.2 | 43.6 ± 13.1 | n.s. |
| Age at onset of eye disease, years | 48.6 ± 15.6 | 41.3 ± 13.1 | n.s. |
| Proptosis, mm | 20.7 ± 3.4[1] | 20.3 ± 3.8[2] | n.s. |
| Thyroid disease (past or present) | 8 (62%) | 62 (81%) | n.s. |
| Age at onset of thyroid disease, years | 47.6 ± 15.1 | 37.4 ± 12.1 | <0.05 |
| Age at onset of eye disease, years | 47.7 ± 15.2 | 40.6 ± 12.7 | n.s. |
| Interval between onset of thyroid and eye disease, years | 0.1 ± 0.4 | 3.2 ± 8.2 | <0.05 |

[1] Affected eye only; [2] mean of both eyes.
Values are mean ± SD. n.s. = Non-significant. From Wiersinga et al. [28].

later respectively. Only 5 patients (4.7%) showed neither signs nor any symptoms of GO [unpubl. data]. Similar data have been generated by other investigators [18–20]. A number of patients with presumed thyroid aetiology of unilateral GO have been shown to have CT and ultrasound evidence of unilateral disease with muscle enlargement without evident abnormal thyroid studies [21]. As already mentioned in previous chapters, there is CT, MRI and/or ultrasound evidence for orbital involvement in almost all patients with autoimmune hyperthyroidism. Clinical evidence of bilateral GO occurs in 80–90% of cases. In unilateral GO clinical signs and symptoms can be found in one orbit only and true unilateral cases are present in 10–20% of patients [22–26]. Variants of different clinical presentations are often called atypical. Among patients referred to a specialized diagnostic ophthalmology unit, the percentage of unilateral cases is even higher. In one study, 11.6% of the patients had apparent unilateral disease [27] and in a study of 90 untreated patients with autoimmune thyroid eye disease referred to a single centre 14% had unilateral findings (table 1) [28]. Many patients with presumed unilateral disease have subtle signs of the other orbit such as increased IOP in upgaze or enlarged extraocular muscles on CT and/or MRI [29]. A study by Enzmann et al. [30] revealed 50% of presumed unilateral GO as having bilateral orbital disease, when evaluated by CT scan. Only 6% were confirmed to be unilateral, all other cases were found to be asymmetric. In patients with unilateral exophthalmos evaluated by ophthalmologists, the aetiology is GO in 10–30% of cases. In a recent (unpublished) retrospective observational case control series of the Orbital Center at the Academic Medical Center, Wiersinga and co-workers

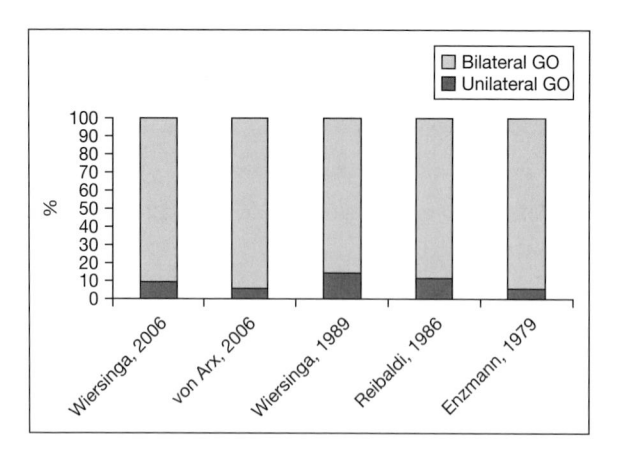

*Fig. 4.* Frequency of unilateral GO.

identified 28 cases with unilateral GO [31]. The prevalence of unilateral GO was 9%. In their series patients with unilateral GO tend to be older than patients with bilateral disease (54 vs. 44 years; p = 0.099) and are euthyroid in a significantly higher number of patients (28.6 vs. 1.8%; p = 0.001). In the majority of their patients with unilateral GO, unilateral extraocular muscle enlargement was found on CT scans. A large number of unilateral GO patients developed bilateral disease after an unpredictable interval of time. Factors that influence progression to bilateral disease remain unknown. They conclude that unilateral GO probably represents an early stage of Graves' disease, initially limited to only one eye and often associated with subclinical thyroid involvement. These data are in support of the view that the less-prominent and clinically less-affected eye is also involved in GO. Thus, although the clinical presentation of GO may often be asymmetric, it is believed to be truly unilateral in a minority of cases, as we may expect in a systemic disease (fig. 4).

## Will Unilateral Graves' Orbitopathy Proceed to Bilateral Graves' Orbitopathy?

In our own series of 105 patients with Graves' disease, 5 of 6 patients with unilateral GO developed bilateral disease. The same phenomenon occurred in the patients of the Amsterdam group, where a large number of unilateral GO patients developed bilateral disease after an unpredictable interval of time. Kalman and Mourits reported a case of late recurrence of unilateral GO on the contralateral side after 7 years. A 44-year-old woman with left unilateral GO underwent two-wall orbital decompression on the left side. After strabismus surgery and left upper eyelid surgery, she was discharged. Seven years later, the patient developed GO on the right side, and she underwent a two-wall orbital decompression on the right side. They concluded that at least in patients with unilateral GO, late recurrence of the disease in the contralateral orbit may occur [32]. Kamminga et al. [33] reported 2 cases with unilateral GO and ipsilateral recurrence after 35 years in the first case and unilateral onset of GO with progression to bilateral disease within weeks in the second case. According to the literature only a small number of patients with presumed unilateral disease (5–11%) do not progress to bilateral disease and have pure unilateral GO [28, 34].

## Is the Clinical Presentation of Unilateral Graves' Orbitopathy Different from Bilateral Graves' Orbitopathy?

According to the literature, the clinical presentation of unilateral or asymmetric GO is not different from bilateral disease relating to symptoms and ocular signs. The hypothesis of a syndrome with an underlying systemic disease as the cause of GO is supported by Werner et al. [14] reporting on 47 patients with consistent bilateral orbital involvement in Graves' disease. Ultrasonic changes, primarily in extraocular muscles, were minimal to moderate in 44 patients, equivocal in 2 and absent in only 1 patient. Saltzman and Mellicker [7] reviewed 8 cases from the literature with exophthalmos preceding thyrotoxicosis and an additional case of unilateral exophthalmos also preceding thyrotoxic symptoms and signs by 20 months. They conclude that unilateral GO might be a forerunner of thyrotoxicosis. In an earlier report on 90 consecutive untreated patients Wiersinga et al. [28] found no differences in 13 patients with unilateral disease. The distribution of age, sex and NOSPECS classes in these patients was similar to those patients with bilateral eye disease, but the interval between the onset of thyroid and eye disease was much shorter in cases of unilateral, than in cases of bilateral eye disease. Patients without clinically evident thyroid disease (n = 20; 22%) were not different from patients with thyroid disease in age, sex or ophthalmological presentation. They concluded that unilateral GO may represent an early stage of the disease, that as a rule already is or develops shortly afterwards into bilateral disease (table 1) [28].

## How Does Unilaterality Affect Treatment?

Unilaterality does not affect treatment, neither of the underlying systemic autoimmune or thyroid disease, nor the orbitopathy itself. On the other hand, it is rather difficult to answer whether patients with active unilateral disease should be treated unilaterally or bilaterally concerning retrobulbar irradiation of the orbit. If we refer to Wiersinga et al. [28] showing that unilateral disease may just precede bilateral disease, a bilateral treatment would be advisable [28, 31]. In true unilateral disease there may be a difference in surgical treatment of the eye changes related to orbital decompression, squint and lid surgery in the sense that only one side has to be operated on. In cases with concurrent degenerative changes of the ocular adnexa, bilateral surgical procedures for aesthetic reasons may become necessary. GO is a systemic disease leading to changes not only of the orbital tissues, but also the entire periorbital area with ptotic eyebrows, dermatochalasis, thickened and altered skin with changes in texture, subbrow and periorbital fat, as well as deep glabellar furrows. In most of these cases, symmetry can only be achieved by bilateral surgical procedures. As already mentioned, unilateral GO is rather rare and most patients are more likely to show asymmetric GO than true unilateral disease. If no comparison with the premorbid state is possible, as it is in most cases, it may be difficult to decide whether Hertel readings of 24–22 represent unilateral disease of the obviously affected side and a normal anatomy of the contralateral orbit or bilateral disease, because Hertel readings before manifestation of the disease were probably 8 on both sides. In these cases, treatment depends on the individual situation and the patient's needs and expectations. Thus, some may wish unilateral treatment only, whereas others find both sides have changed and need bilateral surgery.

## Is Euthyroid Graves' Orbitopathy a Reason to Refrain from Specific Eye Treatment?

GO is an organ-specific manifestation of Graves' disease and needs specific eye treatment independent from the actual thyroid state. In mild disease, symptomatic local treatment with lubricants, sunglasses, prisms or elevated head position while asleep may be sufficient. However, in all cases, whether mild, moderate or severe orbital disease, treatment has to be adequate to the present situation and does not differ from the procedures described in earlier chapters. Special attention has to be paid to the follow-up of these patients. Euthyroid GO is a hardly predictable situation and the clinician should be aware of a possible exacerbation at any time and within a short period of time. Therefore, these patients need an interdisciplinary follow-up by the ophthalmologist and the endocrinologist according to activity and severity of their eye disease. Regular thyroid function tests are strongly recommended in view of the risk to develop hyperthyroidism.

## What Is Globe Subluxation?

Usually the globe is embedded in the orbital tissues and protected by the bony orbit and the lids as described in previous chapters. In normal anatomy about one third of the globe is located behind the intercanthal line drawn on CT scans between the anterior borders of the zygomatic processes about 5 mm inferior to the frontozygomatic suture. Increasing orbital volume in expanding processes of the orbit or a shallow orbit with or without floppy eyelids may consequently lead to protrusion and 'subluxation' of the globe. Although it is relatively uncommon, axial globe 'subluxation' (anterior displacement of the globe equator beyond the orbital rim with lid retraction behind the equator and tethering of the optic nerve) may seriously complicate GO. Rubin et al. [35] detailed the characteristics of patients with spontaneous globe subluxation. Only 4 of approximately 4,000 patients (0.1%) in their practice developed this problem. All 4 had increased orbital fat without significant enlargement of the extraocular muscles on orbital CT. The authors speculated that the increased fat content resulted in more compliance of the soft tissues and that the normal calibre of the extraocular muscles allowed them to become more extensible, permitting globe subluxation. Axial globe subluxation may complicate thyroid orbitopathy. This acute event is an emergency and patients need repositioning of the globe in as short a time as possible. If there are signs of impending or manifest globe subluxation, surgical repair by an experienced oculoplastic and orbital surgeon with orbital decompression and consecutive eyelid surgery is to be considered.

## References

1  Dimai HP, Ramschak-Schwarzer S, Lax S, Lipp RW, Leb G: Hyperthyroidism of Graves' disease: evidence for only unilateral involvement of the thyroid gland in a 31-year-old female patient. J Endocrinol Invest 1999;22:215–219.
2  Drescher EP, Benedict WL: Asymmetric exophthalmos. Arch Ophthalmol 1950;44:109–128.
3  Henderson JW, Campbell RJ, Farrow GM, Garrity JA: Orbital Tumors, ed 3. New York, Raven Press, 1994.
4  Char DH, Norman D: The use of computed tomography and ultrasonography in the evaluation of orbital masses. Surv Ophthalmol 1982;27:49–63.
5  O'Brien CS, Leinfelder PJ: Unilateral exophthalmos: etiologic and diagnostic studies in 82 consecutive cases. Am J Ophthalmol 1935;18:123–132.
6  Rundle FF, Wilson CW: Asymmetry of exophthalmos in orbital tumor and Graves' disease. Lancet 1945;i:51–52.
7  Saltzman SL, Mellicker MC: Unilateral exophthalmos as a forerunner of thyrotoxicosis. Am J Ophthalmol 1951;34:372.
8  Moss HM: Expanding lesions of the orbit: a clinical study of 230 consecutive cases. Am J Ophthalmol 1962;54:761–770.
9  Sattler H: Basedow's Disease. New York, Grune & Stratton, 1952, pp 27–42.
10 Wessely K: Discussion. Ber Ophthalmol Ges 1918;41:80.
11 Purnell EW: B-mode orbital ultrasonography. Int Ophthalmol Clin 1969;9:643–665.

12 Purnell EW: Ultrasonic interpretation of orbital disease; in Gitter KA, Keeney AH, Sarin LK, Major D (eds): Ophthalmic Ultrasound. St. Louis, Mosby, 1969, pp 249–270.
13 Coleman DJ, Jack RL, Franzen LA, Werner SC: High resolution B-scan ultrasonography of the orbit. V. Eye changes of Graves' disease. Arch Ophthalmol 1972;88:465–471.
14 Werner SC, Coleman DJ, Franzen LA: Ultrasonographic evidence of a consistent orbital involvement in Graves' disease. N Engl J Med 1974;290:1447–1450.
15 McNutt LC, Kaefring SL, Ossoinig KC: Echographic measurement of extraocular muscles; in White D, Brown R (eds): Ultrasound in Medicine. New York, Plenum Press, 1977, vol 3, pp 927–935.
16 Shammas HJ, Minckler DS, Ogden C: Ultrasound in early thyroid orbitopathy. Arch Ophthalmol 1980;98:277–279.
17 Pohjanpelto P: The thyroid gland and intraocular pressure: tonographic study of 187 patients with thyroid eye disease. Acta Ophthalmol 1968;97(suppl):11–61.
18 Hodes BL, Stern G: Contact B-scan echographic diagnosis of ophthalmopathic Graves' disease. J Clin Ultrasound 1975;3:255–261.
19 Forrester JV, Sutherland GR, McDougall IR: Dysthyroid ophthalmopthy: orbital evaluation with B-scan ultrasonography. J Clin Endocrinol Metabol 1977;45:221–224.
20 Skalka HW: The use of ultrasonography in the diagnosis of endocrine orbitopathy. Neurol Ophthalmol 1980;1:109–116.
21 Rapoport B, Greenspan FS, Filetti S, Pepitone M: Clinical experience with a human thyroid cell assay for thyroid-stimulating immunoglobulin. J Clin Endocrinol Metab 1984;58:332–338.
22 Grove AS Jr: Evaluation of exophthalmos. N Engl J Med 1975;292:1005–1013.
23 Dallow RL: Evaluation of unilateral exophthalmos with ultrasonography: analysis of 258 consecutive cases. Laryngoscope 1975;85:1905–1919.
24 Lavergne G: Pitfalls in the diagnosis of endocrine exophthalmy. Mod Probl Ophthalmol 1975;14:421–425.
25 Pohjola S: Unilateral exophthalmos with special reference to endocrine exophthalmos with pseudotumor. Acta Ophthalmol 1964;42:456–464.
26 Wende S, Aulich A, Nover A, et al: Computed tomography of orbital lesions. Neuroradiology 1977;13:123–134.
27 Reibaldi A, Avitabile R, Uva MG, Tritto M: Utility of ultrasound in unilateral endocrine exophthalmos. Orbit 1987;6:43–45.
28 Wiersinga WM, Smit T, van der Gaag R, Koornneef L: Clinical presentations of Graves' ophthalmopathy. Ophthalmic Res 1989;21:73–82.
29 Fatourechi V, Pajouhi M, Fransway AF: Dermopathy of Graves' disease (pretibial myxedema). Medicine 1994;73:1–7.
30 Enzmann DR. Donaldson SS, Kriss JP: Appearance of Graves' disease on orbital computed tomography. J Comput Assist Tomogr 1979;3:815–819.
31 Lumera G, Prummel MF, Baldeschi L, et al: Unilateral Graves' orbitopathy: a case-control and retrospective follow-up study (abstract P62). J Endocrinol Metab 2004;8(suppl 1):63.
32 Kalmann R, et al: Late recurrence of unilateral GO on the contralateral side. Am J Ophthalmol 2002;133:727–729.
33 Kamminga N, Jansonius NM, Pott JWR, Links TP: Unilateral proptosis: the role of medical history. BJO 2003;87:370–371.
34 Trokel SL, Jakobiec FA: Correlation of CT scanning and pathologic features of ophthalmic Graves' disease. Ophthalmology 1981;88:553–564.
35 Rubin PA, Watkins LM, Rumelt S, Sutula FC, Dallow RL: Orbital computed tomographic characteristics of globe subluxation in thyroid orbitopathy. Ophthalmology 1998;105:2061–2064.

Dr. med. Georg von Arx
basedow.ch, Interdisziplinäres Zentrum für Endokrine Orbitopathie
Fährweg 10
CH–4600 Olten (Switzerland)
Tel. +41 62 206 8737, Fax +41 62 206 8738, E-Mail georg.vonarx@admedico.ch

# Childhood Graves' Orbitopathy

*Gerasimos E. Krassas*

Department of Endocrinology, Diabetes and Metabolism, Panagia General Hospital, Thessaloniki, Greece

## Is Childhood Graves' Orbitopathy Really that Rare?

The most accurate data on the incidence of Graves' orbitopathy (GO) is derived from a population-based cohort study in Olmsted County, Minn., USA [1]. Only 6 of the 120 incident cases of GO observed in this cohort study were below the age of 20 years. The incidence rates start to increase as of the age of 20 years. Below the age of 20 years the occurrence of GO is a rare event. Incidence rates (cases per 100,000 population per year) are in the age groups 5–9, 10–14, and 15–19 years for females 3.5, 1.8 and 3.3, respectively, and for males 0, 1.7 and 0, respectively, whereas the overall age-adjusted incidence rate was 16.0 cases for women and 2.9 cases for men per 100,000 population per year.

The low incidence of childhood GO might be related to the low incidence of Graves' hyperthyroidism (GH) during childhood. To analyze this further, we compared the prevalence of clinically apparent GO in children and adults with GH. Lid retraction by itself did not qualify for the diagnosis of GO, as this sign can be attributed to the hyperthyroid state, disappearing spontaneously once the euthyroid state has been reached. GO was present in 87 of 286 (30.4%) patients with childhood GH [2–7] and in 118 of 1,050 (18%) adult patients with GH [8–11]. The proportion of GO cases among patients with GH is thus similar between children and adults; it follows that the low incidence of childhood GO can be fully explained by the low incidence of childhood GH.

The data are supported by a recent questionnaire study among members of the European Society for Paediatric Endocrinology (ESPE) and European Thyroid Association (ETA) [12]. The general questions of the questionnaire read:
(1) How many cases of childhood GO (patients up to 10 years old in prepubertal stage) have been seen in your institution in the last 10 years and how many among adolescents (11–18 years of age)?

(2) How many cases of GH (up to 18 years old) have been seen in your institution in the last 10 years?

A total of 1,963 patients with juvenile GH had been encountered by the 67 respondents (23 paediatricians and 44 internists) over the last 10 years, on average 4.6 cases per year by each paediatrician and 2.3 cases per year by each internist. One-third of the patients with GH had GO. Among the patients with GO, one-third were <10 years old (77% of them being seen by paediatricians) and two-thirds were in the age group of 11–18 years (56% of them being seen by paediatricians).

In a recent retrospective study from the Mayo Clinic, Durairaj et al. [13] describes 35 patients 18 years or younger during the 15-year interval 1985 through 1999. There were 27 girls (77.1%) and 8 boys (22.9%). At the time of initial ophthalmic examination, 31 patients (88.6%) were hyperthyroid, 1 (2.9%) was hypothyroid, and 3 (8.6%) were euthyroid. The mean age at diagnosis of thyroid dysfunction was 13.1 years (range 3–18), and the mean age at diagnosis of GO was 15.0 years (range 5–18). Twelve patients (34%) had family members with thyroid dysfunction. The female preponderance, thyroid function at time of diagnosis, the interval of about 2 years between onset of thyroid and eye disease, and the prevalence of a family history of thyroid disease are thus all very similar between childhood and adulthood GO.

## Is the Clinical Presentation of Graves' Orbitopathy in Childhood Different from that in Adulthood?

The available studies suggest that the clinical presentation of GO in children and adolescents is less severe than in adulthood. No race difference has been reported so far regarding thyroid ophthalmopathy in children and adolescents (fig.1). Taking the 77 childhood GO cases from 5 studies published so far [2–5, 13] and contrasting them with 152 new consecutively referred adult GO patients [14], it is clear that soft-tissue involvement and proptosis are the predominant eye changes in childhood GO whereas the more severe manifestations of restricted eye muscle motility and optic dysfunction almost never occur in children (table 1).

## Why Is Graves' Orbitopathy in Children Less Severe than in Adults?

The prevalence of smoking is much lower in children than in adults with GO (4% and 47%, respectively) [5, 14]. Smoking is a risk factor for GO, and the odds increase significantly with increasing severity of GO [15]. One study observes that the manifestation of GO begins to resemble more closely the adult

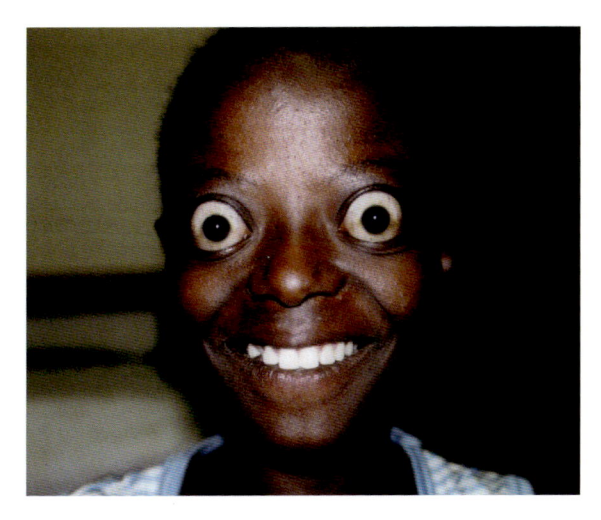

*Fig. 1.* GO in an 12-year-old girl from the Kivu area in the eastern part of Congo. No race difference has been reported so far regarding thyroid ophthalmopathy in children and adolescents. Courtesy of Dr. C. de Clippele and Prof. P. Bourdoux.

*Table 1.* Relative frequencies of eye changes in patients with GO with onset in childhood or adulthood

|  | 77 children and adolescents [2–5, 13] | 152 adults [14] |
| --- | --- | --- |
| Soft-tissue involvement, % | 60 | 75 |
| Proptosis, % | 52 | 63 |
| Extraocular muscle motility defect, % | 6.5 | 49 |
| Corneal involvement, % | 30 | 16 |
| Optic neuropathy, % | 0 | 21 |

findings as adolescence approaches [2]; conceivably, this could be explained by increasing smoking prevalence with age. It is thus plausible to assume that less exposure to tobacco smoke is the reason for the less severe GO in childhood. Indirect evidence supporting this view can be derived from our questionnaire study [12]. When grouped according to smoking prevalence among teenagers in the country of origin, it becomes evident that the proportion of GO patients among children with GH is highest in countries in which teenagers smoke most (table 2). What is striking is that 52% of children with GO in these countries (smoking prevalence ≥ 25%) are 10 years old or younger, whereas this figure (19%) is much lower in countries in which smoking prevalence among

*Table 2.* Occurrence of childhood GO in GH as a function of smoking prevalence among teenagers in their country of origin

| Smoking prevalence among teenagers* | GH | GO | GO, % ≤10 years | 11–18 years |
|---|---|---|---|---|
| ≥ 25% | 644 (100%) | 236 (36.6%) | 52 | 48 |
| 20–25% | 818 (100%) | 223 (27.3%) | 15 | 86 |
| <20% | 452 (100%) | 117 (25.9%) | 24 | 76 |

*Data per country based on WHO Regional Office for Europe, Tobacco Control Database, 2003. Internet:http://data.euro.WHO.Int/tobacco.

teenagers is less than 25%. It is unlikely that children ≤10 years of age smoke themselves; the high proportion of GO in this group is thus best explained by passive smoking as a result of living in an environment in which 25% or more of their peers smoke.

Other predisposing factors for more severe ophthalmopathy are older age and diabetes, which also can explain why GO is less severe in children and adolescents [16].

## What Is the Best Therapeutic Approach for Graves' Orbitopathy in Children and Adolescents?

As the expression of GO in children is, in most instances, both mild and transient, most of the physicians prefer a 'wait-and-see' policy. Indeed, in our recent study [12] 70% of the respondents recommended such a policy for the eye changes. Active intervention (predominantly with steroids) is considered appropriate in case of worsening of eye changes or no improvement of eye changes when the patient has become euthyroid [12]. Doses between 5 and 20 mg prednisone daily are used depending on the severity of the case. Our policy in moderately severe cases is to start with 20 mg daily for 4–6 weeks when a beneficial effect is usually expected, and then tapering the dose accordingly [17]. We are reluctant to use higher doses of glucocorticoids (GC) as well as intravenous glucocorticosteroids. It has to be kept in mind that prolonged prednisone administration, which should be used in some severe cases, is associated with weight gain, immune suppression and growth failure in children [18].

Retrobulbar irradiation has no place in the treatment of juvenile GO in view of the theoretical risk of tumour induction [19].

One important issue is the use of steroids in patients with TED who received radioiodine treatment (RAI) for hyperthyroidism. Two randomized, prospective, controlled clinical trials by Tallstedt et al. [11] and Bartalena et al. [20] clearly demonstrated in adults that radioiodine administration may be associated with a progression of ophthalmopathy in about 15% of patients. Unfortunately, similar data are not available for adolescents for two main reasons. First, RAI as treatment of hyperthyroidism in the paediatric age group is unpopular in Europe and some other continents and second the incidence of GO during childhood is low.

Thyroidectomy, however, might be a suitable option for paediatric GH with GO. In a series of 34 such cases, near-total, total and subtotal thyroidectomy was done in 20, 13 and 1 patient, respectively [6]. At a median follow-up of 53 months, GO had improved in 29 patients (85%) and deteriorated in 1 patient (3%) requiring orbital decompression. Of the 44 patients without eye disease at the time of operation, 2 (5%) developed new GO during follow-up.

It has been shown that somatostatin analogs (SM-as) might be of some therapeutic value. However, most of the initial studies were uncontrolled, not randomized, and included only a small number of patients. We had the opportunity to treat 3 adolescents (2 F, 1 M) with moderate-to-severe TED with SM-as aged 14, 15 and 16 years [21]. All had an increased clinical activity score (CAS 4, 5 and 6, respectively). All were on antithyroid therapy and euthyroid at the time of treatment. They received 20 mg octreotide (sandostatin-LAR) i.m. once every 30 days for 4 months. Their ophthalmopathy improved substantially and CAS decreased in all.

Very recently four double-blind, placebo-controlled clinical studies were published including only adult patients. They demonstrated only a modest improvement in proptosis and lid fissure width [22–25]. The current SM-as targets 2 of 4 somatostatin receptors present in orbital fibroblasts and 2 of 5 receptors found in the lymphocytes of GO patients [26, 27] (table 3). Therefore, there is reason to believe that newer generations of SM-as (like SOM 230) that target a wider range of somatostatin receptors might show better results in the treatment of GO.

It is worth mentioning that in the Mayo Clinic series 31 of 35 children with GO (88.6%) required no or only supportive therapy [13]. No patient received systemic corticosteroids or orbital radiotherapy. One patient (2.9%) required eyelid surgery and three (8.6%) underwent transantral orbital decompression for proptosis that caused discomfort and exposure keratitis. At a mean follow-up of 11 years in 20 of these patients, vision was good in all and 19 had no diplopia.

*Table 3.* Relative abundance of somatostatin receptor mRNA expression in retrobulbar fibroblasts and lymphocytes obtained from GO and control patients

|  | Fibroblasts [26] | | Lymphocytes [27] | |
|---|---|---|---|---|
|  | GO (n = 10) | controls (n = 6) | GO (n = 10) | controls (n = 2) |
| Sst 1 | ++ | − | +++ | − |
| Sst 2 | +++ | +++ | ++ | −/+ |
| Sst 3 | ++ | ++ | + | + |
| Sst 4 | −/+ | − | ++ | −/+ |
| Sst 5 | ++ | − | + | − |

## What About Surgical Decompression of the Orbit in Childhood?

Few cases of orbital decompression in preadolescents and adolescents have been reported so far. Sherman et al. [6] reported that of 34 patients with GH aged <18 years presenting with eye symptoms, one experienced progression of GO requiring orbital decompression. In the 35 GO patients aged ≤18 years reviewed by Durairaj et al. [13], 3 underwent bilateral transantral decompression for exposure keratopathy and correction of disfiguring proptosis; they were all boys 16–18 years of age. It is interesting to note that orbital decompression for GO is not performed in the first decade of life. This seems to be prudent in view of the fact that orbital growth is not completed before the age of 7 years [28, 29].

In conclusion, from all the published data so far, orbital decompression is very rarely performed in children and adolescents, the reason most probably being that GO is less severe and optic neuropathy virtually does not exist at that age.

## References

1   Bartley GB, Fatourechi V, Kadrmas EF, Jacobsen SJ, Ilstrup DM, Garrity JA, Gorman CA: The incidence of Graves' ophthalmopathy in Olmsted County, Minnesota. Am J Ophthalmol 1995;120: 511–517.
2   Uretsky SH, Kennerdell JS, Gutai JP: Graves' ophthalmopathy in childhood and adolescence. Arch Ophthalmol 1980;98:1963–1964.
3   Young LA: Dysthyroid ophthalmopathy in children. J Pediatr Ophthalmol Strabismus 1979;16: 105–107.
4   Gruters A: Ocular manifestations in children and adolescents with thyrotoxicosis. Exp Clin Endocrinol Diabetes 1999;107(suppl 5):S172–S174.
5   Chan W, Wong GW, Fan DS, Cheng AC, Lam DS, Ng JS: Ophthalmopathy in childhood Graves' disease. Br J Ophthalmol 2002;86:740–742.

6 Sherman J, Thompson GB, Lteif A, Schwenk WF 2nd, van Heerden J, Farley DR, Kumar S, Zimmerman D, Churchward M, Grant CS: Surgical management of Graves disease in childhood and adolescence: an institutional experience. Surgery 2006;140:1056–1061.
7 Antoniazzi F, Zamboni G, Cerini R, Lauriola S, Dall'Agnola A, Tato L: Graves' ophthalmopathy evolution studied by MRI during childhood and adolescence. J Pediatr 2004;144:527–531.
8 Werner SC, Coelho B, Quimby EH: Ten year results of I-131 therapy in hyperthyroidism. Bull NY Acad Med 1957;33:783–806.
9 Hamilton RD, Mayberry WE, McConahey WM, Hanson KC: Ophthalmopathy of Graves' disease: a comparison between patients treated surgically and patients treated with radioiodide. Mayo Clin Proc 1967;42:812–818.
10 Kriss JP, Pleshakov V, Rosenblum AL, Holderness M, Sharp G, Utiger R: Studies on the pathogenesis of the ophthalmopathy of Graves' disease. J Clin Endocrinol Metab 1967;27:582–593.
11 Tallstedt L, Lundell G, Torring O, Wallin G, Ljunggren JG, Blomgren H, Taube A: Occurrence of ophthalmopathy after treatment for Graves' hyperthyroidism. The Thyroid Study Group. N Engl J Med 1992;326:1733–1738.
12 Krassas GE, Segni M, Wiersinga WM: Childhood Graves' ophthalmopathy: results of a European questionnaire study. Eur J Endocrinol 2005;153:515–521.
13 Durairaj VD, Bartley GB, Garrity JA: Clinical features and treatment of Graves' ophthalmopathy in pediatric patients. Ophthal Plast Reconstr Surg 2006;22:7–12.
14 Prummel MF, Bakker A, Wiersinga WM, Baldeschi L, Mourits MP, Kendall-Taylor P, Perros P, Neoh C, Dickinson AJ, Lazarus JH, Lane CM, Heufelder AE, Kahaly GJ, Pitz S, Orgiazzi J, Hullo A, Pinchera A, Marcocci C, Sartini MS, Rocchi R, Nardi M, Krassas GE, Halkias A: Multi-center study on the characteristics and treatment strategies of patients with Graves' orbitopathy: the first European Group on Graves' Orbitopathy experience. Eur J Endocrinol 2003;148:491–495.
15 Prummel MF, Wiersinga WM: Smoking and risk of Graves' disease. JAMA 1993;269:479–482.
16 Neigel JM, Rootman J, Belkin RI, Nugent RA, Drance SM, Beattie CW, Spinelli JA: Dysthyroid optic neuropathy: the crowded orbital apex syndrome. Ophthalmology 1988;95:1515–1521.
17 Krassas GE, Gogakos A: Thyroid-associated ophthalmopathy in juvenile Graves' disease: clinical, endocrine and therapeutic aspects. J Pediatr Endocrinol Metab 2006;19:1193–1206.
18 Rivkees SA, Sklar C, Freemark M: Clinical review 99: the management of Graves' disease in children, with special emphasis on radioiodine treatment. J Clin Endocrinol Metab 1998;83:3767–3776.
19 Wiersinga WM: Thyroid associated ophthalmopathy: pediatric and endocrine aspects. Pediatr Endocrinol Rev 2004;1(suppl 3):513–517.
20 Bartalena L, Marcocci C, Bogazzi F, Panicucci M, Lepri A, Pinchera A: Use of corticosteroids to prevent progression of Graves' ophthalmopathy after radioiodine therapy for hyperthyroidism. N Engl J Med 1989;321:1349–1352.
21 Krassas GE: Thyroid eye disease in children and adolescents: new therapeutic approaches. J Pediatr Endocrinol Metab 2001;14:97–100.
22 Dickinson AJ, Vaidya B, Miller M, Coulthard A, Perros P, Baister E, Andrews CD, Hesse L, Heverhagen JT, Heufelder AE, Kendall-Taylor P: Double-blind, placebo-controlled trial of octreotide long-acting repeatable (LAR) in thyroid-associated ophthalmopathy. J Clin Endocrinol Metab 2004;89:5910–5915.
23 Wemeau JL, Caron P, Beckers A, Rohmer V, Orgiazzi J, Borson-Chazot F, Nocaudie M, Perimenis P, Bisot-Locard S, Bourdeix I, Dejager S: Octreotide (long-acting release formulation) treatment in patients with Graves' orbitopathy: clinical results of a four-month, randomized, placebo-controlled, double-blind study. J Clin Endocrinol Metab 2005;90:841–848.
24 Chang TC, Liao SL: Slow-release lanreotide in Graves' ophthalmopathy: a double-blind randomized, placebo-controlled clinical trial. J Endocrinol Invest 2006;29:413–422.
25 Stan MN, Garrity JA, Bradley EA, Woog JJ, Bahn MM, Brennan MD, Bryant SC, Achenbach SJ, Bahn RS: Randomized, double-blind, placebo-controlled trial of long-acting release octreotide for treatment of Graves' ophthalmopathy. J Clin Endocrinol Metab 2006;91:4817–4824.
26 Pasquali D, Vassallo P, Esposito D, Bonavolonta G, Bellastella A, Sinisi AA: Somatostatin receptor gene expression and inhibitory effects of octreotide on primary cultures of orbital fibroblasts from Graves' ophthalmopathy. J Mol Endocrinol 2000;25:63–71.

27 Pasquali D, Notaro A, Bonavolonta' G, Vassallo P, Bellastella A, Sinisi AA: Somatostatin receptor genes are expressed in lymphocytes from retroorbital tissues in Graves' disease. J Clin Endocrinol Metab 2002;87:5125–5129.
28 Haug RH, Foss J: Maxillofacial injuries in the pediatric patient. Oral Surg Oral Med Oral Pathol Oral Radiol Endod 2000;90:126–134.
29 Aret M, Köklü A, Özdiler E, Rübendür M, Erdogan B: Craniofacial growth and skeletal maturation: a mixed longitudinal study. Eur J Orthod 2001;23:355–361.

Prof. Gerasimos E. Krassas
Department of Endocrinology, Diabetes and Metabolism
Panagia General Hospital, N. Plastira 22
GR–551 32 Thessaloniki (Greece)
Tel. +30 2310 479633, Fax +30 2310 282476, E-Mail krassas@the.forthnet.gr

# Prevention

*Luigi Bartalena*

Division of Endocrinology, Department of Clinical Medicine, University of Insubria, Ospedale di Circolo, Varese, Italy

Prevention of a disease is always preferable to its treatment. This is particularly true for Graves' orbitopathy (GO) as approximately one third of affected patients are, at the end of treatment, dissatisfied with their physical appearance and residual functional abnormalities [1].

## What Is Primary, Secondary and Tertiary Prevention?

Prevention may be primary, secondary, or tertiary [2]. Primary prevention of a disease is aimed at avoiding its occurrence by removing risk factors; secondary prevention refers to early diagnosis and treatment of subclinical, asymptomatic disease, to prevent its progression toward clinically overt disease; tertiary prevention encompasses all actions taken after the occurrence of clinical disease, to minimize the risk of disease-related complications and disability. Distinction of these different stages may be difficult and, in some instances, arbitrary. For example, normalization of blood pressure in hypertensive patients may be a secondary prevention of hypertensive heart disease and, at the same time, primary prevention of myocardial infarction or stroke. Nevertheless, classification of prevention into different levels maintains its usefulness, underscoring the need for: (1) modification/abolishment of risk factors, (2) recognition of subclinical disease, and (3) early treatment of initial clinical manifestations.

## Can a General Strategy Be Applied to Prevent Graves' Orbitopathy?

GO is a multifactorial disorder, resulting from a complex interplay of endogenous and environmental factors [3]. The former (poorly understood

*Table 1.* Prevention of Graves' orbitopathy

| Stage | Prevention | Goal | Actions |
| --- | --- | --- | --- |
| Absent disease | primary | to avoid occurrence of disease | refrain from smoking |
| Subclinical disease | secondary | to prevent progression to clinical disease | refrain from smoking, restoration of euthyroidism, prudent use of radioiodine |
| Clinical disease | tertiary | to avoid complications to minimize disability | local measures, medical or surgical treatment of orbitopathy, rehabilitative surgery |

genetic factors, age, gender) are, by definition, non-preventable; the latter (smoking, thyroid dysfunction, and, under certain circumstances, radioiodine therapy for hyperthyroidism) are preventable [4, 5]. It is unknown why only 3–5% of patients with Graves' disease develop severe orbitopathy, about half have only mild eye disease, and the remaining patients apparently have no ocular involvement. This might reflect the fact that environmental factors are more important than endogenous factors. Thus, a general strategy can be devised to act on environmental factors. In other words, medical intervention can effectively influence GO course, by strongly urging patients to refrain from smoking, properly correcting thyroid dysfunction, using radioiodine cautiously, treating moderate-to-severe GO as early as possible [4, 5] (table 1).

## What Can Be Done in the Primary Prevention of Graves' Orbitopathy?

Smoking withdrawal is the only primary prevention measure for GO. Smoking is associated with Graves' hyperthyroidism. In the Nurses' Health Study II on more than 115,000 women aged 25–42 years, cigarette smoking was a predictor of Graves' hyperthyroidism, with a hazard ratio of 1.93 in current smokers, 1.27 in former smokers, and 2.63 in heavy smokers (>25 cigarettes/day) [6]. In a case-control study, the odds ratio of smoking for Graves' hyperthyroidism without ocular involvement was 1.7, but increased to 7.7 for Graves' hyperthyroidism with associated orbitopathy [7]. The odds were even higher in patients with more severe orbitopathy. In a large cross-sectional study, the prevalence of smokers among women Graves' hyperthyroidism *and* orbitopathy (64%) was significantly higher than that in Graves' women apparently without ocular involvement (48%) or in normal controls (about 30%) [8] (table 2). According to a European Thyroid

*Table 2.* Smoking effects on Graves' hyperthyroidism and orbitopathy

---

Increased risk of development of Graves' disease in smokers
Increased relapse rate of hyperthyroidism after antithyroid drug treatment in smokers
Increased prevalence of smokers in adult Graves' orbitopathy patients as compared to Graves' patients without orbitopathy or controls
Increased prevalence of Graves' orbitopathy in children from countries with the highest prevalence of smoking teenagers (with possible role of passive smoking as well)
Graves' orbitopathy tends to be more severe in smokers
Decreased effectiveness of orbital radiotherapy and/or high-dose glucocorticoids for moderately severe Graves' orbitopathy in smokers
Lower risk of developing diplopia and proptosis in past smokers than in current smokers

---

Association (ETA) survey, GO incidence had decreased in the last decade for 43% of respondents and increased for 12%: most respondents in the first group came from European countries with a declining tobacco consumption, while thyroidologists of the second group mostly belonged to countries with an increasing tobacco consumption [9] (table 2).

Whether passive smoking may have the same impact on GO occurrence as active smoking is difficult to ascertain. However, in a recent ETA survey of GO in childhood, the highest proportion (>35%) of Graves' children with orbitopathy was in countries where the prevalence of smokers among teenagers was also highest (≥25%) [10] (table 2). The interesting finding was that in the latter countries the majority (52%) of Graves' children with orbitopathy were ≤10 years of age, suggesting (although not proving) that, owing to their young age and, therefore, the unlikelihood of active smoking, also passive exposure to smoking may contribute to the development of GO [10].

Has smoking withdrawal an impact on the risk of developing GO? Randomized controlled studies on this issue are lacking, but in a prospective study, the relative risk of developing diplopia was 1.8 in current smokers of 1–10 cigarettes/day, increased progressively to 7.0 at a dose >20 cigarettes/day, but decreased to 1.9 in past smokers of >20 cigarettes/day [11] (table 2). This presently is the best, although not conclusive, evidence that quitting smoking may prevent occurrence of the orbitopathy in Graves' patients.

## What Can Be Done in Terms of Secondary Prevention of Graves' Orbitopathy?

Many Graves' patients have subclinical orbitopathy, detectable only by imaging (CT scan, MRI) or other specialist investigations, such as measurement of intraocular pressure in upward gaze, but progression to overt eye disease of different severity may occur. This is probably accounted for, at least in part, by the natural history of GO, because orbitopathy may either precede Graves' hyperthyroidism, occur concomitantly, or follow it even after a long time interval [12]. The latter situation, however, may be due to factors affecting GO course, which can be corrected.

*Thyroid dysfunction* contributes to progression from subclinical to clinically overt GO. In a 5-month follow-up study, orbitopathy remained stable in patients already euthyroid (under antithyroid drug therapy) at the time of first observation; at variance, eye changes progressively improved in patients whose initial hyperthyroidism was subsequently controlled by treatment [13]. In a large consecutive-entry study, prevalence of uncontrolled hyperthyroidism was greater in patients with more severe ocular changes than in those with milder ocular involvement [14]. Hypothyroidism may affect the course of GO as well. In a series of 30 patients referred for severe orbitopathy, half developed eye disease after a period of hypothyroidism [15]. Thus, prompt restoration of normal thyroid function is a required intervention to hinder GO progression and/or contribute to its amelioration, and should be achieved as early as possible both in patients with asymptomatic orbitopathy (secondary prevention) and in those with clinically overt orbitopathy (tertiary prevention). That early diagnosis and treatment of hyperthyroidism probably is effective as secondary GO prevention is indirectly supported (although not proven) by the observation that GO prevalence in newly diagnosed Graves' disease is declining in the last decades [16].

What about the effects of *treatments for hyperthyroidism* on the orbitopathy? Neither antithyroid drugs nor thyroidectomy are disease-modifying treatments. In other words, they do not alter GO natural history [17]. Conversely, radioiodine treatment causes progression of pre-existing orbitopathy (rarely its de novo occurrence) in about 15% of cases [18]. Worsening of eye disease is often transient, is more likely in patients who smoke, have severe hyperthyroidism, high anti-TSH receptor antibody titres, or whose post-radioiodine hypothyroidism is not promptly corrected by L-thyroxine replacement [19] (table 3). Thus, radioiodine therapy is the only treatment for hyperthyroidism associated with a small risk of GO progression. This seems unlikely, if the above risk factors are absent, in patients with no ocular signs prior to radioiodine administration, or whose eye disease is inactive after previous glucocorticoid treatment [20]. In any case, radioiodine, an effective treatment for hyperthyroidism, can safely be used in patients with GO or at risk of developing it, because progression can be prevented by a relatively short-course of oral

*Table 3.* Risk factors involved in radioiodine-associated progression of Graves' orbitopathy

Pre-existing and active Graves' orbitopathy
Smoking
Severity of hyperthyroidism
High TSH-receptor antibody titres
Uncorrected post-radioiodine hypothyroidism

glucocorticoids at moderate doses (25–30 mg prednisone daily, withdrawn over 6–12 weeks) [18, 21, 22].

*Smoking* is associated with a higher relapse rate of hyperthyroidism after antithyroid drug treatment [23]. It is, therefore, conceivable, albeit not proven, that smoking withdrawal may increase the chance for Graves' hyperthyroidism to go into permanent remission (table 2). Because thyroid hyperfunction and related autoimmune reactions have a negative impact on GO, it can be inferred that refraining from smoking in patients treated with antithyroid drugs for hyperthyroidism may be secondary prevention of progression of subclinical to clinically manifest orbitopathy.

## What About Tertiary Prevention of Graves' Orbitopathy?

Once GO is overt, tertiary prevention consists of measures aimed at avoiding complications and minimizing disability. In mild orbitopathy, general measures such as artificial tear drops to lubricate the eyes, eye pads at night to prevent risks associated with exposure keratitis, and prisms to control mild, but invalidating, diplopia may represent effective actions [1]. In moderately severe orbitopathy, either medical treatments (systemic high-dose glucocorticoids and/or orbital radiotherapy) or surgery (orbital decompression) are indicated, the choice of treatment depending on GO severity and activity, to arrest further progression of eye disease and to achieve, if possible, its regression [24]. It is worth underscoring that smoking decreases the effectiveness of glucocorticoids and irradiation [25, 26]; accordingly, smoking withdrawal is also a form of tertiary prevention. In sight-threatening orbitopathy (dysthyroid optic neuropathy), high-dose glucocorticoid treatment or, in case of failure, orbital decompression is urgently required to avoid possible sight loss [1]. In inactive orbitopathy, rehabilitative surgery, i.e. orbit surgery for residual proptosis, eye muscle surgery for strabismus, eyelid surgery for lid retraction, has cosmetic and functional indications to correct residual disability [1].

## What Should One Do when Talking to a Graves' Orbitopathy Patient Who Smokes?

It is evident that smoking is the most important risk factor for GO occurrence and progression. Accordingly, although data on the effects of smoking withdrawal are scant, circumstantial evidence suggests that refraining from smoking is a fundamental intervention in terms of primary, secondary, and tertiary prevention of the disease. Therefore, Graves' patients, independently of the presence or absence of GO and its severity, must be urged to quit smoking. A clear explanation of risks of severe eye disease, profound effects of (not necessarily severe) orbitopathy on daily activities and quality of life, reduced effectiveness of medical treatments (if required), and a strong statement that smoking affects all the above is mandatory. Showing pictures of patients with severe ocular manifestations may help. Physicians should also underscore the fact that if the patient quits smoking, there are good chances that eye disease does not deteriorate, may even improve, and become more responsive to planned treatments. The use of patient's information leaflets containing all the needed information may be useful. However, scaring patients or enhancing their motivations may be not enough to convince them, because refraining from smoking is not easy. Therefore, patients, who are unable to quit smoking by themselves, should be addressed to professional stop-smoking clinics, organizations and groups where they can receive counselling, behavioural therapies or pharmacological treatments.

### Acknowledgements

This work was partially supported by grants from the Italian Ministry of Education, University and Research (MIUR, Rome) and the University of Insubria, Varese, Italy.

### References

1 Bartalena L, Pinchera A, Marcocci C: Management of Graves' ophthalmopathy: reality and perspectives. Endocr Rev 2000;21:168–199.
2 Oberman A: Principles of preventive health care; in Goldman L, Ausiello D (eds): Cecil Textbook of Medicine, ed 22. Philadelphia, Saunders, 2004, pp 44–46.

3 Prabhakar BS, Bahn RS, Smith TJ: Current perspective on the pathogenesis of Graves' disease and ophthalmopathy. Endocr Rev 2003;24:802–835.
4 Wiersinga WM, Bartalena L: Epidemiology and prevention of Graves' ophthalmopathy. Thyroid 2002;12:855–860.
5 Bartalena L, Marcocci C, Pinchera A: Graves' ophthalmopathy: a preventable disease? Eur J Endocrinol 2002;146:457–461.
6 Holm IA, Manson JAE, Michels KB, Alexander EK, Willett WC, Utiger RD: Smoking and other lifestyle factors and the risk of Graves' hyperthyroidism. Arch Intern Med 2005;165: 1606–1611.
7 Prummel MF, Wiersinga WM: Smoking and risk of Graves' disease. JAMA 1993;269:479–482.
8 Bartalena L, Martino E, Marcocci C, Bogazzi F, Panicucci M, Velluzzi F, Loviselli A, Pinchera A: More on smoking habits and Graves' ophthalmopathy. J Endocrinol Invest 1989;12: 733–737.
9 Weetman AP, Wiersinga WM: Current management of thyroid-associated ophthalmopathy in Europe: results of an international survey. Clin Endocrinol (Oxf) 1998;49:21–28.
10 Krassas GE, Segni M, Wiersinga WM: Childhood Graves' ophthalmopathy: results of a European questionnaire study. Eur J Endocrinol 2005;153:515–521.
11 Pfeilschifter J, Ziegler R: Smoking and endocrine ophthalmopathy: impact of smoking severity and current versus lifetime cigarette consumption. Clin Endocrinol (Oxf) 1996;45:477–481.
12 Marcocci C, Bartalena L, Bogazzi F, Panicucci F, Pinchera A: Studies on the occurrence of ophthalmopathy in Graves' disease. Acta Endocrinol (Copenh) 1989;120:473–478.
13 Prummel MF, Wiersinga WM, Mourits MP, Koornneef L, Berghout A, van der Gaag R: Amelioration of eye changes of Graves' ophthalmopathy by achieving euthyroidism. Acta Endocrinol (Copenh) 1989;121(suppl 2):185–189.
14 Prummel MF, Wiersinga WM, Mourits MP, Koornneef L, Berghout A, van der Gaag R: Effect of abnormal thyroid function on the severity of Graves' ophthalmopathy. Arch Intern Med 1990;150: 1098–1101.
15 Karlsson AF, Westermark K, Dahlberg PA, Jansson R, Enoksson P: Ophthalmopathy and thyroid stimulation (Letter). Lancet 1989;ii:691.
16 Kendall-Taylor P, Perros P: Clinical presentation of thyroid associated orbitopathy. Thyroid 1998;8:427–428.
17 Marcocci C, Bruno-Bossio G, Manetti L, Tanda ML, Miccoli P, Iacconi P, Bartolomei MP, Nardi M, Pinchera A, Bartalena L: The course of Graves' ophthalmopathy is not influenced by near-total thyroidectomy: a case-control study. Clin Endocrinol (Oxf) 1999;51:503–508.
18 Bartalena L, Marcocci C, Bogazzi F, Manetti L, Tanda ML, Dell'Unto E, Bruno-Bossio G, Nardi M, Bartolomei MP, Lepri A, Rossi G, Martino E, Pinchera A: Relation between therapy for hyperthyroidism and the course of Graves' ophthalmopathy. N Engl J Med 1998;338:73–78.
19 Bartalena L, Tanda ML, Piantanida E, Lai A, Pinchera A: Relationship between management of hyperthyroidism and course of the ophthalmopathy. J Endocrinol Invest 2004;27:288–294.
20 Peros P, Kendall-Taylor P, Neoh C, Frewin S, Dickinson AJ: A prospective study of the effects of radioiodine therapy for hyperthyroidism in patients with minimally active Graves' ophthalmopathy. J Clin Endocrinol Metab 2005;90:5321–5323.
21 Bartalena L, Marcocci C, Bogazzi F, Panicucci M, Lepri A, Pinchera A: Use of corticosteroids to prevent progression of Graves' ophthalmopathy after radioiodine therapy for hyperthyroidism. N Engl J Med 1989;321:1349–1352.
22 Glinoer D, de Nayer P, Bex M, Belgian Collaborative Group on Graves' Disease: Effects of L-thyroxine administration, TSH-receptor antibodies and smoking on the risk of recurrence of Graves' disease treated with antithyroid drugs: a double-blind prospective randomized study. Eur J Endocrinol 2001;144:475–493.
23 Bartalena L: Glucocorticoids for Graves' ophthalmopathy: how and when. J Clin Endocrinol Metab 2005;90:5497–5499.
24 Marcocci C, Marinò M, Rocchi R, Menconi F, Morabito E, Pinchera A: Novel aspects of immunosuppressive and radiotherapy management of Graves' ophthalmopathy. J Endocrinol Invest 2004;27:272–280.

25 Bartalena L, Marcocci C, Tanda ML, Manetti L, Dell'Unto E, Bartolomei MP, Nardi M, Martino E, Pinchera A: Cigarette smoking and treatment outcomes in Graves' ophthalmopathy. Ann Intern Med 1998;129:632–635.
26 Eckstein A, Quadbeck B, Mueller G, Rettenmeier AW, Hoermann R, Mann K, Steuhl P, Esser J: Impact of smoking on the response to treatment of thyroid associated ophthalmopathy. Br J Ophthalmol 2003;87:773–776.

Prof. Luigi Bartalena
Division of Endocrinology, Department of Clinical Medicine
University of Insubria, Ospedale di Circolo
Viale Borri, 57
IT–21100 Varese (Italy)
Tel. +39 0332 278561, Fax +39 0332 278358, E-Mail l.bartalena@libero.it

# Future Developments

*Mario Salvi[a], L. Baldeschi[b]*

[a]Endocrine Unit, Departments of Medical Sciences, University of Milan, Fondazione Ospedale Maggiore IRCCS, Milan, Italy; [b]Orbital Centre, Department of Ophthalmology, Academic Medical Centre, University of Amsterdam, Amsterdam, The Netherlands

### Is There Evidence that Steroids in Graves' Orbitopathy Act as True Immunosuppressants and Modify Disease Outcome?

Corticosteroid medications have been employed as anti-inflammatory agents for a long time as they are known to act at different levels onto the cascade of the reactions of inflammation [1]. A limited immunosuppressive effect of steroids has also been the rationale for their use in various autoimmune diseases with the purpose to control their chronic course. In GO steroids have been used for many decades as the mainstay of therapy for the moderate to severe forms of the disease [2]. The anti-inflammatory effect of steroids is observed rapidly after the beginning of treatment. Patients report improvement of their eye symptoms while a decrease of the severity of NOSPECS class 2 signs is readily observed and, depending on the degree of involvement, also an improvement of muscle function probably due to edema and volume reduction. Proptosis is the outcome of many intraorbital reactions and its reduction may not only result from decreased inflammation but also from reversal of orbital tissue expansion due to immune infiltration and major involvement of organ tissue. Both the dose-dependent efficacy of steroids and the relationship between time of administration and clinical improvement suggest an important anti-inflammatory effect in GO. As far as the true immunosuppressive effect of steroids, evidence derived from clinical studies suggests that it may be relevant only as a consequence of chronic treatment, perhaps as long as the duration of the disease's active inflammatory phase. Some authors [3, 4] have reported a decrease of serum TRAb levels during the course of treatment with steroids, suggesting a direct effect on the potential immune effector involved in some of the TSH receptor-mediated pathogenic mechanisms of GO [5]. A short course of oral steroids has been successfully administered to prevent GO in patients at high risk, after thyroid ablation with I-131 for recurrent hyperthyroidism [6]. In that study, steroids helped preventing both the initiation of GO or the worsening of pre-existing disease, suggesting their potential immunosuppressive effect on either pathogenic mechanism.

### What Are the Reasons for Exploring the Potential Efficacy of New Immunosuppressive Medications?

Established treating agents in GO such as steroids (which have acceptable efficacy at the cost of relevant side effects [2, 7–9]), and radiotherapy (which is effective mainly in combination with steroids [10, 11] but has a safer long-term side effect profile [12]) have been used for years with different administering modalities and probably limited true immunosuppressive effects. Since we do not yet understand the specific immune mechanisms involved in the pathogenesis of GO, we are only using agents that act as general immunosuppressants, similarly employed in other autoimmune diseases. The need for new immunosuppressive medication is opportune. Lately, a large panel of newly synthesized monoclonal antibodies directed to various molecules expressed on immune cells and involved at different levels in the autoimmune reactions has become available. Some of these have been used in pilot studies and preliminary clinical trials in various autoimmune diseases with promising results.

### Is There Evidence for the Efficacy of New Immunotherapy Agents in Graves' Orbitopathy?

Immunotherapeutic agents in GO have been proposed and employed with only partially satisfying results over the last 20 years but only recently drugs interacting with the action of both Th1 and Th2 cytokines have been made available and tried in GO, although not in controlled studies. Etanercept, a TNF receptor antagonist [13], has been successfully used to treat a patient with severe GO [14] and by Paridaens et al. [15] in a group of 10 GO patients who showed improvement of clinical activity but not of proptosis. The lack of effect on orbital tissue hypertrophy may be due to absent TNF-$\alpha$ receptor expression on orbital fat in active GO [16]. There have been recent reports of significant amelioration of the signs of GO in single patients treated with rituximab, an anti-CD20 monoclonal antibody [17, 18]. Subsequently, Salvi et al. [19] have completed a phase 2 clinical study with rituximab on 10 patients with active GO and different degree of severity and have observed improvement of the CAS, proptosis and motility and stabilization of GO without evidence of recurrence after 12–24 months, when compared to the response to i.v. steroids in a similar group of patients with active GO.

## Which Anticytokine Treatment Would Be the Most Effective in Your Opinion?

Data from the above studies suggest that B cells are key regulators of the immune response in the orbit, perhaps by acting as antigen presenting cells [20] and that rituximab is at the moment the most promising immunomodulating drug in GO. GO pathogenesis is yet unclear, but evidence would support more Th1 cytokine-driven mechanisms, at least in the early stages [21–23]. Specifically, one could hypothesize the use of anti-TNF-α and anti-IL-1 antibodies to be effective in controlling the development of active GO. In vitro evidence that the TNF-α receptor may not be expressed by orbital tissue in the active GO phase [16] and that IL-1 stimulates glycosaminoglycans production and adipogenesis by fibroblasts in tissues derived from either GO patients or controls [24] poses the question of their efficacy until clinical trials are carried out. Other therapeutic targets could be the T cell co-stimulation pathway CTLA4-B7 (abatacept, an immunoglobulin directed against CTLA4, which has shown to be promising in rheumatoid arthritis [25]), and the antigen-presenting capacity of monocytes and inhibition of T cell clones proliferaton by IL-10 [26]. Very recently, Douglas et al. [27] have reported that memory T cells of Graves' disease patients largely express the IGF-1 receptor that could be the target of autoantibodies in GO which stimulate fibroblasts growth and prolong T cell survival, thereby perpetuating the autoimmune process. These data raise the possibility of developing an effective drug to block the IGF-1 receptor. The serum-soluble IL-6 receptor (sIL-6R) has been reported to be elevated in active GO, independently of thyroid autoimmune reactions [28]. Tocilizumab, an anti-IL-6R humanized monoclonal antibody, has been shown to be a promising agent in rheumatic diseases because of its effect on the blockade of the pro-inflammatory cytokine milieu [29].

## What About Rituximab?

Rituximab binds to the CD20 antigen expressed on B cells and blocks the formation of new plasmacells and immunoglobulins [30, 31]. The results of an open trial on rituximab in GO [19] suggest that the drug is effective in modifying the disease course and its clinical impact. A plausible explanation for its effect on GO is that it may affect B cell antigen presentation at the orbital level [20]. On the other hand, evidence for the involvement of autoantibodies directed against the IGF-1 receptor in the initiation of GO [32] suggests that blocking CD20 might

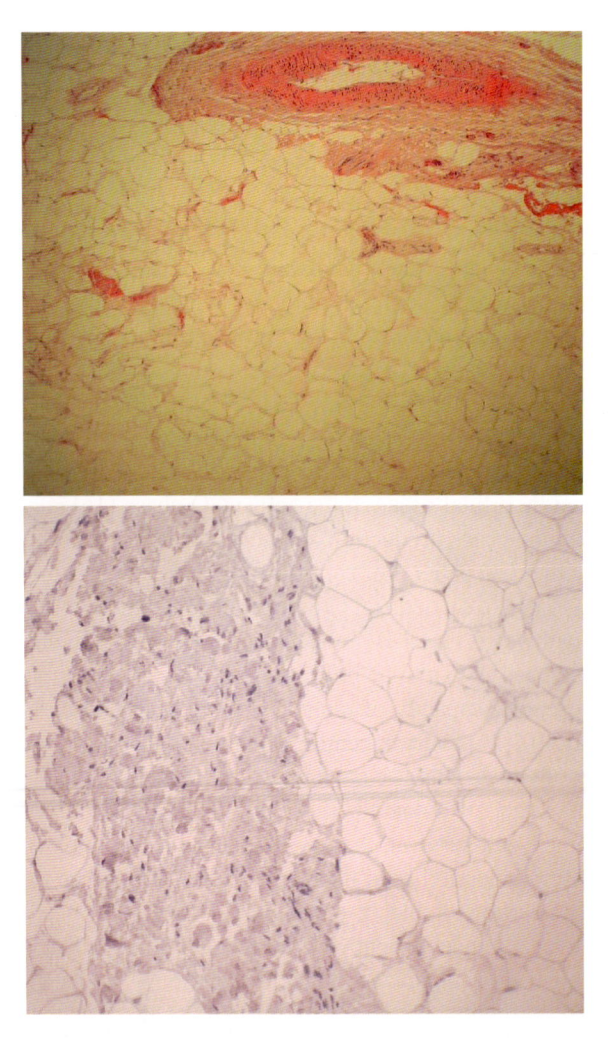

*Fig. 1.* Immunohistochemistry of orbital fat tissue from patients with Graves' ophthalmopathy. Upper panel: Tissue from a patient treated with rituximab that shows the absence of any significant lymphoid infiltrate. Lower panel: Tissue from a patient treated with steroids, with evident lymphocytes. HE.

interrupt the cascade of autoimmune reactions in the orbit. Salvi et al. [17] have indeed reported absence of both B and T cells in orbital tissue specimens after rituximab therapy in 1 patient (fig. 1). In addition, a significant reduction of proptosis measurements was observed after rituximab in 2 patients with Graves' disease and only eye lid inflammation [19]. It is possible that TSH receptor-mediated fibroblast and adipocyte stimulation is also inhibited [22, 33] and this results in the observed decrease of the eye protrusion.

## What About Interfering with the TSH Receptor Pathways?

The pathogenesis of Graves' hyperthyroidism is B cell mediated through TSH receptor binding autoantibodies and there is evidence to support a role of this interaction in fibroblasts and adipose tissue proliferation in the orbit. It is also of interest that TSH receptor mRNA levels in orbital adipose tissue have been shown to be increased in patients with active GO [16]. In addition, early adipogenesis is activated by PPAR-γ ligation [33]. Effective immunotherapy should therefore interfere with TSH receptor expression and binding or with blocking of PPAR-γ ligation [23]. CD20 blocking would be expected to induce a decrease of TRAb in the serum of patients with Graves' disease [34] and perhaps consequent orbital fibroblast stimulation. Interestingly, in the study of Salvi et al. [19] rituximab, while effective on orbital disease, had no effect on serum TRAb and hyperthyroidism (fig. 2), despite the attainment of total peripheral B cell depletion. The lack of effect of rituximab on serum TRAb suggests that this autoantibody, and in general thyroid autoimmune reactions, might be involved in the cross-reactive mechanisms between the thyroid and the orbit but not in the subsequent development of clinical disease.

## Are Technical Developments in Surgical Approaches to Be Expected?

Orbital bone decompression is currently accomplished by piecemeal fracturing with bone nibbing rongeurs and by grinding with high-speed drill equipped with a cutting-burr or a diamond-burr tip. The use of rotary instrumentation in tight spaces, as those available in orbital surgery, carries the not negligible risk of catching soft orbital tissues or damaging the dura. Ultrasonic bone removal recently proposed for orbital surgery represents a promising field of technical development [35]. Hand pieces which transmit 25–29 kHz vibration can easily selectively carve/cut only mineralized tissues. The reliability of ultrasonic bone curettes in orbital surgery, however, still needs to be tested against large numbers, and issues of concern about possible damages to soft tissues when using such devices have been recently aroused in neurosurgery [36].

Technical innovations for decompression surgery are limited as compared with those that are already available and constantly undergo implementation for blepharo- and eyebrowplasty. The reason of this difference is that rehabilitative blepharoplasty and browplasty can benefit from the technical solutions that the most commercial, dynamic world of cosmetic periorbital surgery is offering. These include different types of technologically advanced, incisional, or photo ablative lasers; radiofrequency or laser powered devices aimed at subcutaneous

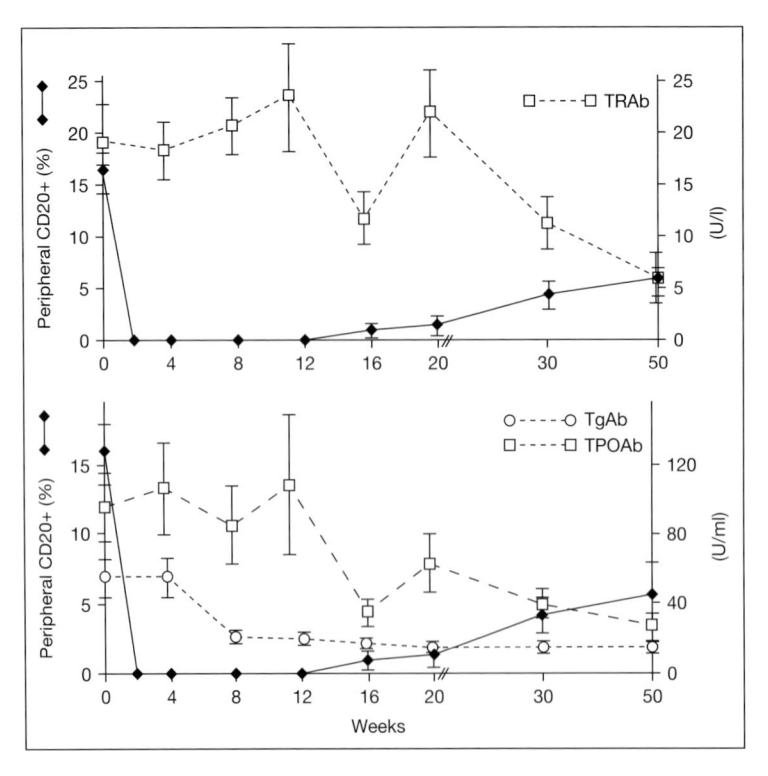

*Fig. 2.* Changes of serum thyroid autoantibodies levels in relation to peripheral depletion of CD20+ lymphocytes after treatment with rituximab in 9 patients with active thyroid-associated ophthalmopathy. Six patients were treated with methimazole, 1 with L-thyroxine replacement and 2 were euthyroid without therapy. TRAb = TSH receptor antibodies; TPOAb = thyroperoxidase antibodies; TgAb = thyroglobulin antibodies. Values are indicated as mean ± SE.

collagen contraction and/or neocollagen genesis; diamond laser scalpels; fillers; endoscopic instrumentation and fixation systems/devices for brow lift.

At present, hard palate mucosa, providing structural and epithelial elements, represents the graft of choice for posterior lamella augmentation in lower lid lengthening, although presenting the disadvantage of not negligible donor site morbidity and surgical time for graft harvesting. Homologous acellular dermal matrix is a processed donor tissue not available in Europe with appropriate consistency for posterior lamella augmentation; one surface is sectioned through the dermis and the other has an intact basement membrane, which provides a structural template that guides conjunctival epithelium migration and repopulation. It is not excluded that in the close future bioengineering (already capable of offering cultured hyaluronan-based dermal autografts) will be able to provide effortless autografts with characteristics similar to homologous acellular dermal matrix with the result of speeding up surgery and eliminating the problem of donor site morbidity.

## Are Conceptual Developments in Surgical Approaches to Be Expected?

Waiting for a specific medical therapy to cure GO, orbital fat and every bone in the orbit have been removed, either alone or in combination, to achieve orbital decompression. Through the years, indications, osteotomies, and incisions for decompression surgery have changed in order to decrease the occurrence of unwanted side effects and possible complications in a simultaneous attempt to maximize satisfaction for an increasingly demanding patient population. At the basis of this type of surgery, however, remains the same conceptual principle of decreasing mechanically, the mechanical contribution to the pathogenesis of GO, or the mechanical sequels of the stable disease, no matter which technique is used [37]. At present, no conceptual departure from this approach has been proposed or explored.

The principles that regulate timing and techniques for surgical correction of restrictive strabismus, primarily due to the orbitopathy itself, are well established, while the pathogenesis of the strabismus consecutive to orbital decompression is not fully understood. A better understanding of the latter may result in conceptual advancements beneficial for its treatment and eventual prevention [38]. Recently, injections of hyaluronic acid gel have been proposed for the treatment of lower lid retraction of various aetiologies. Although its effectiveness still needs to be proven, the layered expansion/reinforcement offered by the hyaluronic acid gel eventually associated to weakening of the retractors may represent a possible conceptual alternative to the traditional autologous, homologous, xenogenic and synthetic spacer grafts which are currently used to provide stiffness and support against gravity [39].

In light of the current literature, no substantial conceptual changes are to be expected regarding blepharoplasty and eyebrowplasty for the near future.

## References

1 Rhen T, Cidlowski JA: Antiinflammatory action of glucocorticoids: new mechanisms for old drugs. N Engl J Med 2005;353:1711–1723.
2 Bartalena L, Pinchera A, Marcocci C: Management of Graves' ophthalmopathy: reality and perspectives. Endocr Rev 2000;21:168–199.
3 Kubota S, Ohye H, Nishihara E, Kudo T, Ito M, Fukata S, Amino N, Kuma K, Miyauchi A: Effect of high dose methylprednisolone pulse therapy followed by oral prednisolone administration on

the production of anti-TSH receptor antibodies and clinical outcome in Graves' disease. Endocr J 2005;52:735–741.
4   Eckstein AK, Plicht M, Lax H, Hirche H, Quadbeck B, Mann K, Steuhl KP, Essen J, Morgenthaler NG: Clinical results of anti-inflammatory therapy in Graves' ophthalmopathy and association with thyroidal autoantibodies. Clin Endocrinol 2004;61:612–618.
5   Bahn RS: Pathophysiology of Graves' ophthalmopathy: the cycle of disease. J Clin Endocrinol Metab 2003;88:1939–1946.
6   Bartalena L, Marcocci C, Bogazzi F, Manetti L, Tanda ML, Dell'Unto E, Bruno-Bossio G, Nardi M, Bartolomei MP, Lepri A, Rossi G, Martino E, Pinchera A: Relation between therapy for hyperthyroidism and the course of Graves' ophthalmopathy. N Engl J Med 1998;338:73–78.
7   Prummel MF, Mourits MP, Blank L, Berghout A, Koornneef L: Randomized double-blind trial of prednisone versus radiotherapy in Graves' ophthalmopathy. Lancet 1993;342:949–954.
8   Marinò M, Morabito E, Brunetto MR, Bartalena L, Pinchera A, Marcocci C: Acute and severe liver damage associated with intravenous glucocorticoid pulse therapy in patients with Graves' ophthalmopathy. Thyroid 2004;14:403–406.
9   Salvi M, Vannucchi G, Sbrozzi F, Del Castello Bottari A, Carnevali A, Fargion S, Beck-Peccoz P: Onset of autoimmune hepatitis during intravenous steroid therapy for thyroid-associated ophthalmopathy in a patient with Hashimoto's thyroiditis: case report. Thyroid 2004;14:631–634.
10  Marcocci C, Bartalena L, Tanda ML, Manetti L, Dell'Unto E, Rocchi R, Barbesino G, Mazzi B, Bartolomei MP, Lepri P, Cartei F, Nardi M, Pinchera A: A comparison of the effectiveness and tolerability of intravenous or oral glucocorticoids associated with orbital radiotherapy in the management of severe Graves' ophthalmopathy: results of a prospective, single-blind, randomized study. J Clin Endocrinol Metab 2001;86:3562–3567.
11  Ohtsuka K, Sato A, Kawaguchi S, Hashimoto M, Suzuky Y: Effect of steroid pulse therapy with and without orbital radiotherapy on Graves' ophthalmopathy. Am J Ophthalmol 2003;135: 285–290.
12  Marcocci C, Bartalena L, Rocchi R, Marinò M, Menconi F, Morabito E, Mazzi B, Mazzeo S, Sartini MS, Nardi M, Cartei F, Cionini L, Pinchera A: Long-term safety of orbital radiotherapy for Graves' ophthalmopathy. J Clin Endocrinol Metab 2003;88:3561–3566.
13  Nash PT, Florin THJ: Tumor necrosis factor inhibitors. Med J Aust 2005;183:205–208.
14  Durrani OM, Reuser TQ, Murray PI: Infliximab: a novel treatment for sight-threatening thyroid associated ophthalmopathy. Orbit 2005;24:117–119.
15  Paridaens D, van den Bosch WA, van der Loos TL, Krenning EP, van Hagen PM: Inhibition of tumor necrosis factor-α activity reduces periorbital inflammation in patients with Graves' ophthalmopathy. Eye 2005;19:1286–1289.
16  Wakelkamp IM, Bakker O, Baldeschi L, Wiersinga WM, Prummel MF: TSH-R expression and cytokine profile in orbital tissue of active vs. inactive Graves' ophthalmopathy patients. Clin Endocrinol 2003;58:280–287.
17  Salvi M, Vannucchi G, Campi I, Rossi S, Bonara P, Sbrozzi F, Guastella C, Avignone S, Pirola G, Ratiglia R. Beck-Peccoz P: Efficacy of rituximab treatment for thyroid-associated ophthalmopathy as a result of intraorbital B-cell depletion in one patient unresponsive to steroid immunosuppression. Eur J Endocrinol 2006;154:511–517.
18  El Fassi D, Nielsen CH, Hasselbalch HC, Hegedus L: Treatment-resistant severe, active Graves' ophthalmopathy successfully treated with B lymphocyte depletion. Thyroid 2006;16:709–710.
19  Salvi M, Vannucchi G, Campi I, Currò N, Dazzi D, Simonetta S, Bonara P, Rossi S, Sina C, Guastella C, Ratiglia R, Beck-Peccoz P: Treatment of Graves' disease and associated ophthalmopathy with the anti-CD 20 monoclonal antibody rituximab: an open study. Eur J Endocrinol 2007;156: 33–40.
20  Drexhage HA: Are there more than antibodies to the thyroid-stimulating hormone receptor that meet the eye in Graves' disease? Endocrinology 2006;147:9–12.
21  Cao HJ, Wang HS, Zhang Y, Lin HY, Phipps RP, Smith TJ: Activation of human orbital fibroblasts through CD40 engagement results in a dramatic induction of hyaluronan synthesis and prostaglandin endoperoxide H synthase-2 expression: insights into potential pathogenic mechanisms of thyroid-associated ophthalmopathy. J Biol Chem 1998;273:29615–29625.
22  Han R, Smith TJ: T helper type 1 and type 2 cytokines exert divergent influence on the induction of prostaglandin E2 and hyaluronan synthesis by interleukin-1 beta in orbital fibroblasts: implications for the pathogenesis of thyroid-associated ophthalmopathy. Endocrinology 2006;147:13–19.

23   Garrity JA, Bahn RS: Pathogenesis of Graves' ophthalmopathy: implications for prediction, prevention and treatment. Am J Ophthalmol 2006;142:147–153.
24   Cawood TJ, Moriarty P, O'Farrelly C, O'Shea D: Smoking and thyroid-associated ophthalmopathy: a novel explanation of the biological link. J Clin Endocrinol Metab 2007;92:59–64.
25   Ruderman E, Pope R: The evolving clinical profile of abatacept (CTLA4-Ig): a novel co-stimulatory modulator for the treatment of rheumatoid arthritis. Arthritis Res Ther 2005;7(suppl 2): S21–S25.
26   Wakkach A, Cottrez F, Groux H: Can interleukin-10 be used as a true immunoregulatory cytokine? Eur Cytokine Netw 2000;11:153–160.
27   Douglas RS, Gianoukakis AG, Kamat S, Smith TJ: Aberrant expression of the insulin-like growth factor-1 receptor by T cells from patients with Graves' disease may carry functional consequences for disease pathogenessis. J Immunol 2007;178:3281–3287.
28   Salvi M, Pedrazzoni M, Girasole G, Giuliani N, Minelli R, Wall JR, Roti E: Serum concentrations of proinflammatory cytokines in Graves' disease: effect of treatment, thyroid function, ophthalmopathy and cigarette smoking. Eur J Endocrinol 2000;143:197–202.
29   Nakahara H, Nishimoto N: Anti-interleukin-6 receptor antibody therapy in rheumatic diseases. Endocr Metab Immune Disord Drug Targets 2006;6:373–381.
30   Tsokos GC: B cells, be gone: B-cell depletion in the treatment of rheumatoid arthritis. N Engl J Med 2004;350:2546–2548.
31   Pescovitz MD: Rituximab, an anti-CD20 monoclonal antibody: history and mechanism of action. Am J Transplant 2006;6:859–866.
32   Pritchard J, Horst N, Cruikshank W, Smith TJ: Immunoglobulin acxtivation of T cell chemoattractant expression in fibroblasts from patients with Graves' disease is mediated through the insulin-like growth factor 1 receptor pathway. J Immunol 2003;170:6348–6354.
33   Valyasevi RW, Harteneck DA, Dutton CM, Bahn RS: Stimulation of adipogenesis, peroxisome proliferator-activated receptor-gamma (PPARgamma), and thyrotropin receptor by PPARgamma agonist in human orbital preadipocyte fibroblasts. J Clin Endocrinol Metab 2002;87:2352–2358.
34   El Fassi D, Nielsen CH, Hasselbalch HC, Hegedus L: The rationale for B lymphocyte depletion in Graves' disease: monoclonal anti-CD20 antibody therapy as a novel treatment option. Eur J Endocrinol 2006;154:623–632.
35   Sival Calcott JA, Limberg JV, Patel S: Ultrasonic bone removal with the sonopet omni: a new instrument for orbital surgery. Arch Ophthalmol 2005;123:1595–1597.
36   Kim K, Isu T, Matsumoto R, Isobe M, Kogure K: Surgical pitfalls of an ultrasonic bone curette (SONOPET) in spinal surgery. Neurosurgery 2006;59:390–393.
37   Baldeschi L: Decompression surgery for thyroid-related orbitopathy: status of the art and unresolved issues; in Guthoff R, Katowitz J (eds): Essential in ophthalmology: Orbit and Oculoplastic. Springer, Berlin, in press.
38   Baldeschi L, Wakelkamp IMMJ, Lindeboom R, Prummel MF, Wiersinga WM: Early versus late orbital decompression in Graves' orbitopathy: a retrospective study in 125 patients. Ophthalmology 2006;113:874–878.
39   Tsirbas A, Jayasundera T, Lee S, McCann J, Goldberg R: Treatment of lower lid retraction with hyaluronic acid gel. Communication at the 24th Meeting of the European Society of Ophthalmic Plastic and Reconstructive Surgery (ESOPRS), London, UK 13–16 September 2006.


Dr. Lelio Baldeschi
Room A2–119, Orbital Center, Department of Ophthalmology
Academic Medical Center, University of Amsterdam
Meibergdreef 9
NL–1105 AZ Amsterdam (The Netherlands)
Tel. +31 20 566 3580, Fax +31 20 556 9053, E-Mail l.baldeschi@amc.uva.nl

# Historical Notes on Graves' Disease

*Maarten P. Mourits*

Department of Ophthalmology, Academic Medical Center – AMC,
University of Amsterdam, Amsterdam, The Netherlands

## Is It Fair to Call Graves' Disease Graves' Disease?

The Welshman Caleb Hillier Parry (fig. 1) gave a detailed clinical description of 13 patients with goitre associated with tachycardia, in one of whom, seen in 1786, protrusion of both eyes occurred. His writings were posthumously published by his son in 1825 [1]. The Dubliner Robert James Graves (fig. 2), in 1835, described in equal detail 3 patients with enlargement of the thyroid gland and palpitations, of whom one also had protrusion of the eyes [2]. The German Karl Adolph von Basedow (fig. 3), in 1840 and 1848, discussed the co-occurrence of goitre, tachycardia and exophthalmos, which has since been called the Merseburger trias [3]. Whereas Graves mainly focused on the general medical aspects of the syndrome, von Basedow had more eye for the ophthalmic implications. Rehn (1884) and Möbius (1887) were the first to point to hyperthyroidism as an essential cause of proptosis [4]. It becomes clear that many early researchers have contributed to our understanding of 'Graves' disease' and the fact we call the condition as such is scientifically not completely correct and fair, no matter what a 'delightful, warm-hearted and enthusiastic' Irishman Robert Graves may have been [4].

More than 200 years have gone by since these first observations were made of proptosis in the context of thyroid gland disease and yet one can just speculate on the causal relationship between the two. It would be attractive to name the disease with reference to its etiology. 'Auto-immune orbitopathy', however, it would be too vague and no exclude other forms of auto-immune orbitopathy. The name thyroid eye disease (TED) neglects the fact that the orbital disease can occur in the absence of any thyroid involvement and underscores the present understanding of a systemic, multi-organ disease, in which other sites such as the legs (pretibial myxedema) and bones may be involved

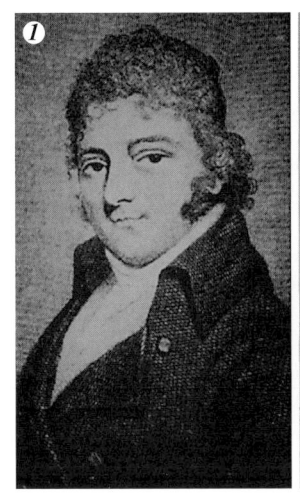

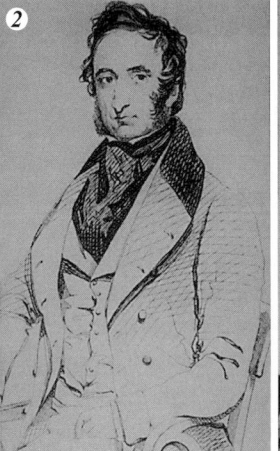

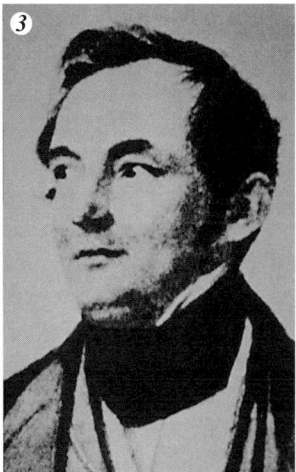

*Fig. 1.* Caleb Parry.
*Fig. 2.* Robert Graves.
*Fig. 3.* Karl Adolph von Basedow.

(Graves' acropachy). For the same reason 'endocrine ophthalmopathy' is a misnomer, because 'endocrine' suggests the cause of the disease to be a change in hormone levels and 'ophthalmopathy' suggests an ophthalmic and not a primary orbital disease. What's in a name? As long as we do not fully understand this 'one of the most puzzling syndromes in ophthalmology' [4], it seems not entirely unfair to call the disease after the person who not only described it for the first time in modern times, but also personally realized the importance of publishing his observations. Therefore, in this book, we speak about Graves' disease, Graves' thyroid disease, Graves' orbitopathy, Graves' dermopathy and Graves' acropachy as a sign of esteem and for the sake of convenience.

### Various Eye Signs Carry Specific Names: Are They Still Relevant?

Several famous clinicians of the 19th and early 20th century have done meticulous observations in patients with Graves' disease. In a time when hard evidence for a diagnosis was often lacking, their signs may possibly have been of great importance. Table 1 has been conceived from Duke-Elder's famous *System of Ophthalmology* [4].

As shown in the chapter by Mourits [pp. 66–77], a diagnosis of GO nowadays rarely is a clinical problem and although one can assess these classical signs in many patients, modern diagnosis is based on other grounds.

Historical Notes

*Table 1.* Eye signs of GO according to late 19th and early 20th century physicians

| | | |
|---|---|---|
| Dalrymple | 1852 | Retraction of the upper lids in primary position |
| Kocher | 1902 | Staring and frightened appearance on attentive fixation |
| Holloway | 1929 | Retraction lower lid(s) |
| Von Graefe | 1864 | Sclera above cornea becomes visible in down gaze |
| Boston | | Jerky movement of upper lid in down gaze not following the globe's movement |
| Joffroy | | Absent forehead creases in upgaze |
| Rosenbach | | Trembling of the lids on gentle closure |
| Stellwag | 1869 | Infrequent and incomplete blinking reflex |
| Enroth | | Fullness of the lids |
| Möbius | 1886 | Weakness in convergence for near objects |
| Gifford | 1906 | Diffilculty in eversion of the upper lids |
| Jellinek | | Abnormal pigmentation of the upper lids |
| Goldzieher | 1900 | Conjunctival hyperaemia |
| Knie | | Inequality of dilation of the pupils |
| Cowen | | Jerky reaction on eliciting the consensual light reflex |

## How Did Old Theories Explain the Relationship between Hyperthyroidism and Proptosis?

The following explanations for proptosis in GO have been given:
- weakness of the EOMs (Cooper, 1849)
- contraction of smooth muscle in the orbit/sympathetic stimulation (Bernard, 1852)
- cardiac neurosis (Filehne, 1879)
- vascular congestion (Von Graefe, 1857; Moebius, 1891; Fründ, 1911)
- edema and fatty infiltration of the orbit (Pochin and Rundle, 1944)
- edema as the result of hydrophilic mucopolysaccharides (Ludwig et al., 1950).

Until recent times, exophthalmos (syn: proptosis; syn: protrusion) has been generally accepted as a significant feature of diffuse toxic goitre, as a sign of thyrotoxicosis [4]. However, this hypothesis could not explain why proptosis persisted or even increased after control of the thyrotoxicosis, nor why some patients had proptosis in the absence of hyper- or hypo-thyroidism. So two types of proptosis were distinguished: a mild form as an expression of thyrotoxicosis (which may have been only lid retraction appearing as proptosis – a condition which is called pseudoproptosis) and a malignant form, that could co-occur with thyroid disease. Means (1945) divided Graves' disease into three types: thyrotoxicosis with and without ophthalmopathy and (Graves') ophthalmopathy with hyper-, hypo- and euthyroidism [4]. Pochin and Rundle hypothesized that this exophthalmos varied in severity following a definite cycle depending on pituitary activity.

After the discovery of the thyroid-stimulating hormone (TSH), secreted by the anterior lobe of the pituitary gland, at the beginning of the 20th century by Loeb and Basset (1928), over-secretion of TSH was considered the cause of Graves' disease and GO. Destruction of the pituitary gland by irradiation was advocated for severe proptosis. However, this theory could not hold when it became clear that in the absence of TSH over-secretion, the proptosis could increase. Next, exophthalmos-producing substance (EPS) was considered the cause of proptosis in GO as it caused proptosis in certain species of fish. However, this fish exophthalmos basically differs from the one in man. Adams, Purves and McKenzie (1956–1958) identified long-acting thyroid stimulator (LATS) or thyroid-stimulating antibody in sera of patients who had undergone pituitary ablation and they believed to have found the substance causing proptosis. LATS is found in 80% of patients with untreated thyrotoxicosis, but severe exophthalmos has been described in patients without detectable LATS. So the etiological role of LATS remains unclear. Today we have arguments that the susceptibility to develop Graves' disease has genetic determinants and that the course of the disease is influenced by exogeneous factors [5, 6].

## Which Are Rundle's Contributions to Our Understanding of Graves' Orbitopathy?

In a series of publications lasting from 1944 until 1960, Rundle and co-workers from Sydney are to be credited for a number of remarkable statements:
- 'the ocular manifestations have emerged as one of the most troublesome features of Graves' disease'
- 'to women of any age, disfigurement of conspicuous eye signs causes acute mental suffering'
- 'purely descriptive notes will not provide a reliable guide during treatment'.

Measuring is knowing must have been one of Rundle's credos. He first measured proptosis, eye movements (e.g. ductions) and lid apertures according to fixed rules on a monthly frequency during 18 months in a cohort of patients [7]. A subset of these patients has been examined by the same observer using identical assessing tools after 15 years [8]. From these observations the – what we now call – 'Rundle's curve' is derived [see fig. 2, p. 80, chapter by Kendall-Taylor]. Rundle assessed that untreated GO runs a course of increasing severity reaching a plateau phase (dynamic phase) followed by a mostly incomplete recessing of symptoms (static phase). He thus concluded that GO to a certain extent is self-limiting. He acknowledged that 'the rate and extent of protrusion and recession, and the incidence of ophthalmoplegia, and therefore of paralytic lid retraction, vary widely (months to years)'. Most patients, however, reach their peak relatively early in the course of Graves' disease and exophthalmos had usually reached its maximum by the time the patient was referred for treatment. In contrast to recent publications [9], no long-term follow-up recurrences were seen. In eyes, static after a year or two, measurements of proptosis 15 years later generally showed little or no change. Nevertheless, 'eye signs had become slight or absent', thanks to a decrease of lid width and an improvement of motility. Already in his early reports, Rundle warns not to correct surgically residual stigmata of the disease before at least 2 years after the peak have been passed. Rundle, therefore, should be honored also as a pioneer of the concept of disease activity and the subsequent treatment implications. But he made more seminal contributions. In a paper from 1945, he writes: 'The average volume of the orbit is approximately 27 cc in males and 24 cc in females. In both sexes normally some 70 percent of the cavity is occupied by retrobulbar and peribulbar structures. The average weight of these structures is 19 g, made up of eye muscles 3.3 g, lacrimal gland 0.65 g, and fibro-fatty residue 15 g. The seven extrinsic eye muscles thus account for approximately 20 percent of the tissue bulk and the fibro-fatty residue and lacrimal gland for 80 percent. The capacity of the orbit can be simply determined by plugging its cavity with plasticine, and then determining the volume of plasticine so used, by water displacement. The degree of orbital filling may be expressed as the ratio between the bulk of orbital tissues (excluding the eyeball and optic nerve) and the capacity of the orbit. There is a linear relationship between the degree of orbital filling and the Hertel exophthalmometer reading. It may be calculated from the regression line relating orbital filling to the exophthalmometer reading that a marked exophthalmos of 6 mm would result from 20 percent increase (4 cc) in bulk of the orbital contents. The average protrusion of the eye in thyrotoxic patients of approximately 2 mm would result from a 6.6 percent increase in orbital filling' [10].

Rundle also notes 'Strands of adipose tissue cells lie between the fibres of the extrinsic eye muscles in both normal and thyrotoxic subjects. The quantity of such adipose tissue is increased in thyrotoxicosis by about 85 percent. No droplets of fat could be demonstrated within the muscle fibres. Comparison of the mean average diameter of the fat globules in eye muscles from normal and thyrotoxic subjects shows the diameter to be decreased in thyrotoxicosis, suggesting that there is proliferation and development of new fat cells. Since in patient with exophthalmos the fat-free weight of the extrinsic muscles is increased, the adipose tissue cannot be simply a fatty replacement of degenerated muscle fibres, but must represent new tissue increasing the total bulk of muscles' [10]. Rundle suggests there is proliferation of adipose tissue cells throughout the

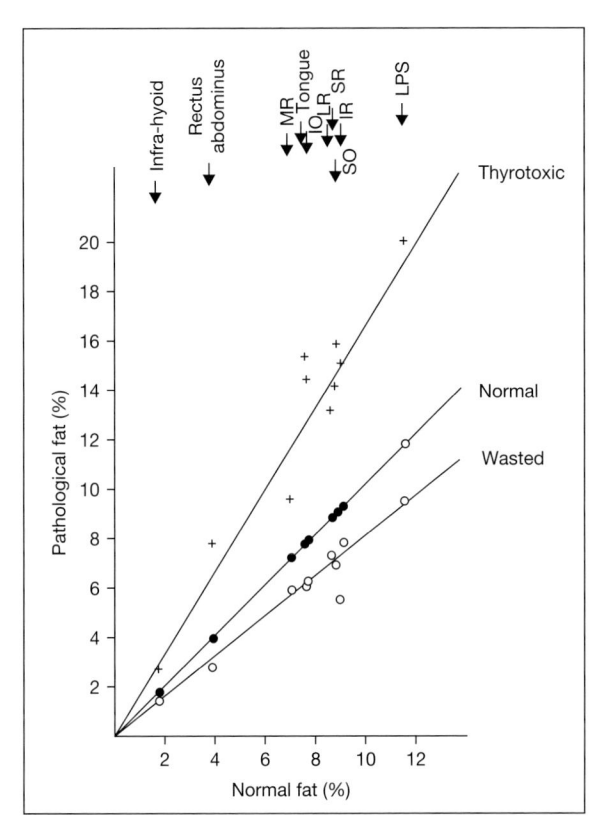

*Fig. 4.* Fat content of eye muscles and other skeletal muscles in thyrotoxic and wasted cases, plotted against the normal fat content of each muscle; each point is based on the mean value for the group of subjects, lines are drawn to fit points for eye muscles. LPS = Levator palpebrae superioris; SR = superior rectus; MR = medial rectus; IR = inferior rectus; LR = lateral rectus; SO = superior oblique; IO = inferior oblique; Tonque = sample from midline; Infra-hyoid = sample from sterno-hyoid; Rectus abdominis = sample from level of umbilicus. By courtesy of the Editor, *Clinical Science*.

orbit, and continues 'It is remarkable that this proliferation of fat occurs in the orbit despite the fact that thyrotoxics coming to post-mortem are generally wasted. Eleven of the 17 thyrotoxic subjects examined by Rundle and Pochin were wasted, four severely. In wasted controls there is marked loss of fat from the extrinsic muscles and residual orbital tissue' (fig. 4). It is only in the last decade that the mechanism behind orbital adipogenesis has been partially classified (see below).

*Table 2.* Criteria for clinical evaluation of effects of orbital irradiation

| | |
|---|---|
| Excellent response | Marked improvement in, or disappearance of, major symptoms and signs |
| | Marked improvement in functional capacity of the individual |
| Good response | Moderate to marked improvement in most symptoms and signs, improved functional capacity, but some persistent clinical manifestations |
| Fair response | Slight to marked improvement in some symptoms and signs, but little or no improvement in that manifestation associated with the greatest disability |
| No response | |
| Worse | Worsening of symptoms or signs after the completion of therapy |

## Which Are Kriss' Contributions to the Management of Graves' Orbitopathy?

Treatment results in a disease with a presentation as protean as GO are hard to evaluate. For instance, how would we score the outcome of a treatment when motility has improved and at the same time proptosis has increased? Kriss and co-workers [11, 12] faced with this problem evaluating the outcome of retrobulbar irradiation, introduced criteria for clinical evaluation of effects of orbital irradiation, which can be used for medical treatment modalities as well (table 2). This concept has been altered into major and minor criteria for the outcome of treatment by Bartalena et al. [13], which in a modified way is used in present studies. Kriss has (co-)authored in almost 30 studies on Graves' disease and developed theories about the origin of the orbitopathy and dermopathy in Graves' disease. In particular, he injected radiolabelled thyroglobulin into the thyroid gland and was able to follow the location of radoactivity, which finally ended up in the orbit. The observation was interpreted as evidence for a direct connection between the thyroid gland and the orbit [12].

## When Was Evidence-Based Medicine Incorporated in Graves' Orbitopathy?

Till the 1980s interpretation of studies on Graves' disease was flawed by the facts that evaluation of treatment outcome was done in incomparable (e.g. hyper- and euthyroid, active and stable) patients, in individuals receiving several therapies at the same time (e.g. radiotherapy and prednisone), whereas no fixed endpoint or sharp outcome measures of the study had been defined. More importantly, the natural course of the disease was disregarded and no control group was used. For these reasons, results were often conflicting. The group of Pinchera, Pisa, Italy, tackled most of these shortcomings in their study in 1983, in which orbital cobalt irradiation combined with systemic corticosteroids was compared with systemic corticosteroids alone [13]. Next came Kahaly's group from Mainz, comparing prednisone and cyclosporine in 1986 [14], followed by the Pisa group again (1987) and the Amsterdam group of Wiersinga in 1989 [15].

## References

1. Parry CH: Collections from the Unpublished Medical Writings of the Late Caleb Hillier Parry. London, Underwoods, 1825, vol 2, pp 111–124.
2. Graves RJ: Newly observed affection of the thyroid gland in females. Lond Med Surg J 1835;7:516–520.
3. Basedov CA: Exophthalmos durch hypertrophie des Cellgewebes in der Augenhohle. Wochenschr Ges Heilk 1840;6:197–120.
4. Duke-Elder S, MacFaul PA: Orbital involvement in general disease; in Duke-Elder S (ed): System of Ophthalmology, vol XVIII, part II. London, Henry Kimpton, 1974, pp 935–968.
5. Hall R, Owen SG, Smart GA: Evidence for genetic predisposition to formation of thyroid autoantibodies. Lancet 1960;ii:187–188.
6. Krassas GE, Wiersinga W: Smoking and autoimmune thyroid disease: the plot thickens. Eur J Endocrinol 2006;154:777–880.
7. Rundle FF: Management of exophthalmos and related ocular changes in Graves' disease. Metabolism 1957;6:36–48.
8. Hales JB, Rundle FF: Ocular changes in Graves' disease: a long-term follow-up study. Q J Med 1960;29:113–126.
9. Kalman R, Mourits MP: Late recurrence of unilateral graves orbitopathy on the contralateral side. Am J Ophthalmol 2002;133:727–729.
10. Rundle FF: Eye signs of Graves' disease. Clin Sci 1945;5:177–197.
11. Donaldson SS, Bagshaw MA, Kriss JP: Supervoltage orbital radiotherapy for Graves' ophthalmopathy. J Clin Endocrinol Metab 1973;37:276–285.
12. Kriss JP, Konishi J, Herman M: Studies on the pathogenesis of Graves' ophthalmopathy (with some related observations regarding therapy). Rec Prog Horm Res 1975;31:533–560.
13. Bartalena L, Marcocci C, Chiovato L, Laddaga M, Lepri G, Andreani D, Cavallacci G, Baschieri L, Pinchera A: Orbital cobalt irradiation combined with systemic corticosteroids for Graves' ophthalmopathy: comparison with systemic corticosteroids alone. J Clin Endocrinol Metab 1983;56:1139–1144.
14. Kahaly G, Schrezenmeir J, Krause U, Schweikert B, Meuer S, Muller W, Dennebaum R, Beyer J: Ciclosporin and prednisone v. prednisone in treatment of Graves' ophthalmopathy: a controlled, randomized and prospective study. Eur J Clin Invest 1986;16:415–422.
15. Prummel MF, Mourits MP, Berghout A, Krenning EP, van der Gaag R, Koornneef L, Wiersinga WM: Prednisone and cyclosporine in the treatment of severe Graves' ophthalmopathy. N Engl J Med 1989;321:1353–1359.

Prof. Dr. Maarten P. Mourits
Department of Ophthalmology, Academic Medical Center – AMC
University of Amsterdam, Meibergdreef 9
NL–1105 AZ Amsterdam (The Netherlands)
Tel. +31 20 566 3518, Fax +31 20 566 9053, E-Mail m.p.mourits@amc.uva.nl

# Author Index

Baldeschi, L. 160, 163, 237
Bartalena, L. 229
Boboridis, K. 88
Boschi, A. 153

Currò, N. 111

Daumerie, C. 34
Dickinson, A.J. 1

Eckstein, A. 188

Kahaly, G.J. XIII, 120
Kalmann, R. 34

Kendall-Taylor, P. 78
Krassas, G.E. 221

Lane, C.M. 153
Lazarus, J.H. 27

Marcocci, C. 100
Marino, M. 27
Mourits, M.P. 66, 246

Nardi, M. 176
Neoh, C. 188

Orgiazzi, J. 41

Perros, P. 88
Pinchera, A. 100
Pitz, S. 57

Salvi, M. 111, 237

von Arx, G. 212

Wiersinga, W.M. XIII, 96, 201

# Subject Index

Activity, Graves' orbitopathy
  clinical assessment 8–11, 83
  definition 6, 7, 81, 82
  laboratory tests 13, 14
  management guidelines 13
Age
  distribution of Graves' orbitopathy 35
  effects on Graves' orbitopathy
    presentation 4
Anterior orbital septum (AOS) 5
Antithyroid drug therapy, Graves'
  orbitopathy outcomes 100, 101, 103
Apical crowding, imaging 59–61
Artificial tears, Graves' orbitopathy
  management 90
Azathioprine, moderately severe Graves'
  orbitopathy management 140–142

Botulinum toxin, Graves' orbitopathy
  management 91, 189, 190

Caroticocavernous fistula, differential
  diagnosis 75
Caruncle, inflammation assessment 10, 11
CD20, therapeutic targeting 238–240
Chemosis, assessment 9
Childhood Graves' orbitopathy
  clinical presentation 222
  epidemiology 222, 223
  severity 222–224
  treatment 224–226
Ciamexone, moderately severe Graves'
  orbitopathy management 140, 142

Clinical Activity Score (CAS) 11, 12, 83
Color vision, assessment 18, 19
Combined thyroid-eye clinic
  definition 96, 97
  fast-track for Graves' orbitopathy patients
    98, 99
  multidisciplinary approach advantages
    97, 98
  patient support groups 98
Computed tomography (CT)
  Graves' orbitopathy diagnosis 71
  orbital imaging 57–59
Conjunctival edema, *see* Chemosis
Conjunctival redness, assessment 8, 9
Corneal ulceration
  Clinical Activity Score 11, 12
  eyelid surgery 190
  Graves' orbitopathy diagnosis 69
  overview 3, 6
Corticosteroids, *see* Steroid therapy
Cosmetic surgery, definition 160
CTLA-4
  Graves' orbitopathy susceptibility locus 86
  therapeutic targeting 53, 239
Cyclosporine, moderately severe Graves'
  orbitopathy management 138, 139

Delayed decompression-related reactivation
  (DDRR) 172
Diabetes, Graves' orbitopathy risks 38, 39
Diagnosis, Graves' orbitopathy
  clinical findings
    corneal ulceration 69

255

Diagnosis, Graves' orbitopathy (continued)
  clinical findings (continued)
    eyeball motility restriction 69
    eyelid retraction 68
    eyelid swelling 67, 68
    proptosis 69
    visual acuity 69, 70
  criteria 70
  errors in complex cases 178, 179
  laboratory tests 70, 71
  overview 66
Differential diagnosis
  caroticocavernous fistula 75
  non-Hodgkin lymphoma 76
  orbital meningioma 72
  orbital myositis 72–74
Diplopia, orbital decompression surgery complication 173
Diuretics, Graves' orbitopathy management 91
Double vision 1, 173
Dysthyroid optic neuropathy (DON)
  apical crowding imaging 59–61
  assessment 18–23, 156
  blindness outcomes 158
  clinical features 2, 3, 6, 154, 155
  definition 153
  evidence-based management 157
  ophthalmological signs 155
  risk factors 22, 153
  surgical management 157, 158
  urgent treatment indications 156, 157
  vision effects 22

Epidemiology, Graves' orbitopathy
  age and sex distribution 35
  childhood Graves' orbitopathy 222, 223
  comorbidity
    non-ocular 38, 39
    ocular 37, 38
  ethnic differences 35
  prevalence 34, 35
  risk factors 35, 36
  trends 34, 35
Euthyroid Graves' orbitopathy, management 218
Evidence-based medicine
  dysthyroid optic neuropathy management 157

historical perspective 252, 253
moderately severe Graves' orbitopathy management 148, 149
Eyelid erythema, assessment 8
Eyelid retraction
  differential diagnosis 68
  Graves' orbitopathy diagnosis 68
Eyelid surgery
  complications 195–198
  debulking and blepharoplasty 198
  indications 188–190
  orbital decompression effects on lid retraction 190, 191
  spacer materials 196, 197
  squint surgery influence on lid configuration 191, 192
  techniques
    lower lid 196
    upper lid 193–195
Eyelid swelling
  assessment 9, 10
  differential diagnosis 67
  Graves' orbitopathy diagnosis 67, 68
Eye muscle surgery
  affected muscle identification 176–178
  complications 185, 186
  expectations and outcomes 182, 183
  indications 179–182
  planning 183–185
  timing 182

Fibroblast, therapeutic targeting 52, 53
Fluorometholone, Graves' orbitopathy management 90
Fundoscopy, optic neuropathy assessment 19

Genetic susceptibility, Graves' orbitopathy 4, 50, 51
Glaucoma, *see* Primary open-angle glaucoma
Globe subluxation 1, 219
Glucocorticoids, *see* Steroid therapy
Graves' disease
  Graves' orbitopathy frequency 29
  localized myxedema 31, 32
  thyroid acropachy 32
Graves, Robert James 246

Subject Index

256

Guanethidine, Graves' orbitopathy management 91

Hyaluronic acid, lower lid injection 243
Hyperthyroidism
  Graves' orbitopathy relationship 27–29, 78, 89
  history of study with proptosis 248, 249
Hypothyroidism
  Graves' orbitopathy relationship 79, 80, 89
  transient hypothyroidism after hyperthyroidism treatment 105, 106

Insulin-like growth factor-1 (IGF-1) receptor
  antibodies and Graves' orbitopathy 47
  therapeutic targeting 239
Interleukin-1 (IL-1), therapeutic targeting 53, 239
Interleukin-6 (IL-6), therapeutic targeting 53, 239
Intravenous immunoglobulin (IVIg), moderately severe Graves' orbitopathy management 139, 140, 142, 143

Ketorolac, Graves' orbitopathy management 90

Lantreotide, *see* Somatostatin analogs

Magnetic resonance imaging (MRI)
  Graves' orbitopathy diagnosis 71
  orbital imaging 58, 59, 63
Mild Graves' orbitopathy
  antioxidant therapy 116, 117
  intra-orbital involvement 111
  oral steroid therapy 114
  progression 111, 112
  radiation therapy 115, 116
  treatment versus wait and see 112, 113
Moderately severe Graves' orbitopathy
  azathioprine therapy 140–142
  ciamexone therapy 140, 142
  combination steroid and radiotherapy 135–138
  cyclosporine therapy 138, 139

evidence-based therapeutic recommendations 148, 149
  immunosuppression indications 120, 121
  intravenous immunoglobulin therapy 139, 140, 142, 143
  intravenous steroid therapy
    adverse effects 130
    outcomes 126–130
  oral steroid therapy 121–125
  radiation therapy
    outcomes 131–133
    protocol 133, 134
    safety 134, 135
  retrobulbar injection of steroids 130
  somatostatin analog therapy 144–147
Myasthenia gravis (MG), Graves' orbitopathy risks 39
Myxedema, Graves' disease association 31, 32

Natural history, Graves' orbitopathy
  'burn' out 84, 85
  euthyroidism restoration 78, 79
  hyperthyroidism 78
  hypothyroidism 79, 80
  mild disease progression 111, 112
  modifying factors 85, 86
  recurrence 85
  return to normality 84, 85
  Rundle's curve 80
  treatment guidance 83, 84
  typical course 80, 81
Non-Hodgkin lymphoma, differential diagnosis 76
NOSPECS classification
  class frequencies 14–16
  overview 14, 15
  severity assessment 14, 16–20, 83

Octreoscan, orbital imaging 62
Octreotide, *see* Somatostatin analogs
Ocular motility impairment
  affected muscle identification 176–178
  Graves' orbitopathy diagnosis 69
  mechanisms on Graves' orbitopathy 176
  presentation 3
  surgery, *see* Eye muscle surgery

Optic neuropathy, *see* Dysthyroid optic
  neuropathy
Orbit
  imaging
    apical crowding 59–61
    computed tomography 57–59
    indications 57
    magnetic resonance imaging 58, 59,
      63
    octreoscan 62
    positron emission tomography 64
    ultrasonography 61, 62
  immune reactions 48–50
  thyroid autoimmunity and orbit
    pathology 47
Orbital decompression surgery
  aims
    functional aims 164, 165
    rehabilitative symptomatic aims
      165–167
  childhood Graves' orbitopathy
    management 226
  complications
    delayed decompression-related
      reactivation 172
    prevention 172, 173
  dysthyroid optic neuropathy management
    157, 158
  lid retraction effects 190, 191
  overview 163
  prospects 241–243
  technique
    fat removal 167, 170, 171
    osteotomy 167, 170, 171
    rehabilitative surgery 168, 169
Orbital meningioma, differential diagnosis
  72
Orbital myositis, differential diagnosis
  72–74

Parry, Caleb Hillier 246
Pathogenesis, Graves' orbitopathy
  clinical manifestation mechanisms 5, 6,
    44, 45
  orbital tissue pathology
    adipogenesis 43
    early inflammatory changes 42, 43
    glycosaminoglycan production 43, 44

  overview 41, 42
  triggers 45–47
Patient support groups 98
Pentoxifylline, mild Graves' orbitopathy
  management 116
Perimetry, optic neuropathy assessment
  19
Photophobia 1
Plica, inflammation assessment 10, 11
Positron emission tomography (PET),
  orbital imaging 64
Prevalence, Graves' orbitopathy and trends
  34, 35
Prevention, Graves' orbitopathy
  general strategy 229, 230
  primary prevention 230, 231
  primary, secondary, and tertiary
    prevention definitions 229
  secondary prevention 231–233
  tertiary prevention 233, 234
Primary open-angle glaucoma (POAG),
  Graves' orbitopathy risks and
  management 37, 38
Proptosis
  assessment 20
  differential diagnosis 69
  Graves' orbitopathy diagnosis 69
Ptosis 3
Pupil response 19

Quality of life (QoL)
  definition 201
  Graves' orbitopathy
    GO-QoL questionnaire
      components 204–206
      findings 206
      recommendations 209, 210
      therapeutic outcome measurement
        207, 208
    health-related quality of life 203,
      204
    response shift 206, 207
    restoration after treatment 208, 209
    usefulness of measurements 201–203

Race
  effects on Graves' orbitopathy
    presentation 4

epidemiology of Graves' orbitopathy 35
Radiation therapy
  mild Graves' orbitopathy management 115, 116
  moderately severe Graves' orbitopathy management
    combination steroid and radiotherapy 135–138
    outcomes 131–133
    protocol 133, 134
    safety 134, 135
  response classification 252
Radioiodine
  childhood Graves' orbitopathy management 225
  Graves' orbitopathy outcomes 101–104
  Graves' orbitopathy trigger 45
  guidelines 106
  risk factors in Graves' orbitopathy progression 233
  total thyroid ablation 107, 108
Rehabilitative surgery
  definition 160
  orbital decompression surgery, see Orbital decompression surgery
  patient selection 161, 162
  steps 161
  timing 161
Rituximab, Graves' orbitopathy management 238–240
Rundle, F.F. 249–252
Rundle's curve 80, 249

Severity, Graves' orbitopathy
  assessment 14, 16–20, 83
  childhood Graves' orbitopathy 222–224
  definition 6, 7, 82, 83
  treatment guidance 92, 93
Sex distribution, Graves' orbitopathy 35, 36, 86
Signs, Graves' orbitopathy
  common signs 1, 2
  history of study 247, 248
  severity assessment 14
  unusual signs 2, 3

Smoking
  cessation
    benefits 89
    promotion 234
  Graves' orbitopathy risks 36, 51, 52, 85, 86
  primary prevention of Graves' orbitopathy 230, 231
  secondary prevention of Graves' orbitopathy 233
Somatostatin analogs
  childhood Graves' orbitopathy management 225
  moderately severe Graves' orbitopathy management 144–147
Steroid therapy
  mechanism of action 237, 238
  mild Graves' orbitopathy 114
  moderately severe Graves' orbitopathy
    combination steroid and radiotherapy 135–138
    intravenous steroid therapy
      adverse effect 130
      outcomes 126–130
    oral steroid therapy 121–125
    retrobulbar injection 130
Strabismus, see Ocular motility impairment
Surgery, see Eyelid surgery; Eye muscle surgery; Orbital decompression surgery; Rehabilitative surgery
Symptoms, Graves' orbitopathy 1

Thyroglobulin, antibodies in Graves' orbitopathy 46
Thyroid acropachy, Graves' disease association 32
Thyroidectomy
  childhood Graves' orbitopathy management 225
  Graves' orbitopathy outcomes 102, 103, 107, 108
Thyroid-stimulating hormone (TSH) receptor
  antibodies and Graves' orbitopathy 30, 31, 46, 47, 50, 70, 71, 85
  therapeutic targeting 241
Trauma, Graves' orbitopathy trigger 45

Subject Index

259

Tumor necrosis factor-α (TNF-α),
 therapeutic targeting  53, 238, 239

Ultrasonography, orbital imaging  61, 62
Unilateral Graves' orbitopathy
 clinical presentation  217
 mechanisms  212–216
 progression to bilateral disease
  216, 217
 treatment  217, 218

Very severe Graves' orbitopathy, *see*
 Dysthyroid optic neuropathy
von Basedow, Karl Adolph  246